A First
Materia Medica
for Homoeopathy

The Principles of Homoeopathic Philosophy

A self-directed learning text

Margaret Roy

A4 • £19.95 • 151 pages • illustrated • paperback • 0443 048215

An understanding of the principles of homoeopathic philosophy is fundamental to the successful practice of homoeopathy. For ease of study, this text presents key ideas in homoeopathy in the form of a self-directed study programme which can be followed in its entirety or read selectively.

Key features
The reader is introduced to:
- basic concepts and laws in homoeopathy
- how to read and record symptoms homoeopathically
- the use of Repertories of symptoms
- how to interpret and analyse a case.

Additional features throughout the text
Suggestions for:
- further reading
- learning activities
- self-testing questions.

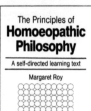

This excellent resource can be used as a companion volume to *A First Materia Medica* and will be invaluable to all students of homoeopathy and readers coming to the subject for the first time.

Churchill Livingstone

A First Materia Medica for Homoeopathy

A self-directed learning text

Margaret Roy

Principal, The Scottish College of Homoeopathy and Practising Homoeopath

Foreword by

Vassilis Ghegas MD

CHURCHILL LIVINGSTONE
EDINBURGH LONDON MADRID MELBOURNE NEW YORK AND TOKYO 1994

CHURCHILL LIVINGSTONE
Medical Division of Longman Group Limited

© Longman Group Limited 1994

First published 1994

ISBN 0 443 04820 7

British Library Cataloguing in Publication Data
A catalogue record for this book is available from the British Library.

Library of Congress Cataloging in Publication Data
Roy, Margaret.
    A first materia medica for homoeopathy: a self-directed learning
    text/Margaret Roy.
        p.   cm.
    Includes bibliographical references and index.
    ISBN 0-443-04820-7
    1. Homeopathy—Materia medica and therapeutics. I. Title.
    [DNLM: 1. Homeopathy—programmed instruction. 2 Materia Medica-
    programmed instruction. WB 18 R888f 1994]
    RX601.R59 1994
    615.5'32--dc20
    DNLM/DLC
    for Library of Congress   94–4032

Illustrator: **Nicola Percy**
with assistance from:
John Logan and the staff at Botanical Gardens, Glasgow
Geoff Hancock and Richard Sutcliffe, Science Department, Glasgow Museums

For Churchill Livingstone

Commissioning Editor: Inta Ozols
Senior Project Controller: Neil A. Dickson
Project Controller: Nicola S. Haig
Copy Editor: Linda Pica
Design: Keith D. Kail, Type Area, Falkirk
Sales Promotion Executive: Hilary Brown

Produced by Longman Singapore Publishers (Pte) Ltd.
Printed in Singapore

Contents

Foreword

I am honoured to preface this book by Margaret Roy, as fate has chosen us to be members of the same family of homoeopathic therapists – those therapists who are found midway between materialism and a more spiritual approach, as witnessed by the author's knowledge and personal experience.

We hope that with this book, therapists will be stimulated to guide their patients not only to a well balanced life, but also to the harmony which conforms to the laws of purity, and the presence of which is proof of the existence of health.

Athens, 1994   V. G.

How to Use this Text

The following information will help you to make the best use of this self-directed learning text. Please read the Introduction before starting the first lesson, to set the rest of the book fully in context. Each lesson adds progressively to the previous, bringing in more and more philosophical concepts and widening the scope with which we study each remedy. The idea is not to learn lists of symptoms but to build up an image of the patient. Using the philosophy we can understand the importance of the symptoms, first in order to match the remedy accurately and secondly to understand the level of disease and therefore the process of cure.

The technique in studying the early remedies can be repeated in later remedies whilst the early remedies can be revised using the approach used in the later remedies.

Here is a summary of the stages:

- Memorize keynote and characteristic symptoms
- Study how keynote, characteristic symptoms and modalities reflect the essence of the remedy
- Build the keynotes, characteristics and modalities into typical acute symptom pictures
- Note the exciting cause and study the different symptom pictures (remedies) it can give rise to
- Not all symptoms occur in the patient. Disease occurs at different levels, as do some symptoms. Put symptoms into groups of greater or lesser severity, e.g:

> acute illness
> local acute – eye, ear, etc.
> functional disturbance in system – digestive, respiratory, etc.
> chronic disease
> constitutional disturbance, i.e. temperament.

Note which symptoms occur at all levels.

- Build up personality pictures of the essence expressing temperament. To what factors is the temperament sensitive? How does this patient act in certain situations?
- Connect the temperament with the illnesses to which it predisposes the patient. What exciting and maintaining causes is the patient sensitive to? What is the characteristic symptom picture at the acute and chronic level?
- Study how the miasmic taint of the remedy is reflected in the symptoms or how it affects the symptoms.
- Study how the nature of the original substance may give greater understanding of the essence of the remedy.
- Similar symptom pictures have a completely different aetiology depending on the remedy, e.g. grief, pathologies such as hypertension.

The recommended textbooks will help with different aspects of the above. The exercises within each chapter and the cases at the end of the text will further develop the themes above and aid the memory. Ultimately only a study of the provings (the original investigation which gave the remedy to healthy people) will show you the full extent of the symptom and the conditions under which it arises. Allen's *Encyclopedia of Materia Medica* is invaluable here.

In studying the recommended texts, pay particular attention to the cases so you learn how the symptoms present. Remember a full symptom has five aspects: time, location, sensation, modality and intensity. Look always for that which is unique and individual as this will enable you to match the symptom picture of remedy and patient most closely. Here, we are speaking of philosophy. The success of your work with patients will depend on how well your understanding of Materia Medica *and* philosophy can throw light on the state of the vital force. It is the vital force you must cure and it is this you must study. This is the study of the patient and his/her susceptibilities.

Biggar, 1994   M. R.

Key to 'Activity' Symbols

The following symbol denotes an activity which involves ...

... reading

... writing

... observing

... further research

... self-test questions

Note on type used

Bold and roman type is used in each section on keynotes and characteristics to emphasize the more commonly occurring or distinctive symptoms. These have been borrowed from texts such as Von Lippe, Tyler, Nash and Allen.

Italic type occurs in some sections of the text to draw attention to the use in context of the keynote or characteristic symptom.

Introduction

The Remedies

Types of Remedy

A homoeopathic medicine is called a remedy. There are over 2000 of them derived from plants, minerals, metals, acids and alkalis, from animal venoms and from diseased human tissue.

The bulk of homoeopathic remedies used every day are derived from plants. Indeed the homoeopath took over the pharmacopoeia of the herbalist in many countries and different cultures, e.g. European, American Indian, and Indian. However, the resemblance to herbal medicine ends here. Whilst both would agree to the natural and holistic approach of the other, the homoeopathic concept of disease is radically different from most forms of herbalism.

The next largest group of remedies comes from the mineral kingdom and includes organic and inorganic chemicals, salts, acids and metals, such as Carbo vegetalis (wood charcoal), Sulphur and Phosphorus, Natrum muriaticum (sodium chloride), Nitric acidum, Aurum (gold), Stannum (tin) and Cuprum (copper). Many of these remedies are produced from the pure chemical. Many of the metals are produced from their nitrate salts – all nitrate salts being soluble. Some well-known polycrests (see Glossary) are unknowable as to their constituents! Causticum is perhaps one of the best known of these. It was prepared by Samuel Hahnemann himself, the founder of homoeopathy as we know it today, and, because its exact ingredients are unknown and cannot be reproduced, dilutions of his original preparations are still in use over 100 years later. Some minerals are amongst the most valuable remedies, having a profound effect on the body's metabolism and on the psyche.

The mystique of homoeopathy often surrounds those remedies that are derived from animal venoms, especially those from snakes and spiders. Other animals are less exotic – Apis mellifica (honey bee), Cantharis (Spanish fly), Pulex (common flea). There is little mystery and even less barbarity. Only two Lachesis snakes were killed and that over 100 years ago. The remedy prepared from the venom is still in use, doing a great deal of good to many people. There have only been two Tarantula spiders killed. As the bottle of Tarentula Cubensis was dropped, no-one knows what was scraped up from the floor, so the remedy cannot be repeated.

The homoeopath does not experiment with animals. No homoeopathic provings are done on animals, because their body and psyche is different from that of a human. No animal can show the range of mental and constitutional symptoms of a human, or speak precisely of subjective sensations, or of what makes his/her symptoms better or worse.

The effects of animal venoms are usually known from cases of poisonings. Allen's *Encyclopedia of Materia Medica* collects symptoms of both the proving and the poisoning as the homoeopathic remedy is not proved on the physiological level. However, since the field of action of the remedy will include these same physiological areas on which the poison acted, information is required. In homoeopathy there is a bonus! You will find it fascinating to study the animal's behaviour, then compare it with the character and temperament of the patient.

The fourth group of remedies is rather special. It contains the nosodes which are potentized from the product of disease, such as Tuberculinum from diseased tuberculoid lung, or Morbillinum from measles. They are used in special situations, e.g. when the organism has not been able to completely recover from disease, or when the offspring are devitalized by inherited traits. Before going into practice there will be a need to study them in detail, but they will not be dealt with here, as this is an introductory text book.

The Essential Character of a Remedy

In studying the text, it is important to understand how the *essence* of the remedy gives rise to the characteristic nature found in any ailment the remedy may cure.

At this first level of study, it is important to ask which *keynotes* are most distinctive of that particular remedy, though one or two may be shared by other remedies. Keynote symptoms help us to separate the remedy from all others and this simplifies matters at the beginning. In an otherwise healthy individual these are also the symptoms we are most likely to notice in a first aid situation, or an acute situation.

1

In deep chronic illness today, keynotes may be absent because the patient either does not have the energy to produce them, or many of the symptoms have been suppressed by bad habit or drugging. In these cases, much more skill is required to identify the essence pattern of the remedy and to link it to a character study, or a constitutional pattern.

We are thus reminded that a homoeopathic remedy can be understood at many different levels, just as the homoeopath recognizes disease appearing at different levels of seriousness. *Acute disease* is (usually) 'a healthy explosion which is a process of self-corrections'.* *Chronic disease* is in response to an underlying weakness or predisposition which has been exposed by trauma, continual stress or poor habits, or old age with its weaker energy.

Some remedies are very well suited for acute disease, whilst others are better suited to chronic disease. In this text we will pay more attention to acute disease. Underlying all treatment, the homoeopath has a concept of improving health permanently, by constitutional treatment, through which the underlying weaknesses, or predispositions, are removed or strengthened. At some level, almost all remedies can act constitutionally.

Studying the Remedies

There are probably as many different approaches to the study of remedies, as there are homoeopaths. In the lessons that follow, I will, of necessity, take only one approach in each lesson, but I will introduce enough approaches to enable you to make a choice when you go on to a thorough study of other remedies yourself.

One of my aims is to link the study of Materia Medica firmly with philosophy, so this has determined some of the different approaches. In general I have attempted in my choice and selection of symptoms to ground the student firmly in homoeopathic thought, thus I have emphasized the individuality of the remedy – its keynotes and characteristics.

The beginner to homoeopathy often emphasizes and gathers lists of particulars. Although the physical symptoms are important to the homoeopath, the individuality of the remedy is found first in the Strange, Rare and Peculiar, then in the Mental and Emotional symptoms, then in the General symptoms. This does not mean the homoeopath negates the common pattern of disease, or its prognosis. The emphasis in homoeopathy is in finding the best-fit remedy – the similimum that can produce the same symptoms and therefore cure.

Also in homoeopathic philosophy you will find that disease presents on the sensation and dysfunction level before it reaches structural change on the physical level. If we can treat on this level, it means we can correct the pattern of disease earlier. Symptoms of sensation and dysfunction are often more individualized, whilst disease on the physiological level has less individuality of expression, so to treat disorder before it reaches this level, when it is still individualized, allows for a more accurate prescription.

The study of disease in homoeopathy is the study of the expression of the life force. The varieties are infinite. Each remedy has a unique symptom picture.

The Homoeopathic Approach to Disease

The Vital Force and Role of Symptoms

The homoeopath recognizes only one disease, the disturbance of the vital force. Put simply, the human being is an amazing organism of body, mind and soul functioning in total harmony. The vital force acts to perpetuate and correct the balance to remain in that harmony we call health. A healthy organism will keep itself healthy and if injured will act to speedily repair damage. Not one part can be affected without affecting the whole. Any action to repair a part involves the re-orientation of the whole. The term given to this concept of the human organism is holism – the adjective, holistic, is more common.

* J T Kent *Lectures on Homoeopathic Philosophy.*

The homoeopath goes further than this holism to say that in the process of self-correction, the organism produces *symptoms*. As in Laing's psychiatry these are not the signs of ill health, but an indication that the healing process has begun. Symptoms are like the ripples in a pool that spread outwards, dissipating the energy of disturbance after a stone has been thrown in. To the homoeopath, the symptoms are a guide as to how well the healing process is proceeding. Hering's* Law of Cure shows a pattern to the movement of symptoms if cure is occurring:

- Symptoms should move out of vital organs into less vital organs
- Symptoms should generally move outwards, e.g. as discharges, or from mucous membrane or gut to skin
- Symptoms move from above downwards, e.g. in skin diseases
- Symptoms will reverse themselves as the disease goes to surface, so the last to appear are the first to disappear and the first group of symptoms may even reappear at the end of the illness.

This understanding of the role of symptoms is fundamental to the homoeopath. Samuel Hahnemann, the founder of homoeopathy as we know it, stated that nothing can be known about disease except what is seen in the symptoms and nothing can be cured except the symptoms. These symptoms do not show the affliction, or disease, but the pattern of disturbance it produces. We cannot see the disease because we cannot see the vital force.

If you have no other knowledge of homoeopathic philosophy, recommended reading is George Vithoulkas's book *Homoeopathy & The New Man*, or Harris Coulter's book *Homoeopathic Science & Modern Medicine* (see bibliography). The companion text to this is *Principles of Homoeopathic Philosophy* (Roy 1994) which will give you a thorough and systematic introduction to the subject.

To the homoeopathic mind, in order to cure, a medicine must be capable of enhancing the pattern of symptoms already produced by the organism in the process of cure. If the homoeopathic remedy can do this, it will work *with* the organism to restore health more speedily. This is natural medicine. To use a homoeopathic medicine, it becomes necessary to know what symptoms it can produce, so it is given to healthy individuals until it produces symptoms. This process is called a 'proving'. When these symptoms are collected together in books called Materia Medicas, they form the 'symptom picture' of the remedy – which we will be studying.

Homoeopathy derives its name from the principle 'like cures like'. In practice, this means that when we see a patient we collect the symptoms in minute detail, then administer a medicine which has been shown to produce exactly these same symptoms. The closer the match, the better the cure.

Hahnemann stated that *every* medicine has two actions, the first being opposite to the second. In the case of homoeopathy, the first action is selected to enhance the symptom picture of the patient, so the second action is to cure the patient 'gently, rapidly and permanently'. The reaction stage, the enhancement of the patient's symptoms, is controlled by the selection of a potency to fit the energy level of the patient.

The Minimum Dose to Start a Reaction

Potency is perhaps the most complicated of all homoeopathic concepts and only concepts in modern science have attempted to explain it. Put simply, potency is the energy of the remedy which is matched to the energy of the patient. The object of the homoeopathic medicine is to stimulate the organism to create movement. It is the movement of the symptoms outwards that indicates cure, but once this process has started, unless it is slow and hampered, or too violent, the medicine is not needed because cure is taking place. The role of the medicine is only to start the process and, as in hormone or enzyme reaction, very little is needed, so the homoeopathic remedy is much diluted and usually only one dose is used.

Potentization refers to the creation of potency by repeatedly diluting and succussing (a violent jarring shake) a remedy. Thus, although the homoeopathic remedy may be obtained as

* Dr Constantine Hering set out to disprove homoeopathy in the late 19th century. Like many others he ended up being converted. He produced a 10-volume encyclopedia, *Hering's Guiding Symptoms*, and of course he developed his Laws of Cure.

pills, pillules, powders, tablets or tincture – the difference in these forms is convenience, or the preference of the prescriber – but always the name of the remedy is followed by a number which refers to the potency. This number refers to the number of times the medicine has been diluted then succussed. If X follows the number, it has been diluted on a scale 1:10 (D on the continent of Europe); or if C, or *no letter*, follows the number, the medicine has been diluted on the scale of 1:100. The more diluted the medicine, then the more powerful it is. Hahnemann saw such a powerful medicine as acting on the dynamic plane. Today one view or paradigm for this might be to say the medicine is liberated energy, capable of acting directly on the energy body of the human and therefore of creating very deep change.

The common potencies used are 6, 12, 30, 200, 1M(1000), 10M. From 200 is considered a 'high potency', below that a 'low potency'. The terms are relative. In health stores, usually only the 6C potency is available and the use of a potency above 30C is not recommended without more knowledge. The 46 remedies in this textbook are the most common, with a very wide field of action, from first aid, or acute situations, to deep chronic problems. The purpose here is to study the symptom picture of the remedy and to look at its common usage, therefore we will not deal with the technicalities of prescription in any depth. (This is dealt with in *The Principles of Homoeopathic Philosophy*, see bibliography.)

The Hierarchy of Symptoms

When the symptoms are collected in the case-taking, they are ordered into a hierarchy of:

- Strange, Rare and Peculiar
- Mental and Emotional
- General
- Particular.

The first of these groups is most unusual and therefore enables rapid and accurate selection of a remedy. The second group, Mental and Emotional, refers to the subjective state of the patient which may be regarded as the most evolved, or individualistic level. To select a remedy that will cover this level is to reach the constitutional level, where deep, long-lasting change may be expected. Likewise, the General level covers the whole of the being (I am hungry, I am cold, I am strongly affected by draughts) and therefore the constitutional weaknesses.

J T Kent would never have considered a case properly diagnosed unless either, or both, of these two levels were included in the symptom picture. Particular refers to what is happening in the separate parts and, as such, could be relatively insignificant unless such a symptom was strongly characterized by peculiar sensations or modalities (better or worse from . . . .). When a homoeopath takes a case, always he/she is looking for what is most individualistic and special about the symptoms.

When the proving is done, the symptoms are divided into three groups:

- Black-type symptoms, in darkest type, refer to those symptoms found in all provers
- Italic type symptoms refer to symptoms found in a large group of provers and known through clinical experience to yield to that particular remedy
- Ordinary type symptoms occurred in the proving uncommonly, and there is, as yet, poor validation in clinical experience.

When the symptom picture of a patient is taken, the symptoms may be underlined according to their intensity (see Vithoulkas' *The Science of Homoeopathy*).

When a remedy is selected, attention is also paid to the balance of the symptoms, the importance of one compared to another. This may lead to a different choice or remedy, so it is necessary in studying Materia Medica to acknowledge which symptoms are most important, common or intense (black-type symptoms) in each remedy. It is useless in homoeopathy to have simply a list of symptoms. In advanced study it is important to recognize how the symptoms came about, which came first and why, then how the picture proceeded to develop and why. When we see the patient, we ask how he/she got into this state, at what point the symptoms appeared and how the situation escalated.

So the study of Materia Medica is the fascinating study of human dynamics, what forces make each individual into the person he/she is and as we grow what effect such strains and stresses have on the body and psyche.

Advanced Studies

In the main, this text will look at basic characteristics and keynotes of remedies, building up a symptom picture. However, remedies are more complex than this, and so are people. In homoeopathy, we are dealing with a dynamic living organism, which functions on many different levels, and is constantly changing. In yet more advanced study it is necessary to look at how the remedy breaks down at each stage of the disease process. Here I have put an intermediate step at the end of each lesson, taking the remedy a little into action to see what situations arise and how it copes with these. I have set down questions to guide further study to begin the comparison with other remedies. To answer the questions you will have to do some research on your own, using the recommended texts and some of the textbooks from the advanced category of the booklist.

Recommended Further Reading

In different parts of the text interesting passages from specific books will be drawn to your attention. For Lessons 1–6, where the emphasis is on keynotes, characteristics and modalities and the presentation of the acute or typical symptom picture, valuable further reading might be:

J H Allen	Keynotes and Characteristics with Comparisons
Adolf von Lippe	Keynotes and Redline Symptoms
Douglas Gibson	Studies of Homoeopathic Remedies
M Tyler	Homoeopathic Drug Pictures
E B Nash	Leaders in Homoeopathic Therapeutics

For information on the physiological action of the medicine read:

E A Neatby and T G Stonham A Manual of Homoeopathic Therapeutics

From Lesson 7 onward you will find the essence character of the remedies in:

J T Kent	Lectures on Homoeopathic Materia Medica
C Coulter	Portraits of Homoeopathic Medicines, Vol 1 and 2
W Gutman	Homoeopathy
Edward C Whitmont	Psyche and Substance
George Vithoulkas	Any Materia Medica

LESSON ONE

The ABC Remedies

Aconite, Belladonna, Chamomilla

Aim: To define the relationships between the exciting cause, the symptom picture produced by the remedy and the characteristic weaknesses of this type of constitution.

Objectives: To identify the exciting cause in a case of Aconite, Belladonna and Chamomilla.
To describe the characteristic symptoms in a case of Aconite, Belladonna and Chamomilla.
To distinguish between the symptoms of:

    turmoil in circulation
    turmoil in brain
    turmoil in temperament.

To identify the grades of symptoms in a symptom picture.

Headings: INTRODUCTION
ACONITE: Origin; Essence; Keynotes and Characteristics; Characteristic Presentation of Symptoms; Turmoil in Circulation; Fear; Similar Remedies
BELLADONNA: Origin; Essence; Keynotes and Characteristics; Characteristic Presentation of Symptoms; Turmoil in Brain; Belladonna in Rage; Similar Remedies
CHAMOMILLA: Origin; Essence; Keynotes and Characteristics; Characteristic Presentation of Symptoms; Turmoil in Temper; Similar Remedies
SELF-TEST QUESTIONS
FURTHER STUDIES

Introduction

These are known as the ABC remedies. In so naming them it was recognized that they are common remedies in children's ailments which tend to be sudden and often violent, having inflammation or temperature. Their characteristic symptom pictures may be found also in the early stages of illness where inflammation is common, i.e. before the suppurative stage or structural change sets in.

In this type of acute illness, vitality is not lowered but there is a strong disturbance, exciting cause, that causes a swift and powerful reaction from the vital force. The exciting cause is therefore strongly marked in the symptom picture. Each body responds along its lines of weakness producing a characteristic and individual symptom picture which the homoeopath then labels by the name of the remedy that cures. The pattern produced is an individual response repeated whenever this vital force is disturbed because the weaknesses are the same. We say the patient has a certain constitutional type which is also labelled with the same name as the remedy, hence an Aconite or Belladonna patient or disease pattern.

What follows will show that Aconite works on the autonomic nervous system producing a symptom picture that is described as *turmoil in circulation*, Belladonna draws the blood into the head producing *turmoil in brain*, whilst Chamomilla works more on the emotional level producing *turmoil in temperament*.

There is much similarity in the symptoms produced, so at this stage it is important to enhance their differences and to identify their uniqueness, or individuality. Thus we will emphasize

7

the keynotes and characteristics. Keynote symptoms are like the signature tune of the remedy. Characteristic symptoms are trends that run through the symptom picture in any ailment.

Aconite

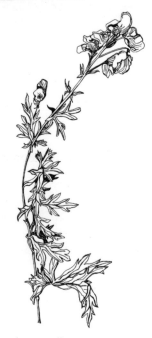

Aconitum napellus

Latin name: Aconitum napellus
Common name: Monkshood, wolfsbane
Botanical family: Ranunculaceae
Habitat: Damp and shady forests

Origin

The original proving was done by Hahnemann who took the juice from the plant as it started to flower (see Hahnemann, Samuel, *Materia Medica Pura*. B Jain Publishers, New Delhi). The separate effects of roots, flowers, etc. are unknown.
Caution: Since Aconite is a deadly poison it is never used below the third decimal potency (3X).

Essence

When we speak of the 'essence' of a remedy, we are describing the character of the energy that runs through the symptom picture. The state of the Aconite patient is described as *tension*, like a coiled spring he/she is ready for action, so the explosion is violent or he/she is paralysed by fear. These opposites will be present at different stages in the disease or in the overall history of the patient's symptoms. *The more healthy the more reactive.*

Keynotes and Characteristics

- **Fear**

- **Convinced he/she will die at a specific hour**
- **Pupils contracted to pinpoints**
- **< fright**

- **< cold dry exposure**
- < midnight
- Left sided
- **Hot, swollen redness of affected part**
- **Full bounding pulse**
- Redness of face becomes deathly pale on sitting up
- **Restlessness**
- **Pains** – tearing
            intolerable
            like knives
- **Sensation of a tingle**

- Convulsions with jerking and twitching of single parts such as an arm or leg
- **Paralysis**

- Retention of urine in the new born
- **Copious drenching sweats at the time of crisis**

It can be so great it is seen in the face of the patient.
This is connected to their fear of death.

The eyes are particularly noticed in the fear state.
The debility may continue for many years.
Exciting cause.
Exciting cause.
This is a modality to many of the ailments.
Though not always so there is a distinct trend.

Especially in fever, also in high blood pressure.
This is most commonly found in fever.

Toss and turn all night, e.g. after fright or with pain.
Because the nerves are affected.

May come with pain because of nerve involvement.
This is most likely to be found in childhood fevers.

Especially after fright, may affect only single parts, such as an arm or leg.
Is a form of paralysis after fright.
This is a robust animal reaction!

- Sweats on uncovered parts
- **Thirst – especially for bitter drinks**

- Everything tastes bitter except for water
- Apex left lung

- Dry, hard cough on respiration

- Trigeminal neuralgia on left side, after exposure to cold dry winds.

Strange, Rare and Peculiar.
This is most useful to distinguish Aconite from Belladonna.
Strange, Rare and Peculiar symptoms found in serious febrile states.
Is affected when inflammation reaches this vital organ as in pneumonia.
As we will see later this remedy often occurs in croup, or in children after exposure to cold dry winds.

ACTIVITY 1

Keynote and characteristic symptoms are so labelled because they occur commonly in cases denoting Aconite. They help us to identify the remedy. Note that they still fall into the categories of symptoms:

Strange, Rare and Peculiar
Mental and Emotional
General
Particular
Common.

List the keynotes and characteristics above and assign them to one of the five categories of symptoms.

ACTIVITY 2

Symptoms tell the homoeopath the depth of disturbance of the vital force. Symptoms on the level of sensation may occur long before serious pathology so to recognize the remedy at this level may prevent the development of serious pathology.

From the keynotes and characteristics list those symptoms describing *sensation*. All of these symptoms are experienced subjectively. Example: *pain feels intolerable.*

ACTIVITY 3

Symptoms of causation are invaluable as they describe weaknesses or susceptibility characteristic of this vital force. A symptom of causation is also called an exciting cause. What are the two major causations in the Aconite Patient?

Characteristic Presentation of Symptoms

Not all the keynote symptoms will be available in every Aconite case. Some will appear as the illness becomes more serious, but each and every Aconite case will have a characteristic pattern.

The causation will be found in most cases. Cold, dry exposure will usually give rise to inflammation. Fright produces a deeper pattern which will be dealt with separately.

In a very healthy situation, the vital force *reacts suddenly* and with *violence. On exposure to cold dry conditions*, sneezing with watery discharge may commence before an hour has passed. Fever may follow, with *hot dry* skin and *restlessness. The pulse will strengthen* and the temperature continue to rise depending on degree of exposure. A warm drink, a hot water bottle and a good night's sleep and the patient may be right as rain in the morning – especially if helped by a dose of Aconite.

A slightly less healthy vital force or more particular exposure may produce more local symptoms, e.g. in an ear, in the throat or the trigeminal nerve of the face. The part will be *red, hot and dry. The pain tearing* but *better for warmth. The left* is more likely to be affected. There may be *thirst* or *anxiety* which in turn produces *restlessness.*

More severe exposure may affect the vital organ, in this case, the lung, as in pneumonia or

9

pleurisy. There may be local *heat* and *tearing pain* plus general *fever*. Now we may see the *white face on sitting up*, *the sweat on uncovered parts*, *the bitter taste* and even the *pinpoint pupils* with *anxiety*. The *upper left* of the chest will be more affected. There may be an *aggravation around midnight* and such a *fear* they may *predict their death*.

ACTIVITY 4

Describe the symptoms of:

Earache
Pain in the throat
Neuralgia in the face.

Pay attention to which symptoms come first and then how they develop; describe each stage in sequence. This pattern of development will later help you to differentiate between remedies.

ACTIVITY 5

Modality symptoms are usually present in a case. These refer to what makes the patient's condition better or worse. The pain in each of the three cases in Activity 4 is better with warm applications. This is an example of modality. Modalities are important as they help us to differentiate remedies. From the text books list more modalities of Aconite, separating those which are aggravations from those which are ameliorations.

Turmoil in Circulation

Aconite has a powerful effect on the circulatory system, through its action on the autonomic nervous system which produces the *fight or flight* response – we either run with fear or we are paralysed by it. As adrenaline enters the system, blood vessels contract and the heart beats faster. The *tension* this gives rise to can be seen in the arousal (excited/excitable) state called panic.

This same tension can be seen in some forms of high blood pressure (hypertension) brought on by anxiety. The blood vessels contract, the heart beats faster, the pulse is full and bounding, and as the blood moves to the head there is a red face and bursting sensation. Often this will end in a nosebleed. The patient may fear for his/her life!

It is the fear of the Aconite patient and the action of Aconite to dilate contracted blood vessels that makes it of excellent use as a first aid remedy in some heart attacks.

In an acute anxiety attack, palpitations create even more fear and panic as the patient senses the abnormal, the uncontrollable or irrational, and fears for his or her life. The blood flow is upset, tending towards the head, as in the overwrought patient who develops apoplexy. The bounding pulse and fullness in the head are strongly felt symptoms. In the Aconite patient this happens with a speed which is frightening.

The fullness of the arteries easily produces bright red haemorrhage in any injury but if Aconite is the best remedy to cure, fear and the autonomic nervous system play a big hand too, producing some of the symptoms above, e.g. restlessness, anxiety for recovery, pinpoint pupils, cold sweat.

The fullness of the arteries produces such individualized symptoms as:

- as if the head would burst
- parts feel enlarged.

On the more local level it is possible to see a need for Aconite in an acute inflammatory case of rheumatism where the part is hot, dry and so swollen it feels large or as if it will burst. There is anxiety, of course. This may still fit the symptom picture of other remedies but if the best choice is to be Aconite, drenching sweats soon occur. Causation provides another pointer to Aconite – this acute condition started after exposure to a dry, cold situation.

Inflammation may be seen as local circulatory disturbance. The activity of the blood is increased to the injured part bringing more oxygen, nutrients, white blood cells to remove debris and platelets to plug gaps. This may also happen in response to a chill – in the ear, throat, tonsils, or in the lungs. The part responds rapidly with heat, swelling and pain. If a general fever follows, the cold drenching sweats and thirst may appear. The restlessness may show in moaning over their pain or they may toss and turn all night. This will be familiar to the mother of the small child. The child illustrates well the Aconite patient's reaction to illness. How can you explain illness to a child? Its intellect cannot understand so it is distressed and fear shows as anxiety. What will happen to me now?

ACTIVITY 6 List those symptoms from your Materia Medica textbooks that correspond to 'Turmoil in Circulation'. Differentiate between mental, general and local disturbance.

Fear

The fright side of the arousal equation needs special attention. It gives other characteristic pictures of the Aconite patient.

In illness the adaptations of the patient are affected. The mechanism does not work correctly. In the Aconite patient this means too much contraction (tension) or the lack of it.

First a paralysis is created in which the part is held rigid. We talk of being paralysed with fear. A good example is a rabbit held rigidly immovable waiting on the frightening object passing by. The paralysed bladder sphincter causing retention of urine in a newborn baby can be treated by Aconite when fear is the cause. Since Aconite works through the autonomic nervous system it is usually involuntary muscles that are affected. Often the breath is held in, for example.

After fright, the child may appear stunned and unable to respond, may run away blocking out the experience. The shock may be so great that the fear is carried for years, even a lifetime. If it cannot be put into words, which is often the case, it may produce blindness, deafness, dumbness or paralysis of the offending part. The key is locked in the unconsciousness because the person has not been able to react. In fear the patient holds him/herself away from the experience. The response is rigid and irrational. This irrationality can be seen in the child who is doing something for the first time, riding a horse, or a bike, diving off the high board in a swimming pool. The body may stiffen, the breath is held, the heart beats faster, the pulse bounds, the face may be red, but the mind is paralysed so it cannot go beyond this point, cannot give the orders to the muscles. If the situation is serious, the cold sweat and pinpoint pupils occur. Once the thing is done, the unknown dissolves so there is no further problem, but taking that first step is an ordeal.

If there is a sudden fright, the opposite may occur. The bladder or bowels may open involuntarily. This is a well-known reaction to fright. Tension, contraction and palpitations may then follow. Think of the experience of a haunted house!

In the child the fright may go on to produce an inflammatory illness or a cough that stays persistently. This cough is usually worse at midnight – the witching hour or the time of irrational fears!

ACTIVITY 7 Describe in detail the appearance and circumstance of an Aconite child riding a bike for the first time.

Similar Remedies

There are no end of possibilities here and we will deal only with the more common, following up in more detail in the advanced work.

Arsenicum is a remedy of fear and restlessness after midnight. Unlike Aconite, it would rather die than face the unknown. Arsenicum also has a very profound effect on circulation. It has a fastidious and organized personality, fearful of its social position.

Rhus toxicodendron is a remedy of restlessness and inflammation. It is even more physically restless than Aconite. It is much more irritable than fearful.

Causticum suffers from coughs in cold dry weather. The cough is worse on expiration and also tends to be left-sided. The fearful character of Causticum is more complex and pessimistic than

Aconite. A well Aconite patient is ruddy and healthy.

Hepar sulphuris suffers from coughs on exposure to cold dry weather. Its right-sidedness may not be apparent in the cough, but again like Rhus toxicodendron it is more irritable than fearful. Hepar sulphuricum is one of the chilliest remedies in the Materia Medica, very sensitive to draughts.

Spongia develops a cough after exposure to cold dry weather but the patient is worse on inspiration. Similar to Aconite the cough gets worse up till midnight.

Phosphorus is a remedy of irrational fear which sees monsters in the wallpaper. There is much imagination in Phosphorus and like Aconite it is a left-sided remedy that produces chest problems. The Phosphorus fear of death is calmed by company. Phosphorus patients are more frivolous in nature and much more easily diverted from their fear than Aconite.

Belladonna

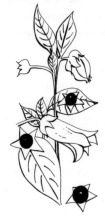

Atropa belladonna

Latin name:	Atropa belladonna
Common name:	Deadly nightshade, common dwale
Botanical family:	Solanaceae
Habitat:	Dry soils throughout Europe

Origin

Originally it was proved by Hahnemann from the tincture of the whole plant. Details of the proving are found in Hahnemann's *Materia Medica Pura*. Allen's *Encyclopedia of Materia Medica* contains information from poisonings after eating the berries.

Essence

Conflagration is a great consuming fire. Fire rises upwards, so many Belladonna symptoms move up to the vulnerable head. Almost all conditions requiring Belladonna involve inflammation producing:

- burning heat
- bright redness and dryness
- violent pains that throb, pulsate or shoot
- swelling.

Even on the mental and emotional level the most characteristic Belladonna state is rage, hot-headedness.

Keynotes and Characteristics

• **Sudden, violent conditions**	Describe all Belladonna cases.
• **Bright redness**	This is the increased local activity of the blood in inflammation, bringing nutrients, oxygen and the repair units of red and white blood cells.
• **Radiating heat**	Indicates the excessive presence of the blood. So hot is the face, says Kent, that you can feel the heat even without actually touching it. The Belladonna temperature is very high.
• **Dryness**	The heat is so severe the part is quite dry.
• **Throbbing pains**	Indicate congestion of the blood in that part.
• **Shooting pains**	Move along the tract of the nerve, often from a local spasm.

• **< heat**	Both of which increase the activity of the blood and movement to the head.
• **< sun**	
• **< right side**	This is very marked in this remedy.
• Pains move upwards	Like Hypericum they move back to the brain along the nerves.
• Red streaks along the lymph vessels	Are present in severe local inflammation such as mastitis.
• **Upward movement to head**	Of the blood, gives the fiery red colour and heat to the face.
• **Visible throbbing of carotid artery**	Since this supplies the head it indicates the very great movement of blood to the head and reflects the bounding pulse found in all arteries.
• **Dilated pupils**	This symptom gives Belladonna its name – beautiful lady. Belladonna works opposite to Aconite, dilating rather than contracting.
• **Aversion to strong light**	The dilated pupils are very sensitive to light.
• **Sensitivity to noise**	There is a strong action to over-sensitize all sense organs.
• **< jar**	This is particularly noted in the headache, but the sensitivity to touch is present in all affected localities.
• **Violent spasm**	This is intense throb or violent contraction of muscular tissue. It may be seen in the non-striated muscle of ducts – bile, pancreatic, urethra, uterus – or in jerkings or voluntary muscles in convulsions, etc.
• **Lack of sweat**	Until the crisis breaks, then the sweat brings down the temperature.
• **Convulsions**	Such is the heat in the Belladonna fever and since the head is so vulnerable, convulsions occur as the temperature rises.
• **Delirium**	The heat in the head creates turmoil in the brain. The patient sees monsters and has mania – *see the following symptoms.*
• Wild staring look	The pupils are dilated and the brain not focused with the eyes.
• Outbursts of wild laughter	This is the mania stage when all is out of order.
• Bites and strikes bystanders	More common in children in delirium. Hahnemann used Belladonna on the insane.
• Rips pillows	As above.
• **Rage**	The fear disappears so quickly to appear as rage. There is too much heat in the head!
• **Fear of dogs**	It shares this symptom with two related remedies, *Tuberculinum* and *Pulsatilla. Stramonium*, another remedy from the Solanaceae, has a marked presence of animals in dreams.
• **Fear of water**	Belladonna is one of the main remedies in rabies with its hydrophobia. The mania is then also present.
• Sensitivity to getting head wet	This is the chill factor, so it even applies to getting the hair cut. The head of Belladonna is very sensitive. Colds or worse ensue. **Exciting cause.**
• **< 3 p.m.**	There are several arguments for some of these time modalities. Frankly we do not know why the Belladonna patient should be < 3 p.m.

ACTIVITY 8

List the keynotes and characteristics of Belladonna and assign them to one of the five categories of symptoms:

Strange, Rare and Peculiar
Mental/Emotional
General
Particular
Common.

ACTIVITY 9

List all the keynotes and characteristics which you can think of to describe sensation.

ACTIVITY 10

What are the major causations of Belladonna? How might this apply to a case of epilepsy? Use your Materia Medica textbooks to find the characteristic symptoms of the Belladonna patient's epilepsy and describe how these develop from the causation.

ACTIVITY 11

List as many modalities of Belladonna as possible, using your textbooks. Separate aggravations from ameliorations.

Characteristic Presentation of Symptoms

Belladonna can be of use anywhere in the body where the activity of the blood is increased to cause inflammation.

Inflammation is the body's first line of defence. It is the increased activity of the blood to a locality bringing oxygen, nutrients and the repair units of red and white blood cells. This is a very swift action so the energy of Belladonna can be described as *sudden* and *violent*. This characterizes all Belladonna situations. Locally, on the site of an injury such as insect bite or the accidental blow from a hammer, there is *bright redness* and *heat*. The heat is so fierce that the part is *dry*. The local congestion of the blood causes *throbbing pains* locally but so severe is the congestion that *pains shoot upwards*. The modality is *better for cold applications*. This is not highly marked but is a useful distinction between Belladonna and Hypericum which has the same local inflammation. Where nerves are damaged it produces the keynote of *shooting pains along the tract of the nerve*. Belladonna produces a *red streak along the lymph vessels* from the wound. This is most often seen when the breast is inflamed as in mastitis. There are characteristic red streaks radiating from the nipple, accompanied, of course, by throbbing pains and heat.

On the acute general level, inflammation is *fever*. Chill and damp especially cool the head producing a fiery heat and congestion which shows a *red face*. The Belladonna child can have a very high temperature. Blood moves in the direction of the head producing a *visible throbbing of the carotid artery*, in the angle of the throat under the jawbone. The temperature is so great, *heat radiates* from the patient. Kent says that 'you want to withdraw your hand' or even that 'the sensation of heat remains in your finger afterwards'. The face may feel tight as it dries and burns. Internally, *the head feels full* – an intense throbbing pain may result. The fever may burn itself out after sleep or the pain and congestion may continue. There is a *lack of sweat until the crisis breaks*. We can tell that the remedy has acted when it produces sweat. If the sweat does not appear the temperature can soar. The eyes become glazed and *the pupils dilate*. The patient is noticeably *thirstless*. Delirium or even convulsions may appear if the vital force cannot localize the disturbance outwith the brain.

If the disease can be localized the tonsils, throat, or ears, may be affected. The Belladonna patient has *a great sensitivity of the sense organs*. The eyes are affected when there is congestion in the head, so the pupils dilate and there is an *aversion to strong light*. This is seen commonly in the headache. If the ears are affected there is a great heat, fullness and throbbing and, of course, *a sensitivity to noise*. Always the *right side is worse*. When a part is congested there is a *sensitivity to touch*. When the head is congested the keynote symptom *< jar* can be seen. There is a strong reaction producing *rage* when the bed is accidentally knocked. Any sudden movement increases discomfort in the affected part. When the head is very sensitive *each step reverberates through the head*.

A local inflammatory condition characterizing Belladonna can be found on the organ level in gallstone colic or where searing pains are associated with passing kidney stones. Such cases need expert attention. However, let us look more closely. In *violent spasm* (intense throb) the local part is very sensitive contracting spasmodically. If only we could cut the patient open we might surely see the swelling and fiery redness. To the homoeopath, all symptoms are part of the whole individual so we do not see the need of Belladonna in a case of gallstone colic without the presence of other more general symptoms. So, we do not need to cut the patient open to find the remedy if we can observe the whole case.

When the sweat breaks the crisis is over and the temperature drops. When the cold breaks the nose runs copiously. Belladonna is not well known as a remedy that goes down into the vital organs. It is able to produce a very high temperature instead.

ACTIVITY 12 Describe the Belladonna symptoms produced after a bee sting, sunstroke or throat pain.

Turmoil in Brain

This title applies to Belladonna as a fever remedy. A really healthy vital force reacts with speed and thoroughness so that a fever may be over and done with more rapidly than the act of externalization to the periphery, e.g. production of spots in measles – the fever comes before the spots.

Hahnemann used Belladonna as a specific in scarlet fever where the fire in the blood rushes out to the surface of the skin to produce large patches of fiery bright red rash. Once the wave – the disease process – reaches the skin the crisis is over.

The danger arises when the wave does not break. The vital force produces the fever and cannot stop. The temperature frequently rises to 103°+ in measles and scarlet fever, and the pattern of the energy flow in Belladonna is to the head! All the heat moves to the head often causing convulsions or delirium.

Anything that causes an increase of blood flow to the head will produce the turmoil in the brain. This may appear after a chill to the head, classically after getting the head wet, but also after getting the head too hot as in sunstroke.

As Belladonna affects the brain and the central nervous system the senses are disordered. This patient is very sensitive to all impressions producing exaggeration, so frightening nightmares and delusions are seen. Hideous faces appear. Monsters and animals, especially dogs, reach out to devour the patient. There is fear. The eyes stare and the pupils dilate. There is much excitement at first but as the fear is rapidly changed to anger the patient strikes out, bites, or rips up the bedclothes or anything else within reach. Clarke says they even growl and bark like dogs. He/she may prattle on or withdraw into stupefaction. Belladonna is very closely associated with Hyoscyamus and Stramonium which are also remedies of inflammation and mania. Each has differing proportions of atropine and hyoscine.

This fire exhausts the patient so they withdraw, avoiding company. As the excitement burns itself out on the level of the sensorium, activity ensues on another level – the motor nerves and vasomotor centre of the brain are stimulated, so muscles jerk and twitch in convulsions. Collapse and paralysis follow so eventually the breathing fails as the pneumo-gastric nerve is paralysed. Neatby and Stonham's *Manual of Homoeo-therapeutics* has an interesting and very full account of Belladonna affecting the central nervous system.

ACTIVITY 13 List those symptoms from your Materia Medica textbooks that correspond to turmoil in the brain. Differentiate between general and local disturbance and note those symptoms showing on a mental level.

Belladonna in Rage

The fire of Belladonna on the mental level can only produce consuming rage. This can be typified as hot-headedness. The image of rage is with steam coming out of the ears! We talk of blowing off steam and the concept is of a sudden explosion which is over and done with when it is out. This is the nature of the Belladonna rage. It is the type that produces apoplexy, but apoplexy is also associated with pomposity and being a windbag. Behind this is the idea of something very different from rage. Fear is close behind the Belladonna rage but the rage comes very quickly to defend the patient from the fear. Remember the hideous monsters 'getting at' the patient. This is the unconscious fear which remains.

There is no limit to the Belladonna outburst. They are capable of much destruction whilst externalizing the rage. Hence the biting and striking. This patient can lash out. He/she consumes people, tears them apart in the mind and then it is gone, just as quickly as it came.

ACTIVITY 14   Describe the temper tantrum of the Belladonna child. What do you think caused it?

Similar Remedies

Nux vomica has the rage of Belladonna that strikes out. It also has the heat moving up to congest the head but it has little of the delirium as most of its activity is in the digestive system. Nux vomica has the spasms of Belladonna.

Phosphorus has similar delusions to Belladonna and the movement of heat to the head but in Phosphorus the fear remains. It is a very fearful remedy.

Hypericum has similar red, throbbing swellings with shooting pains upwards in local inflammation. Belladonna is < heat whereas Hypericum < cold.

Chamomilla

Latin name:	Matricaria chamomilla
Common name:	Chamomile, corn feverfew
Botanical family:	Compositae
Habitat:	Found throughout Europe in cornfields and waste ground. The Victorians and earlier ages grew chamomile lawns where the sweet scent clung to the hems of ladies' dresses.

Origin

A tincture is made from the whole plant gathered when in flower. It was Hahnemann who first proved the remedy.

Today it is common to find the herb formed into a tea to calm nerves. It has been used for a long time as an anti-narcotic especially against the effects of overuse of coffee and opium.

Matricaria chamomilla

Essence

The main feature of Chamomilla is nervous excitability leading to irritability and *over-sensitivity*. Hahnemann states Chamomilla 'is unsuitable for persons who bear pain calmly and patiently'.

On a deeper level of physical disorder, it is described as 'suitable to nervous, bilious constitutions, and to the choleric temperament' – Hamilton, Edward, 1852 *The Flora Homoeopathica*, London.

Keynotes and Characteristics

• **< teething**	Because the child is so sensitive to pain. It cries piteously with rage and helplessness.
• **Temperamental** – rage	Temper tantrums. Throws things and bangs its head off the floor.
– nothing satisfies	Nothing is right and the patient is vexed and helpless, so rages at nothing, the injustice of it all.

- **Capricious**

The patient throws away what is asked for. There is not enough direction to tackle the problem and come to terms with it, yet nothing will distract either.

- **Contrary**
- Sends the doctor from the room
- Quarrelsome and rude

A better description of temper as the patient gets older. He/she cannot speak a civil word. This often applies to the woman during menstruation or pregnancy.

- **> being carried** (passive motion)

This matches the restless helplessness of the child. It shrieks as soon as it is put down so the parents end up walking the floor all night.

- **Restlessness**

The patient moves around a great deal in pain or emotional distress.

- Rocks back and forth

Usually in pain or distress. This is a way in which the older child or adult can express the passive motion. Nothing eases his/her plight.

- **Vexation**

Exciting cause.
This has a strong effect on the digestive system producing colic rather than diarrhoea. The baby derives colic from the mother's milk after she has been angered.

- **Hypersensitive**
- **< chagrin**
- **< humiliation**
- **< bad news**
- **Nerves over-stimulated**

All three of the next symptoms are **exciting causes** that play on the hypersensitivity. The expression may be depression rather than anger. She sits separate from others looking into herself. Usually this arises from a state of constant and continual pain. The patient tends to be overexcited, even hysterical and suffers insomnia. Pains out of proportion.

- **Intolerable pains**
- **Over-sensitive to pain**

The pain threshold is very low, so the child suffers terribly in teething and colic.

- **Numbness with pain**

The pain totally dominates consciousness and they cannot escape it.

- **Sweats with pains**
- Cutting, tearing pains
- < warm drinks

This is uncommon.
Because of the strong effect on the nerves.
A most unusual modality to pain, it is found most clearly in toothaches.

- < warmth in general
- Pains < open air
    < strong winds
    < night
    < touch
    < 9 a.m. and 9 p.m.
- **Convulsion**

This remedy is an acute of Lycopodium, which has the wind aggravation strongly marked. Lycopodium also has 'numbness in spots' and may drive the poor patient to despair because they are so sensitive.
The nerves are a major field of action of this remedy, so are over-stimulated as the temperature rises.

- Twitching, especially of calves, during pregnancy
- **Lienteric stools**

Digestion, like everything else about this patient is not completed. Hence the next three symptoms too.

- Green stool like chopped egg or spinach.
- Stools and vomit smell sour.
- **Flatus smells of rotten egg**

Is present in toothache/teething especially.

17

• Copious salivation	When colic or flatus disturbs digestion.
• > pressure on the abdomen	This child is thus often carried over the shoulder when it has digestive problems.
• One side of the face hot and red	This is easily seen in fever, toothache and affections of the facial nerves.
• Face sweats after eating and drinking	**Strange, Rare and Peculiar.**
• **Thirst**	This may be incessant with fever and pain.

ACTIVITY 15 List the symptoms above under the headings Strange, Rare and Peculiar, Mental and Emotional, General, Particular.

ACTIVITY 16 List the symptoms of sensation.

ACTIVITY 17 List the modalities of Chamomilla. Separate into aggravations and ameliorations.

Characteristic Presentation of Symptoms

The most notable facet of this remedy is the temperament, the *contrariness* and *capriciousness*, that arises out of being crossed. Being crossed is the **exciting cause**. It may be present as *vexation*, *chagrin*, *humiliation*, *bad news* or *intolerable pain*. This patient's nervous system is very sensitive. There is a very clear mental and emotional picture of *irritability* which in turn has a strong effect on the digestive system.

In teething the pains are intolerable. The poor mite wrestles helplessly, *calmed only by walking the floor with him/her*. As soon as he/she is put down he/she screams piteously. There is *copious salivation* and *the affected side of the face becomes red and hot*. *Colic* frequently accompanies teething, although it may arise on its own if the child is thwarted or may be passed in the mother's milk if she is of the Chamomilla type and becomes vexed. In colic, pain centres on the *umbilical area* and since it is *ameliorated by pressure*, the young child is often carried about the floor with parent's shoulder pressing into the abdomen, fireman style! The digestion is so disturbed it is uncompleted. *Sour vomit or eructations* come up; *sour-smelling lienteric stools* go down. The *stools are often green* in the young child, like chopped spinach. They may be *full of mucus*. Much *flatus* is produced that *smells of rotten eggs*.

When the child is older and more active Chamomilla may be of use in the 'terrible twos' who are often still *teething*. At this age the child is developing a concept of self, so is often *wilful*. Here we will see the exciting cause, vexation, chagrin or humiliation giving rise to the digestive symptoms. In the teething, we will see the child *rocking back and forth, crying with frustration*. We will also see the capriciousness – won't eat this, but when that is given it is thrown away. In temper tantrums and infantile rages, when he/she does not get what is wanted, *things are thrown, feet are stamped, screams of rage* accompanying banging his head off the floor. In this state many mums will tell you there is a point reached where the object is forgotten and the state of rage is perpetuated for itself. The child tires itself out, but is now so *overexcited* it is impossible to relax, to change gear into another state. This is a good example of **turmoil in temper**. Everything is now *out of all proportion*.

Turmoil in Temper

Hypersensitivity describes the Chamomilla state. Almost all the exciting causes are mental and emotional, thwarting the will of the individual. Even the oversensitivity to pain thwarts the will. There is a helplessness in which the patient is overwhelmed and irritated. As he/she exacts their will on blind fate, anger and frustration result.

It is easy to see this as a children's remedy because the young child is both omnipotent and helpless, so frequently ends up thwarted. It is a remedy of the spoiled child or of the young woman who is flattered and pandered to but effectively is not taken seriously, so has little bouts of 'hysteria' or temper.

In the adult, this remedy very much resembles Staphysagria but the stimulus in Staphysagria comes from without whereas I would say that of Chamomilla is from within. The Chamomilla patient cannot negotiate or come to terms. On the one hand he/she would not conceive of the need to do so, so is piqued. On the other hand, the pains are intolerable. There is no calm within. Nothing satisfies. They cannot see reason. They become argumentative and rude, with no civil word for anyone. A woman is often worse at times of hormonal change.

ACTIVITY 18 Describe in detail the symptoms of the minor ailments below in a Chamomilla patient.

Earache
Toothache
Headache.

ACTIVITY 19 Describe the behaviour of the three year old Chamomilla child at the tea table with the family.

Similar Remedies

Coffea has oversensitive, overexcited nerves and intolerable pains. They are restless and irritable and throw things. But they are > warmth and are < for nice surprises and joy.

Staphysagria has the frustration, helplessness and < anger of Chamomilla. The nerves and teeth are also strongly affected. A major exciting cause is < insult. Once again this remedy is > warmth, i.e. opposite to Chamomilla.

Nux vomica has frustration and is < anger. Nux is more impatient than helpless. It is out of order rather than out of proportion.

Calendula has the intolerable sensitivity to pain and is better for movement but there is more fear than anger in Calendula.

Colocynthis is a remedy of vexation that affects the digestive system with colic which is > hard pressure on the abdomen but Colocynthis is > for warmth, unlike Chamomilla.

ACTIVITY 20 Below is a table of comparison between Aconita, Belladonna and Chamomilla. Fill in the gaps from your notes and textbooks.

Aconite	*Belladonna*	*Chamomilla*
Turmoil in circulation	_____	Turmoil in temper
Fear – intangible (ghosts/dark)	**Fear** becomes **anger**	**Cross** and _____
Fear of _____	Fear of water	_____
Restless	_____	Restless
_____	Pupils dilate	_____
_____	Strikes out and bites	Capricious
< midnight	_____	< 9 a.m. and 9 p.m.
< fright	**< jar**	< _____
< cold dry winds	< sun	< _____
> _____	> rest	> being carried
	> lying on abdomen	
Thirst for bitter things	_____	Thirst for cold acid drinks
Pain tearing and cutting	_____	_____
_____	Sweats after crisis	_____
Bright face alternates with paleness		_____

SELF-TEST QUESTIONS

Find your answers in the text and then compare with the answers in the answer section.

1. Which remedy sweats with pain?
2. In which remedy does pain shoot along the nerves?
3. In which remedy is the sensation described as a tingle?
4. In which remedy will you find numbness with pain?
5. Which remedy is:
   a) right-sided?
   b) left-sided?
6. What are the fears of Belladonna?
7. Name three symptoms that accompany the Aconite fear.
8. State the modalities of:
   a) Aconite
   b) Belladonna
   c) Chamomilla.
9. Which remedy thirsts for bitter things?
10. Which remedy sweats on uncovered parts?
11. Which remedy sweats after eating?
12. Which remedy does not sweat in fever?
13. Which remedy has a cold sweat?
14. Name four exciting causes of Chamomilla.
15. Name two exciting causes of Belladonna.
16. Name two exciting causes of Aconite.
17. Describe the stools of Chamomilla.
18. How does paralysis affect the Aconite patient?
19. Describe the delirium of Belladonna.
20. How can Aconite help the heart patient?
21. Describe the capriciousness of the Chamomilla patient.
22. What relieves the colic of the Chamomilla patient?
23. What is peculiar about the heat in the Belladonna fever?
24. What is peculiar about the coloration of the face in the Aconite patient?
25. Describe the mastitis of the Belladonna patient.

Further Studies

Aconite

1. Compare the fear of Aconite to that of Phosphorus, Arnica, Causticum, Silicea and Argentum nitricum.
2. Compare the manifestation of fever in the Aconite patient and in the Baptisia patient.
3. Aconite is frequently used in haemorrhage – compare its use to that of Phosphorus and Ipecacuanha.
4. Compare the effects of cold, dry weather as it manifests in the following remedy pictures – Aconite, Causticum, Hepar sulphuricum and Nux vomica.
5. Compare the remedy picture of Aconite in pain with that of Chamomilla and Coffea.
6. Aconite, Belladonna and Ferrum phosphoricum are commonly seen in inflammatory problems. Compare their use.
7. Tyler uses Aconite and Spongia commonly in croup. Compare the manifestation of these two remedies in this inflammatory illness.
8. How do you think Aconite, Belladonna and Nux vomica are used to help hypertension?
9. Describe the heart attack case which may respond to the use of Aconite.
10. Describe the digestive system of the Aconite patient and determine when this system is likely to be disturbed.

Belladonna
1. Compare the fever symptoms of Belladonna, Stramonium and Hyoscyamus.
2. What relationship do you see between the deadly nightshade and the woody nightshade?
3. Describe the headache of Belladonna and compare it to that of Glonoine and Bryonia.
4. Name one childhood illness when the patient may be liable to convulsions and explain how Belladonna can be of use.
5. Name at least one inflammatory condition in an organ to which Belladonna may be applied. Describe this patient in detail.
6. How does the symptom picture of Belladonna compare with that of Phosphorus? Give similarities and differences.
7. Describe an acute affliction of a Calcarea patient that might respond to Belladonna as an acute remedy.
8. Is Belladonna only an acute remedy?
9. Compare the symptom picture of Belladonna and Pulsatilla in earache.
10. When might you use Belladonna in a first aid situation? Describe the symptom picture.

Chamomilla
1. Compare and contrast the symptom picture of Chamomilla and Nux vomica.
2. Distinguish between the symptoms of Chamomilla, Aconite and Belladonna in common cold.
3. Compare the capriciousness of Chamomilla, Ipecacuanha and Pulsatilla.
4. Name six remedies worse for anger and distinguish between them.
5. Describe the Chamomilla baby with colic. Compare this to the Lycopodium baby.
6. Describe a scenario at Chamomilla's first dancing class.
7. Chamomilla aggravates 9 a.m. and 9 p.m. Bryonia aggravates 9 p.m. to 3 a.m. Would you ever confuse these two remedies?
8. How does Chamomilla resemble Calendula?
9. What effects might you expect from drinking too much chamomile tea?
10. When is Chamomilla of use in insomnia?

First Aid Remedies

Arnica, Symphytum, Calendula, Hypericum, Ledum, Bellis Perennis

Aim: To demonstrate how the essence particular to these remedies makes them curative in specific first aid situations.

Objectives: To relate the essence of these six remedies to first aid cases.
To describe the characteristic symptoms of these six remedies in first aid cases.
To select a suitable remedy for some common first aid situations.

Note: To select a suitable potency you should study Lesson 8 in *The Principles of Homoeopathic Philosophy,* Margaret Roy.

Headings: INTRODUCTION
ARNICA: Origin; Characteristics of the Plant; Essence; Keynotes and Characteristics; Centralizing Action; Some First Aid Situations; Similar Remedies
SYMPHYTUM: Origin; Essence; Keynotes and Characteristics; Characteristic Presentation of Symptoms; Eye Injuries; Similar Remedies
CALENDULA: Origin; Characteristics of the Plant; Essence; Keynotes and Characteristics; Characteristic Presentation of Symptoms
HYPERICUM: Origin; Characteristics of the Plant; Essence; Keynotes and Characteristics; Some First Aid Situations; Similar Remedies
LEDUM: Origin; Characteristics of the Plant; Essence; Keynotes and Characteristics; Sluggish Circulation; Punctured Wounds; Eye Injuries; Similar Remedies
BELLIS PERENNIS: Origin; Characteristics of the Plant; Essence; Keynotes and Characteristics; Characteristic Presentation of Symptoms; Similar Remedies
SELF-TEST QUESTIONS
FURTHER STUDIES

Introduction

Homoeopathic remedies are of immense worth in first aid situations because:

- they can stop bleeding
- they can minimize shock.

In homoeopathy *any* remedy can act to stop bleeding because it stimulates the vital force which preserves life as its first priority. The organism has a procedure to isolate the outside world, plug gaps, clean out the debris and recreate the protective skin barrier. The homoeopathic remedy stimulates this process.

In first aid situations many die or recover poorly because of shock. Shock takes many forms. It is a state in which the vital force has been so disturbed that it cannot start the healing process. Of course, the homoeopathic remedy is ideal here because it works directly on the vital force.

However, a remedy will only work on the vital force if there is susceptibility, i.e. if the remedy can resonate with the predisposing weaknesses and the individual way in which these are expressed. Since there are limits to the ways in which the organism can malfunction when damaged from without on the physical level, there are 'specifics' which are of great value in first aid situations. We will look at these and at how their symptom picture facilitates this.

A word of caution. Homoeopathic remedies will work very effectively to cut the healing time to about one third but these results will be elusive if the remedies are prescribed routinely. The basics of a homoeopathic prescription remain always to carefully match the symptom picture of the patient with that of the remedy.

You should also be aware that basic first aid practices are indispensable. For example, pressure and elevation of parts can be carried out easily to relieve many haemorrhages.

Arnica

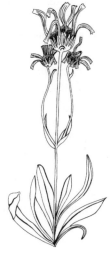

Arnica montana

Latin name:	Arnica montana
Common name:	Leopard's bane, mountain daisy, fallkraut
Botanical family:	Compositae
Habitat:	It grows in mountainous areas throughout Europe

Origin

Hahnemann prepared this remedy from juice extracted when the fresh plant was pressed.

Characteristics of the Plant

It is a perennial herb very like the daisy but much taller, one foot, which grows in cold high altitudes near the snow line. Gibson says it is conspicuous by its bright yellow flowers that 'are in such untidy disarray as to give the impression that the head of the plant has been bashed, perhaps by the mountain gusts'.

Gibson also tells us that, before the tincture is prepared from the root, flowers and leaves, the larvae of the arnica fly must be removed. Apparently these are commonly found on the plant. Before antiseptics and modern hygiene, larvae (maggots) were commonly found on wounds! Arnica is a remedy par excellence for wounds.

Miranda Castro tells us that '. . . its flowers, if inhaled when freshly crushed, cause sneezing – hence one of its nicknames, sneezewort'. There are many who take this remedy at the first sign of a cold!

Essence

Arnica is a deep constitutional remedy which works on the heart and circulation, so it has a profound effect on blood flow, on bleeding and, in physiological shock, on centring the volume of blood on the vital organs. In an accident Arnica helps the patient to regain equilibrium *from the centre*, from the heart.

Keynotes and Characteristics

• **Parts feel bruised, or as if beaten**	This may be actual external damage or due to a toxic internal state, as in 'flu'.
• **Parts lain on feel bruised**	So the patient moves constantly looking for the soft spot.
• **The bed feels hard**	
• **As if hit by a blunt instrument**	As in a fall or blow. This is the sensation of Arnica injuries.
• **Leave me alone, I'm alright**	Says the patient taking space to centre him/herself.
• Bruising	Blue-black in this remedy.
• Haemorrhagic tendency	Seen in most injuries.
• **Shock**	The organism is knocked out of alignment. Look at the mental symptoms!
• **Fear of being touched or approached**	A mental and physical need for space.
• **Wake up suddenly in the night with thoughts of the accident**	Frightened and then can't sleep. Stuck in groove they can't get out of.
• Terrible dreams of an accident or being harmed	This is part of the constitutional symptom picture as well as of the acute accident.

• In a coma he answers questions then falls off again	He is able to align and converse but with great effort.
• Forget quickly what is said to them	On a constitutional level this indicates he/she is losing a grip on reality.
• Cold extremities	The blood 'centres' in the chest and abdomen.

ACTIVITY 1   Once again order the symptoms into the following categories so you are aware of the relevant importance.

Strange, Rare and Peculiar
Mental and Emotional
General
Particular.

ACTIVITY 2   List those symptoms which are sensations.

ACTIVITY 3   Find the modalities of Arnica, separating those which are aggravations from those which are ameliorations.

Centralizing Action

The strong centralizing action of Arnica can be seen most clearly where there has been severe blood loss.

The organism has to use the volume left to nurture vital organs which are all centrally situated so the walls of arteries contract allowing less blood to the extremities which are pale and clammy, with a thready pulse.

Arnica acts to restore integrity to the whole. No other anatomical system has such immediate contact with all the parts as the circulatory system through which Arnica acts. As well as blood volume, it acts on the clotting factor which seals off the body when its physical integrity is breached. This is often a first stage in repair. Arnica is a remedy of haemorrhage and bruising par excellence.

On the local level the keynote symptoms are:

• parts feel as if bruised, or as if beaten
• as from a blow by a blunt instrument
• parts lain on feel bruised
• the bed feels hard.

If given immediately after the fall or blow, bruising does not develop because the vital force is able to react to correct the effect before the reaction goes too far. In one sense it is as if the walls of the blood vessel do not leak their contents but maintain their integrity. The opposite is also true when Arnica is able to dissolve a blood clot in stroke, coronary thrombosis or pulmonary embolism. Each medicine has its opposite reaction often at a different stage of the disease process. Here the action of Arnica is still to maintain the integrity of the whole and protect the vital organs.

The action of Arnica on the nervous system makes it invaluable as a pain killer. Pain accompanies the majority of injuries. It is the organism's signal that all is not well, that something is out of alignment and needs rebalanced. One type of pain peculiar to Arnica, *pricking from without inwards*, shows the pattern of movement to the centre. *Tingling of the extremities* occurs when the blood is limited or when nerves are affected as in some injuries.

The mental symptoms of Arnica show distinctly the centring action when we consider that the patient experiences a hiatus or space before reaction sets in. On the physical level this is expressed in the *numbness* that follows many injuries. It is a suspension of feeling before the pain occurs. In shock this may be a gasp, an open-eyed wonder, a brief speechlessness, or a jolt after an event that needs a little time to sink in. How long does it take to realize what has happened? At the scene of the accident the patient may need to create this space as others rush in to help before he/she has re-centred enough to react. So the Arnica patients *send help away saying there is nothing wrong*. They drag themselves from the scene and may take a while to realize the extent of their injury. Or in severe shock the patient may refuse to admit any damage. On the other hand, the patient may be only too well aware of injury, over-protecting self or the part, by *reacting strongly to the approach of others* or any *attempt to touch the part*.

When unconsciousness follows an injury, there is a bizarre situation when the patient *answers when spoken to* then sinks immediately back into unconsciousness. How can this be, except the patient draws together enough energy to function then disintegrates again immediately.

ACTIVITY 4   List the keynote and characteristic symptoms that illustrate lack of integrity.

Some First Aid Situations

There are many who would use Arnica routinely after any injury or shock. Here are some common first aid situations which specifically fit the Arnica symptom picture.

Bruising

Any damage to soft tissue causes bleeding below the surface, present in the Arnica patient as a blue-black coloration and accompanied by a bruised sensation. The bleeding and pain do not appear immediately. Instead there may even be numbness or a tingle before the pain appears. Arnica not only removes the pain, it also prevents the discoloration.

Tooth Extraction

Here there is shock to the disengaged nerve. A part is removed creating an opening into the body interior. The surrounding tissues are bruised. Blood vessels are damaged. Arnica is a great help to minimize the shock and bruising, to stop bleeding and pain.

Head Injury

Arnica is used almost specifically in head injury because there is no room within the skull for swollen soft tissue or bruising. Any excess matter puts pressure on space which ultimately affects the brain and consciousness so accommodation of the trauma must be speedily accomplished.

Should concussion develop and the patient recover consciousness to answer questions then Arnica is well indicated as a choice of remedy.

Concussion

Usually we use this term to refer to head injuries but it is possible to see concussion as any impact or physical shock to the bones – any injury from a blunt 'instrument'. Whilst bruised pains arise in the surrounding soft tissues, the afflicted periosteum of the bone may give rise to tearing pains. Horses often suffer concussion to the leg bones after trotting too much on hard surfaces. Humans may suffer concussion of the spine after mis-stepping or jumping onto a hard surface – the vertebrae are compressed.

Sprains and Strains

When a part has been overstretched or overused, a bruised ache often results. This may occur after heavy lifting, digging the garden for the first time in the spring, an extra long walk – any unusual use of muscles and tendons. As in the Rhus toxicodendron condition, the pain is increased at the first movement after rest but is better as the movement is continued. The ache is caused by stagnation and build-up of lactic acid in the muscles. The first movement increases the congestion. Further movement drains the tissues. The part is > for heat which improves circulation.

Hoarseness of the voice from overuse falls into this category too, when we remember that the vocal cords are connective tissue like the tendons and ligaments.

Broken Bones

Broken bones are a special situation that almost always requires Arnica. When a bone is broken there is usually damage to blood vessels and nerves, as well as bruising in the surrounding tissue. The periosteum of the bone which is rich in nerves is damaged. Arnica acts as a painkiller and stops bleeding so preventing a great deal of the physiological shock and trauma that surrounds broken bones.

After Operations

Operations are accompanied by bruising, bleeding and shock, so Arnica given before an operation can speed up recovery. It helps the nervous system recover from the shock of a general anaesthetic.

After Childbirth

During childbirth several things may happen which Arnica can help. There is a lot of bruising to the soft parts of the vagina and surrounding tissues. There is, frequently, overstrain of the muscles of the uterus and abdomen. There is usually bleeding. After childbirth the volume of blood reduces rapidly – this is one of Arnica's major fields of action – so given at this time it can ease change and prevent complications such as embolisms.

Given to the mother, it will also help the baby recover from the shock of birth and aid the recovery of the baby's head from being squeezed through the birth channel. If the child is breast fed it will get the remedy through the mother's milk without any need for separate medication.

ACTIVITY 5

Arnica acts to dissolve the clot in coronary thrombosis. It is a major heart remedy. Using one of the recommended textbooks, list the heart symptoms of Arnica.

ACTIVITY 6

Picture the Arnica patient at the scene of an accident. How do you think they will act?

Similar Remedies

Rhus toxicodendron has a similar action to Arnica in sprains and strains. Both have the same bruised pains and the same modalities. < first movement, > continual movement, > massage, > heat. Both can be just as irritable.

Symphytum is similar to Arnica in bone damage. The bone pains are tearing and persist long after the injury.

Aconite Arnica acts like Aconite to stop bleeding, Aconite by altering the dilation of the blood vessels. Both are remedies of fright that will dream of the ordeal or wake in the night disturbed by its memory.

Hypericum resembles Arnica in its effect on the nerves. Both produce numbness in nerves after concussion.

Symphytum

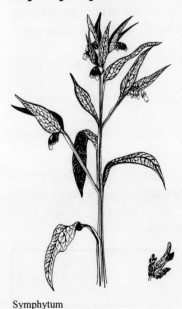

Symphytum

Latin name:	Symphytum officinalis
Common name:	Comfrey, knitbone
Botanical family:	Boraginaceae
Habitat:	Found in Europe in damp, low-lying fields, ditches and pond banks

Origin

This plant has long been used as a herb to heal bones and for bronchial problems. A potage of the leaves was used for the latter. The homoeopathic remedy was prepared from a tincture of the fresh root collected before flowering and in autumn but the proving was insufficient to produce a full picture so what follows is dependent on homoeopathic and herbal clinical experience.

Essence

The remedy *brings objects together*. Clarke quotes from Gerarde, the ancient herbalist, ' ... The same (leaves) bruised and laid to in manner of a plaister, doth heal all fresh and green wounds, and are so glutinative, that it will solder and glue together meat that is chopped in pieces, seething in a pot, and make it in one lump'.

Keynotes and Characteristics

- **Prickling pains in bones**

- **Bone pains after the fracture has healed**
- **Irritability at point of fracture**
- **Spasmodic jerkings of injured part**

- Cannot bear anyone to approach
- Pain in eye as if from a blunt instrument
- **Sensation as if the eye lid passed over a lump when the lid was closed**
- **Eyelid closes spontaneously of its own accord**
- Eyelid appears to droop all the time
- As if the ears were stopped up

- Back pain from sexual excesses
  < touch
  < motion
  < pressure
  > warmth

These three symptoms are all found in bone injuries or where bone injuries have failed to heal.

This is a little like tetanus! You may need to differentiate between Symphytum and Ledum. As in Arnica.
As in Arnica. It often cures where Arnica fails in eye problems.
Strange, Rare and Peculiar.

Due to spasm. As when someone tries to touch your eye unexpectedly.
After spasm, overactivity, comes, collapse.
This remedy produces a lot of mucus but here we have a sensation.

ACTIVITY 7

Order and list the symptoms above under the categories:

Strange, Rare and Peculiar
Mental and Emotional
General
Particular.

Characteristic Presentation of Symptoms

There is little individuality recorded for this remedy. It has a strong effect on *bones that fail to heal*. Its particular attributes in these situations include:

- prickling pains
- irritability over the site of the fracture
- jerks and spasms in the injured part.

The last, spasm, can be seen in other affected parts. It is spasm in the muscle that causes *the eye to suddenly droop* or to *fail to open* in the morning. The herbalists used it for coughs with copious mucus – one would expect the cough to be spasmodic.

The *lump sensation in the eye* reflects 'lumpiness' elsewhere. Lumps appear on poorly healed bones. At other times the remedy has been known to cure cancerous tumours. J H Clarke quotes a case in which Symphytum healed a protuberance that appeared on the spine *after a blow* to the back. Herbalists also used the remedy for caries of the bone.

Once again we see that each medicine has two actions, the first being opposite to the second.

Eye Injuries

One could not leave this remedy without commenting on its remarkable efficiency in eye injuries caused by a blow of almost any kind. You will note that when a foreign object is poked into the eye, it often responds by involuntarily blinking rapidly – spasmodically. Hence, when Symphytum is indicated in eye injury there is spasm and the sensation of a lump.

ACTIVITY 8

Read about the herbal use of Symphytum.

Similar Remedies

Arnica has a similar effect on bone tissue, especially where pain persists after the injury appears healed.

Ledum has jerkings and twitching around the site of a wound.

Calendula

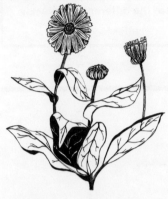

Calendula officinalis

Latin name:	Calendula officinalis
Common name:	Marigold
Botanical family:	Compositae
Habitat:	Found throughout Europe in cultivated parts

Origin

A tincture is prepared from the leaves and flowers.

Characteristics of the Plant

Calendula is a plant of the sun. The petals are a vivid orange glow. As the sun rises it opens these and when the sun sets the petals close. When the weather is wet or cloudy, the petals remain closed. Calendula is described as sun-loving; we could also say life-loving.

Essence

This remedy is a vulnerary with amazing aseptic properties. It has a specific action on epithelial tissue.

Keynotes and Characteristics

- **Pains out of all proportion**   As in Chamomilla.
- **Pains as if beaten**   As in Arnica
- Pains sting if there is fever
- Exhausted by pain
- Abscesses and suppurating wounds
- **< cloudy weather**   The flower closes as the sun passes.
- **> warmth**   The movement of the life blood is enhanced.

Characteristic Presentation of Symptoms

Calendula is a truly valuable remedy in first aid. Its specific action to repair epithelial tissue, as occurs in skin, makes it ideal for many kinds of wounds. It promotes granulation and prevents suppuration.

Ragged wounds such as grazes are ideally treated with Calendula. Some tell us we should have known this because the ragged leaves of the Calendula plant resemble the ragged skin that hangs down limply from the wound. This is The Doctrine of Signatures which was used by old herbalists, such as Culpepper, to give ideas as to the possible use of a plant suggested by its appearance.

It is near the surface of the skin (or organs), where Calendula has its strongest action, that we find the endings of sensory nerves. Therefore, we should not be surprised to find in the provings of Calendula the symptom *pain out of all proportion*. Applied neat to a wound, the Calendula tincture can sting severely so it is usually diluted 1:40. The action on the nerves may be further illustrated when used to help the patient who is *exhausted by pain* and *very chilly*. In this case Calendula is very similar to Chamomilla.

Perhaps the most impressive action of Calendula as a vulnerary is its *asepsis*. Since no micro-organisms can grow in its presence it heals wounds cleanly. It is used to bathe wounds when the tincture is diluted 1:40. It is recommended to use warm water to dilute as this promotes healing further – Calendula is > *heat*. After childbirth it is ideal to wash the vulva with a warm cloth soaked in Calendula to prevent sepsis and to soothe bruised soft tissue. After tooth extraction a warm mouthwash of Calendula will have the same effect of preventing sepsis and soothing pain.

ACTIVITY 9

Read up on Calendula in:

J H Clarke *Dictionary of Materia Medica*
Edwin Hamilton *Flora Homoeopathica*
Adolf von Lippe *Keynotes and Red Line Symptoms*.

ACTIVITY 10

Leave a few morsels of minced meat in a solution of Calendula. Expose another few morsels of minced meat with no Calendula solution. Compare the difference at weekly intervals.

Hypericum

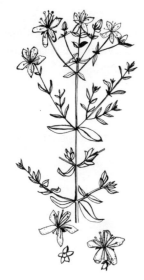

Hypericum perforatum

Latin name:	Hypericum perforatum
Common name:	St John's wort
Botanical family:	Hypericaceae
Habitat:	Open woods and hedgebanks in temperate Europe

Origin

The remedy has a long history of use by herbalists for healing wounds. The homoeopathic remedy is prepared from a tincture of the whole fresh plant. It was proved by several sources including Muller.

Characteristics of the Plant

This bush has a buttercup-type yellow flower in late summer. The bark is smooth like the myelin sheath of nerves. By nature the plant belongs to the most evolved type – the angiosperms. In action the remedy has a profound effect on nerves, the most evolved animal tissue. A characteristic symptom is pain along the tract of the nerve, also appearing symmetrically in the other limbs – just as the leaves appear in pairs on opposite sides of the stem. When held up to the light the leaf shows perforations which Gibson states are tiny oil glands. If we consider the dermis of the skin it too contains many secretory sweat glands.

The redness of the veins and the lance-shaped leaves have traditionally associated the remedy with bleeding.

Essence

The main action of Hypericum is on the nerves. It acts as a prophylactic in tetanus because it so strengthens the nerves that the bacilli cannot attack. As in Arnica, movement is to the centre of the nervous system, i.e. along the tract of the nerves to the brain itself, hence the vertigo after mis-stepping because the concussion travels all the way along the spine.

Keynotes and Characteristics

• **Pain shoots along the tract of a nerve**	Towards the centre of the nervous system.
• **Pain shoots upwards or towards the spinal cord**	
• **< moving the affected part**	The nerves must be activated to move any part.
• Shooting pains recur if the part is touched	
• Pains < movement, touch, pressure	Because the sensory nerves are activated.
• **Redness, swelling, throbbing**	As in Belladonna. The inflammation is found where parts rich in nerves traumatized.
• **Numbness** (After Injury)	As nerves are damaged. It may persist long after.
• **Vertigo – as if being lifted into the air**	This often occurs in head injury.

• Persistent buzzing in the head	May appear after head injury.
• Pain in phantom limbs	Where the nerve endings have been damaged by amputation.
• **Depression following injury or operation**	The central nervous system is depressed or suppressed and cannot recover.
• Asthmatic respiration after injury	This is as a result of total shock to the system.

ACTIVITY 11   List further individualistic symptoms after reading the chapters on Hypericum in:

J T Kent   *Lectures on Homoeopathic Materia Medica*
Adolf von Lippe   *Keynotes and Red Line Symptoms*
M Tyler   *Homoeopathic Drug Pictures.*

Some First Aid Situations

Injury to Nerves

Hypericum is often called for in injury to parts rich in sentient nerves, e.g. fingertips, toes, bed of nail, coccyx and periosteum. It is used especially for mechanical injury to nerves. If a finger is crushed, as when accidentally hit by a hammer, or shut in a door, there will be *redness, throbbing, numbness* and perhaps *pain shooting up the arm*. In this injury the bone of the finger is involved so the periosteum is bruised causing prolonged pain since it is rich in nerves. Later numbness may set in as the nerves are so excited they can no longer respond. *Shooting pain* may occur again *if the part is touched*, otherwise numbness may persist.

Hypericum may be called on especially when the spinal nerves are damaged usually by concussion but also by a direct blow. After the injury the patient may find that greater pain shoots upwards along the spine and into the brain *when he/she tries to move a part, e.g. an arm*. In childbirth the coccyx is often damaged and headaches may result or sensitivity when the part is touched.

Where there is head injury, Hypericum may be indicated in two ways which both suggest nerve involvement. First is *vertigo* with a peculiar sensation of *being lifted into the air*, and second is a *persistent buzzing in the head* especially at night. If either of these symptoms are present after head injury Hypericum is a better remedy than Arnica. It may be given in a 30th or 200th potency and repeated as the sensation recurs.

When nerves are damaged after amputation, pain persists in phantom limbs on occasion. Hypericum may be of value here to repair nerves. It may also be of use to promote integrity and aid healing when a limb or part is almost severed from the body in an accident.

Punctured Wounds

Hypericum is most commonly called for in first aid situations involving deep wounds or burns. In the punctured wound there is a risk of dirt and bacteria being sealed into the wound as it heals and closes over the surface. This is especially likely to happen if Calendula is used as it heals the epidermal layer very rapidly. The interior muck then produces a suppuration. This often happens to horses when medication is put on a punctured foot wound to seal it. Modern medicine dislikes such a wound to be closed as tetanus bacteria multiply in such anaerobic situations and these attack nerves.

Hypericum in the 30th potency speeds the repair of deep dermal tissue, prevents suppuration and strengthens the nerves so tetanus cannot attack. Even Kent suggests this routinely as it is such a life-saver. However, it is still best to have the indicated symptom picture of throbbing, redness, burning with shooting pains extending towards the spine. If these are present, it does not matter what caused the punctured wound – a nail, a wasp, a knife, a snake. Hypericum can be used to treat snake bites especially when the venom attacks the nerves – a much higher potency may be required of course!

Burns

Hypericum is well used as a remedy for burns because of its effect on healing the deep dermal layer of the skin. Its action to prevent suppuration is invaluable in burns when one of the major complications is sepsis. Homoeopathic treatment of burns uses bandages soaked in Hypericum.

Over a two-week period more Hypericum solution may be applied to the bandage, but the bandage is *not* removed. It may be covered by a second bandage which is changed as it gets dirty. Using Hypericum the homoeopath has no fear of sepsis so there is no need to continually change the bandage ripping off the newly formed skin in the process. Thus Hypericum heals burns without scarring.

Burns are often accompanied by much pain because the deep layer, the dermis, is damaged. This is where the sensitive nerve endings lie. Use the pain as an indicating symptom and repeat the 30th potency of Hypericum each time the pain returns.

It is of especial use in electric burns which often penetrate into the body and exit again after shooting along a pathway. The character of shooting along a pathway makes Hypericum homoeopathic in such incidents.

Other Uses

Toothache believed by some to be worse than childbirth because it is a nerve pain. It may respond well to Hypericum if the symptoms agree!

Corns and bunions often involve pressure on underlying nerves. When this happens Hypericum can be useful.

ACTIVITY 12 Describe in detail the symptom picture of a burns patient who might respond to Hypericum. Pay particular attention to the pains.

ACTIVITY 13 Read up on the poisoning effects of cobra venom. How might Hypericum prove a similimum?

ACTIVITY 14 List the modalities of Hypericum, separating those which are aggravations from those which are ameliorations.

Similar Remedies

Belladonna shares the throbbing, red swellings after local trauma. It even has the red streaks striking in towards the centre from the wound. However, Belladonna is < warmth.

Apis has red swellings as in Belladonna and Hypericum. It also has the stinging pains of Hypericum and may share oedematous swellings around the wound.

Staphysagria has a profound effect on nerves especially the spine. It has cutting pains that persist after the injury. It is also used for injuries from sharp implements.

Ledum

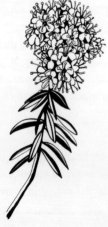

Latin name:	Ledum palustre
Common name:	Marsh tea, wild rosemary
Botanical family:	Ericaceae
Habitat:	Cold, marshy peat bogs of Northern Europe and America

Origin

There is a long history of use as a herb in Northern Europe. Hahnemann proved the remedy homoeopathically after preparing a tincture from the dried twigs.

Characteristics of the Plant

This plant is a member of the heather family. It grows in northern climes in cold, wet surroundings. It survived the ice age. One of its adaptations is said to be the downy hairs on the undersurface of the leaf which conserve heat. Indeed Gibson says the name is derived from the Greek 'ledos' meaning a woollen garment.

The dark green of the leaf enables better use of the sun for photosynthesis in northern latitudes. Is it coincidence that the patient is dark haired and prefers the cold?

This is a remedy of sluggish conditions, of alcoholism and biliousness. The odour of the plant is described by Gibson as akin to hops, whilst the taste is bitter.

Essence

This is a very deep remedy of circulation. The constitution is sluggish and congested. Flow of blood to extremities is so poor blueness is common locally. Patients often have a rheumatic diathesis and are prone to gout. The furthermost extremities are affected so it looks as if symptoms begin below and travel upwards.

Keynotes and Characteristics

• **Coldness of part > more coldness**	Truly a **Strange, Rare and Peculiar symptom** when a wound is cold and > cold.
• **Blueness**	Because there is not enough oxygen.
• **Numbness**	Because there is little circulation of blood locally.
• Twitching around the wound	The nerves are affected locally. This is also a major symptom of tetanus.
• Ecchymosis – greeny-yellow	The bruising occurs in first aid situations and where blood flow is sluggish. Because circulation is slow it remains a long time.
• **Left sided moves to right**	
• **Upper left, lower right sidedness**	The lower part has already shifted to the right. Difficult to recognize. This is a general symptom shared with Rhus toxicodendron.
• **Symptoms appear to start below and travel upwards**	In fact sluggish flow first cuts off the extremities.
• Swollen hot joints << heat.	Because circulation is activity which increases heat.
• **Lack of vital heat**	Is the general state of the first keynote, cold > cold.
• **Desires alcohol**	It is interesting we crave what makes us worse, in this case alcohol makes us more sluggish.
• Boils	Because of poor circulation and build-up of toxins.
• Stiffness of muscles	Because of sluggishness and toxic build-up.
• Bruised feelings in muscles	One stage on from the above.
• Intense itching of feet and ankles	This build-up of toxins under the skin starts in the lowest extremities and proceeds upwards.

ACTIVITY 15   List the symptoms above under the appropriate headings:

Strange, Rare and Peculiar
Mental and Emotional
General
Particular.

ACTIVITY 16   List those symptoms which are sensations.

ACTIVITY 17   List the modalities of Ledum, separating them into aggravations and ameliorations.

Sluggish Circulation

What does this mean?
How does it affect constitutionally?
How does it apply to a first aid situation?

Although it is possible that the organism is so shocked after trauma that it slows down, it should be apparent to you that there is a deeper state here. The situation that produces coldness and blueness in a wound did not appear suddenly. It is often present in alcoholics after long abuse of the drug. The heart is certainly affected in the end and many characteristic symptoms of Ledum relate to this stage. However, before the vital organs decay there is a multitude of more local symptoms of congestion – the dull hue that increases to *discoloration* as circulation fails, *boils*, *itching of feet and ankles, irritable rash under the skin, acne-like eruption, stiffness* and *bruised feelings in the muscles*.

Consciousness is affected so *irascibility* and *dissatisfaction* may indicate a toxic state. The discontented escape to the bottle! This leads on into *sobriety* then to isolation as the patient *prefers his/her own company*. You could say the Ledum patient is cold emotionally.

This same shutting out is to be seen in the extremities. First the over-acid metabolism isolates and irritates joints such as the big toe in **gout**. Neatby and Stonham tell us Ledum seeks out the small joints because 'they are less cellular'. Later the whole foot is irritated and itchy, then coldness and discoloration set in. If bruised muscles come first, the *soles of the feet may be tender to stand on* or, more likely, the muscles higher up the leg may ache. There are *itchings* and *cramps* and *oedematous swellings* so the whole symptom picture is usually described as rheumatism constitutionally.

ACTIVITY 18 Describe in detail the symptom picture of a Ledum patient with gout. Use as many keynotes and characteristics as you can.

Punctured Wounds

When a deep wound occurs, the integrity of the organism is broken so it must react to re-establish itself. This is done primarily through the actions of the blood bringing nutrients, oxygen, white blood cells and platelets.

In the Ledum patient the circulating system is slow to perform the task. The heat does not occur – indeed vitality and more heat are lost so *the part affected becomes cold*. The blood that does leak into the surrounds of the wound is venous. *Blueness persists* long after the injury has healed because the circulatory system is so slow to mop up the debris.

Irritability is shown by *twitching*. The affected part could not cope with heat. It would only irritate further because there is not enough flow. Indeed the injured part is *cold, blue, numb and better for cold applications*. The numbness is the lack of vitality so even the nerves are stunned.

In such a lifeless situation the anaerobic tetanus bacilli can thrive to create further twitching and numbness by attacking the nerve.

Where bleeding does occur, *the blood may be black*. This half-congealed, half-coagulated state of the blood should remind you of the effect of venom from the viper type of snake. This poison acts through the circulatory system slowing down the blood and causing it to coagulate. It comes as no surprise, therefore, that snake bites are also punctured wounds which respond well to Ledum.

Eye Injuries

This is a useful remedy for black eyes. This part of the body is easily bruised as the surrounding skin is so thin. When an injury involves bleeding into the vitreous humour of the eyeball this resembles the Ledum situation because there is no blood circulating there to clear the debris, the blood vessels being outside the ball of the eye itself.

The peculiar affinity of Ledum for the eyes can be seen in the *headache* which may be *accompanied by bursting eyeballs*.

ACTIVITY 19 Find out more specific details of the Ledum patient's type of headache.

Similar Remedies

Lachesis is a snake venom with a profound effect on the circulatory system. It produces blue discoloration, alcohol craving, sensitivity to touch and is averse to anything like heat which increases circulation.

Rhus toxicodendron is very similar to Ledum in the way it creates an itchy rash under the skin and the effect it has on muscles and joints. Muscles ache, joints are swollen and sore.

Symphytum in eye injuries resembles Ledum. Both may twitch though Symphytum feels a lump under the lid that is little different from the sand felt in the eye of the Ledum patient.

Bellis Perennis

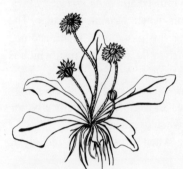

Bellis perennis

Latin name:	Bellis perennis
Common name:	Daisy, wound-wort, bruisewort
Botanical family:	Compositae
Habitat:	Grassland throughout temperate climes

Origin

The proving was done from a tincture of the whole fresh plant.

Characteristics of the Plant

Like the marigold, the daisy opens and shuts its petals with the sun. This gives rise to another name, 'the day's eye'. It is a hardy perennial as those who mow lawns will attest. When trodden on, it bounces back. In homoeopathy it is used to revitalize bruised soft tissue.

Essence

This is a remedy of stasis where weak soft tissue is often engorged with venous blood so there is a bruised sensation.

Keynotes and Characteristics

- **Venous stasis** — May cause varicose veins in engorged soft tissue.

- **Bruised sensation**
- **Effects of blows to soft tissue**
- **< sudden cold soaking** — **Exciting cause**.
- **< cold drinks when overheated** — The stomach is especially affected by cold.
- **Tired, desires to lie down** — This is a general level interpretation of stasis and worn-down tissue.

- **Left sided**
- **Sleeplessness at 3 a.m.** — Links this remedy to a group of tuberculoid remedies such as Tuberculinum and Pulsatilla.

- Wakes too early and cannot sleep again
- Stitches in spleen — This hints at the potential depth of Bellis perennis.

- Head pain from occiput to sinciput. — As in Pulsatilla another remedy of venous stasis.

ACTIVITY 20

Arrange the above symptoms into a list under the headings:

Strange, Rare and Peculiar
Mental and Emotional
General
Particular.

ACTIVITY 21

Make further notes on the remedy after reading:

J H Clarke *Dictionary of Materia Medica*
M Tyler *Homoeopathic Drug Pictures*

Characteristic Presentation of the Symptoms

The remedy is often used after accidents involving soft tissue (e.g. abdominal organs) or after operations or childbirth. It could be described as the Arnica of soft tissue because it is used for *bruising*. In such events we do not see the bruising but know it has taken place and may be led to the remedy by the *bruised pain*. I have also noticed a tendency in the patient to support the part which is *sensitive to touch*. This symptom picture may be found in overweight venous stasis types *before menstruating* when the reproduction *organs are engorged*. Similarly the remedy is used for problems in pregnancy such as piles, varicose veins, a bruised and *tired uterus*.

Overworked muscles may respond well to Bellis perennis when *weakness* results. The elderly will often produce tired, sore muscles and surrounding soft tissue after unaccustomed exercise. Both of these symptom pictures may include the *desire to lie down* and rest, which is not refreshing, and *sleeplessness*.

Generally the bruised part is *soothed by rest and warmth*. *After a soaking* the situation may be brought on, on a general level, with aching and tired muscles all over. More specifically, *the stomach will feel weak* and *nauseated after cold drinks chill it* when overheated.

The constitutional type will produce the typical headache when stressed. The remedy is seldom used constitutionally because it is poorly proved.

Similar Remedies

Arnica resembles this remedy in bruising but the Arnica type is more likely to be irritable than weak.

Rhus toxicodendron resembles Bellis perennis in muscular strain. However, Rhus toxicodendron does not have the weakness. Instead of resting Rhus patients will be restless.

Pulsatilla shares the venous stasis of Bellis perennis. A bruised sensation is characteristic of Pulsatilla. It also affects the reproductive organs. The Pulsatilla patient produces varicose veins and a tired womb in pregnancy and has bruised pelvic organs before menses. Even the headache is similar but Pulsatilla is right-sided whilst Bellis perennis is left-sided.

ACTIVITY 22

Construct your own reference table of a first aid situation in which you could use these remedies. Pay particular attention to the characteristic symptoms and keynotes that would guide you to select each remedy.

SELF-TEST QUESTIONS

Answers can be found in the answer section.

1. Which remedies you have studied in Lessons 1 and 2 fit the situations given below?
   a. A child has just been bitten and the wound has started to swell. As yet there is no colour but there is a numbness creeping up the arm into the elbow.
   b. The little boy flicked the collar of his shirt into his eye. It is very painful to touch and in fact feels as if there is something in it but you can see nothing.
   c. Jean fell off her bike and has skinned her knee. It is very sore.
   d. Tom was hit by a football and the white of the eye is starting to show bloodshot after only ten minutes. The eyelid twitches and is cold.
   e. Vincent picked up his father's soldering iron. There is a deep indent across the palm which is red on either side. He is screaming. The pain is throbbing.

f. The old lady is complaining about a funny noise in her head. After careful questioning you learn that she fell and hit her head yesterday.

g. After falling off a ladder the patient has numbness in the hip which feels very stiff. After rubbing it and encouraging her to move it she seems to feel better.

h. The child awakes from a nightmare bathed in sweat and obviously in a very frightened state.

i. Jenny's abdomen feels bruised and sore. She rubs it gently. She had some ice cream after her sauna this morning.

j. Mum has very sore arms after struggling home with the Christmas shopping. The next day her muscles are stiff and sore when she gets up in the morning. They are better after a while when she gets going.

k. The patient accidentally shuts her hand in a drawer. It is throbbing violently and has gone red. The pain shoots upwards but is better when she waves it very gently in the air.

l. The little girl fell down when rushing towards her mother for a sweet. She is distraught and screaming and seems inconsolable until her mum picks her up and rocks her gently to and fro.

m. Old John dropped a brick on his foot whilst gardening. It is now black and blue and very sore. The only relief he gets at night is sticking it out of the covers to keep it cool.

n. Uncle Fred was stung by one of his bees. The pain is hot and stinging and the wound is red and throbs.

o. Mary stubbed her toe on the pavement. It is now considerably swollen and throbs. She does not want anyone to touch it and gets fearful if anyone approaches too quickly. Her family laugh at her caution.

2. What is the difference between Belladonna and Hypericum in a bite from a gnat?

3. After a child fell out of its pram what different symptom pictures might develop if the remedy was:
   a. Aconite?
   b. Arnica?
   c. Symphytum?

4. In what kind of injury might you compare Arnica, Ledum and Symphytum?

5. In a burns case, how would you distinguish Hypericum as the remedy?

6. What is the similarity between Chamomilla and Calendula?

7. When would you choose Hypericum rather than Calendula for a cut?

Further Studies

Arnica

1. Compare the heart symptoms of the Arnica patient with those of the Lachesis and Aconite patient.
2. Describe the flu symptoms of the Arnica patient.
3. Describe the behaviour and symptoms of the Arnica patient who has just broken a leg falling down a cliff.
4. List and explain the modalities of Arnica.
5. How do the skin problems of Arnica resemble those of Rhus toxicodendron and Arsenicum?
6. Compare Arnica, Bellis perennis and Ledum.
7. Read Neatby and Stonham's chapter on Arnica.

Symphytum

1. Compare Symphytum, Arnica and Ruta in bone pains and affections.
2. Make notes on the type of bronchial symptoms aided by Symphytum.
3. Compare the use of Symphytum, Mercurius and Causticum in bone tumours.

Calendula

1. Compare the effects of different bacteria which affect surface wounds.
2. Compare the pains of Calendula, Chamomilla and Coffea.
3. Compare Calendula, Hypericum, Ledum and Hepar sulphuris calcareum in suppuration.
4. How does the action of Calendula on epithelial tissue affect its use as a remedy in cancer conditions?

Hypericum

1. 'Hypericum is to the nerves what Arnica is to the blood and circulation.' Discuss.
2. Tyler begins to tell us of Hypericum and the Doctrine of Signatures. From your knowledge of this plant, and first aid, expand on this theme.
3. How is Hypericum to be recognized in head injuries?
4. Give three distinctive symptoms by which you would recognize Hypericum in an illness.
5. Compare Hypericum and Staphysagria in spinal damage.
6. Research the effects of tetanus and its presentation.
7. Make notes on the effect of Hypericum in asthmatic conditions.

Ledum

1. What is the difference between the symptoms of Ledum and Hypericum in punctured wounds?
2. Compare Ledum with at least three other remedies you might use in first aid for insect bites.
3. Compare the use of Ledum with that of Hypericum, Ruta and Rhus toxicodendron in injuries of the fingers and toes. See Tyler, *Drug pictures* p.502, if you have problems.
4. Compare the symptoms of Ledum with those of Lachesis and Carbo vegetalis in dropsy of old people.
5. Compare Ledum, Sulphur and Lachesis in alcoholics.
6. What are the similarities between the Ledum and Lycopodium symptom picture?
7. When is Ledum a better remedy than Arnica in bruising?
8. When is Ledum a better remedy than Aconite or Symphytum in eye injuries?

Bellis Perennis

1. Compare the bruising of Bellis perennis and Arnica. Which would you use for a traumatic injury of the testicles? Give reasons.
2. When would you use Bellis perennis for injury to the spleen?
3. Compare the symptom picture of Bellis perennis and Pulsatilla.
4. Bellis perennis, Rhus toxicodendron, Dulcamara and Pulsatilla are all worse after getting soaked. Compare the symptom picture that arises.

The Solanaceae – a Botanical Grouping

Hyoscyamus, Stramonium, Tabacum, Dulcamara

Aim: To discover how plants from the same family, even with alkaloids in common, have distinctive symptom pictures.

Objectives: To identify the keynotes and characteristics of each remedy.
To describe the difference in the symptom picture of each.

Headings: INTRODUCTION
HYOSCYAMUS NIGER: Origin; Characteristics of the Plant; Essence; Keynotes and Characteristics; Characteristic Presentation of Symptoms; Spasm; Similar Remedies
STRAMONIUM: Origin; Characteristics of the Plant; Essence; Keynotes and Characteristics; Disturbance in the Brain; In Fever; Similar Remedies
TABACUM: Origin; Characteristics of the Plant; Essence; Keynotes and Characteristics; Characteristic Presentation of Symptoms; The Neurasthenic Type; Similar Remedies
DULCAMARA: Origin; Characteristics of the Plant; Essence; Keynotes and Characteristics; Characteristic Presentation of Symptoms; Nervous Affections; Similar Remedies
SELF-TEST QUESTIONS
FURTHER STUDIES

Introduction

In this lesson we will look at four members of the Solanaceae family which also includes Belladonna, Mandrake, Tomato and Potato. A few members of the family are edible. A few like Belladonna are so poisonous they can kill. It reminds us that some naturopaths do not consider potatoes to be a healthy food and that, in our own practices, we often take tomatoes out of the diet of certain types of patient – the rheumatic, acid type – because they increase irritability in the system.

Whilst each plant is unique even within the family group, there are similarities in family groups. Homoeopathy brings out the relationships between plants in developing the full symptom picture in the provings.* You should find it interesting to compare the similarities and differences in these remedies.

Before beginning you may find it of use to review the information you collected on Belladonna.

Hyoscyamus Niger

Latin name:	Hyoscyamus niger
Common name:	Henbane, hogbean
Botanical family:	Solanaceae
Habitat:	It is found throughout Europe and in some parts of North America on road sides and rubbish heaps.

*It opens a whole new perspective for your study of plants.

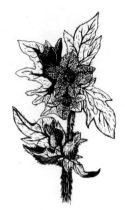

Hyoscyamus niger

Origin

Hahnemann proved the remedy from a tincture prepared from the whole plant.

Characteristics of the Plant

In Antiquity, three varieties were known and used medically – except the black henbane, Hyoscyamus niger, which was considered too poisonous. It is a prickly biennial. The yellow trumpet-shaped flowers have a huge purple eye at the centre. The leaves are of two types – one year a simple oval leaf occurring as a rosette at the base, then the next year the pale leaves appear on a stem that rises to 3 feet to carry the flowers aloft. All is covered in hairs which secrete a resin that gives the leaves a sticky, clammy feel. The whole plant has a heavy oppressive odour. Gibson quotes Scherk as saying it lives 'exclusively on human refuse, on the corpses in the cemetery or the offal that lies around human dwellings.' This is not a nice plant!

Essence

The remedy has such a strong effect on the mind, the person is 'out of it'. He/she retreats to their own inner world. The personality changes. It is a remedy of delirium, of grief and disappointed love, and of insanity. There is a niggle that all is not as it seems and *they* are out to get him/her. This drives them to deceitfulness as a defence. It is a very provocative remedy. Like the plant the person exists in two worlds and there is *conflict at the point of interchange* between the two.

Keynotes and Characteristics

• **Spasm**	Parts may jerk and twitch. Jerk and twitch with worms. Can't swallow fluids. Epilepsy – attacks end in sleep. **All** muscles twitch, even eyes.
• **< fright**	**Exciting cause** of some of the jerking.
• **Dry hacking cough as if a dry spot in the throat**	< cold air.
• **Spasm without consciousness**	As in epilepsy.
• **Prattles**	As if delirious!
• **Hands move constantly, picking at bedclothes**	There is a restless spirit here.
• **Eyes stare**	As in Belladonna fever. They bump into things because they do not see them.
• **Jaw drops**	As in a corpse.
• **Jealous**	**Exciting cause**.
• **< disappointed love**	**Exciting cause**.
• **< rage**	Will reduce the patient to an apoplectic speech-lessness.
• **Bite and strike out**	As in Belladonna.
• **Incoherent speech**	As occurs after fright or apoplexy.
• **Paranoia**	That someone is out to get them.
• **Fear poisoning**	They often won't take the medicine.
• Fear of being alone	What might others be plotting? What might attack them?
• Fear of running water	Surely not as in witches?
• **Sleepless**	Because brooding.
• **Starts awake again**	Once again a restless spirit.
• **Suddenly sits up in the middle of the night**	But not conscious. Usually when mentally disturbed.
• **Restless in sleep**	Twitches or cries, showing mental disturbance.
• Cruelty	They can be sly and vindictive.
• **Imbecility**	Eventually the mind cuts out.
• Expose themselves	In insanity they are sexually depraved.

• **Sing lewd songs**	They do not need to be depraved to do this. Think of some senses of humour.
• Make gestures	Usually having sexual connotations.
• **Cunningly deceitful**	They are very suspicious and play games with you.
• Sees dead loved one sitting in a chair, or standing in the room. They talk as if the vision were still alive.	Here is an example of their two worlds.

ACTIVITY 1   Separate the symptoms and list under the categories:

Strange, Rare and Peculiar
Mental and Emotional
General
Particular.

ACTIVITY 2   List the symptoms produced by spasm.

ACTIVITY 3   List the modalities and the exciting causes to show you know the difference. Separate modalities into aggravations and ameliorations.

Characteristic Presentation of Symptoms

This is seldom a remedy for minor problems. When the Hyoscyamus patient succumbs it is with violence as in Belladonna. It is a remedy of change – as when the leaf-type changes from one year to the next.

In illness there is a *great sinking of strength*. Consciousness is affected. In the eye there is no focusing, though they *spasmodically open and close the lids*. There can be *deafness* in the ear because the nerve is affected. This pattern occurs in all disorders. As energy sinks there is *spasmodic activity but no consciousness*.

In fever they will *prattle* and *pick at the bedclothes*, but there is no relationship to the real world. The *eyes stare*, the *jaw drops*. Speech becomes *incoherent* as they fail to get it together. If forced into the outer world they become irritated and *spit*, metaphorically or in reality, *bite* and *lash out*. They feel unsafe. If this gets worse, the paranoia may lead to *fear of being poisoned*. There is such a difference between the inner and outer world.

In the constitutional picture they are *jealous*, *suspicious* types, but do not present this overtly. They are *covetous* since they fear that someone who knows too much about them has power over them. Thus they are *sly*. They may avoid questions, or *lie*, smiling at you as if innocent. They may try all sorts of subtle ways of escaping the interview, and the remedy. It is often the relatives that bring them because they are worried about them suddenly *sitting bolt upright in bed* in the middle of the night, with no consciousness whatever. When speaking to you they may have a *nervous tic* when they are worried or defending themselves. This symptom picture may arise after *grief*, the loss of a loved one, or *disappointed love*. It is the mind underneath that is trying to speak of its disturbance in the middle of the night. It cannot get out. The feelings are locked in. The tic is a sign of conflict between their inner reality and outward expectations.

These patients can feel so threatened in their loss that they become truly paranoid. The *mania* of Hyoscyamus is horrific to behold. It may be simply prattling, *talking to the loved one that is not there* and suspicious of you because you do not share their world or they lose touch with reality. If there is any foundation for their fears, real or imagined, they may *retaliate subtly*, but most *vindictively*. In the end they may *rage* and storm violently. When they are totally insane and out of themselves the *sexual depravity* may become evident as there are no ties with the norms of society. This can be most distressing. One lady I knew of lost her husband to another woman. She appeared eventually to have accepted this but disappeared every so often and came back, to the shock of her very religious family, with her clothes in tatters and obviously the worse for wear. During the interview she behaved perfectly normally and said she did not know what they were talking about. Did she know?

ACTIVITY 4 Using the *Mind* section of Kent's Repertory, find out the different ways in which mania might be represented.

ACTIVITY 5 Check the entry in the Repertory for Hyoscyamus under the rubrics for the mental and emotional symptoms given here. In what grade of type do they appear?

Spasm

This characteristic of Hyoscyamus needs special mention. It occurs on an acute and chronic level and as a result of the exciting cause or trauma.

Where there is acute inflammation the part may go into spasm. During an acute illness, it may appear on the general level as involuntary diarrhoea or micturition. These always come with restlessness and fearfulness. The child does not want to be alone. When they catch cold there is usually a cough. This is spasmodic and characterized by a dry patch in the throat which reacts to cold air.

When Hyoscyamus is indicated in many diseases of childhood there are convulsions where all the muscles twitch but there is no consciousness. This is a remedy of epilepsy in which fits often occur in sleep. If not, it is followed by sleep. The spasms are described as angular, tossing the body around. Interestingly, the face is purple – remember the flower?

The exciting causes, even in such as epilepsy and St Vitus' dance, are usually marked. Fright is a major exciting cause, giving rise to spasms. The child may be frightened into a cough, may start from sleep, or sit bolt upright without consciousness in the night, may develop a tic, St Vitus' dance or epilepsy.

ACTIVITY 6 Describe the symptoms of the epileptic fit of the Hyoscyamus patient.

ACTIVITY 7 Read the account of Schenk's poisoning on page 245 Gibson, Douglas 1987 *Studies of Homoeopathic Remedies*, Beaconsfield. Note how the feet are different from the vertical body as in the plant!

Similar Remedies

Causticum produces spasms from fear. It is more a depressed, reserved type.

Drosera has the spasmodic cough, as if something were stuck in the throat. It is irritable and reactive.

Phosphorus is one of the few remedies outside the Solanaceae that resembles Hyoscyamus. It is a fearful remedy that produces symptoms after fright. It can also be a remedy of sexual depravity and disappointed love. Both have hoarseness too. It is a remedy of imagination and clairvoyance rather than spasm.

Stramonium

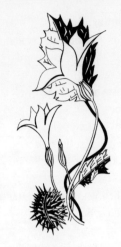

Datura stramonium

Latin name:	Datura stramonium
Common name:	Thorn apple, devil's apple, devil's trumpet, stink weed.
Botanical family:	Solanaceae
Habitat:	It grows throughout Europe, Asia, North America 'where a rank soil is created by deposits of refuse from human habitation.'

Origin

The proving was done by Hahnemann from tincture prepared from the fresh plant before flowering. Powdered seeds are also used to prepare the mother tincture.

Characteristics of the Plant

This is a most striking plant with enormous leaves. These give off a heavy, nauseating odour with narcotic properties. The sweet-smelling white flowers cause stupor if smelled for too long. The flowers open at night to attract night-flying insects – this is most unusual. The seeds are especially poisonous. Gibson has a keen sense of the hostility of the plant. He says the fruit '. . . explodes like a hand grenade, scattering black seeds of death.'

Essence

Terror runs through the Stramonium symptom picture. Inflammation affects nerves and brain, creating much disturbance. Like Belladonna, Stramonium contains a higher proportion of atropine than hyoscyamine alkaloid, hence the greater influence of inflammation in the symptom picture than in that of Hyoscyamus.

However, Stramonium is also a remedy of *alienation*. Here the terrors of the inner world invade the conscious world, so they are still in the nightmare when sleep has ended.

Keynotes and Characteristics

• **Terror**	It is visible on the face as in Aconite, but it is imaginary in origin.
• **< fright**	Gives rise to spasms and convulsions.
• **See animals jumping about in the dark**	This remedy has the imagination of Phosphorus.
• **Scream in nightmares**	There is so much terror in this remedy.
• **Rigid with fear on waking**	The young child is rigid like a board. 'They shrink in fear from the first object seen.'
• **Eyes stare**	As in Belladonna.
• **< looking at glistening objects**	Sensory nerves are much excited. Bright objects cause delirium, spasm and convulsions.
• **Small objects look large**	Another example of the distressed sensory nerves.
• **Cannot bear to be alone**	Because of the fear.
• **Want their hand held**	To be in touch with the real world which eludes them.
• **Rave**	This occurs in delirium brought on by all sorts of fevers – measles, scarlet fever, etc.
• **Desire to escape**	In delirium.
• **Talks incessantly**	In fever or when ill.
• **Struck speechless**	With fright.
• Calls things by the wrong name	The cognitive faculties are also disturbed.
• **<< alcohol**	It can be used for alcoholics when they see things and frighten themselves.
• **Hot, red face, cold hands and feet**	Blood and heat move upwards to the head. Unlike Belladonna they sweat with heat.
• Cannot bear to be uncovered in sweat	
• Speech incoherent with headache	Because the nerves are disturbed.

• Painlessness	Where pain would be expected.
• Spasm	Is as highly marked in this remedy as in Hyoscyamus.
• Spasm in top half of the body only	**Strange, Rare and Peculiar.**
• Voluntary muscles more mobile, involuntary muscles slow down	Stramonium is known for gracious movement as opposed to Hyoscyamus' angular, awkward movements.
• Consciousness in convulsions	It is the opposite of Hyoscyamus.
• Suppressed eruptions	Cause nervous disturbance.
• Moods swing between joy and sadness	This is a movement between two poles, one outward moving and the other reflective.
• Pray all the time	When stuck in the reflective world.
• Sing all the time	When outward going.
• Obsessive	Rather than paranoid. They want a lot of attention. Note, obsession is a holding-on.
• Lewd	As in Hyoscyamus.
• Fumble genitals	Similar to Hyoscyamus' gestures but note the fixation with one area is more marked.

ACTIVITY 8   List the symptoms under the categories:

Strange, Rare and Peculiar
Mental and Emotional
General
Particular.

ACTIVITY 9   List the exciting causes and modalities of Stramonium, showing you know the difference between these two terms.

ACTIVITY 10   List all the symptoms that show a disturbance of the sensorium.

Disturbance in the Brain

Hyoscyamus shows disturbance of the passions, the emotions. In Stramonium it is the brain that is disturbed, affecting perception and cognition.

Stramonium was sacred to the Navajo Indians who used it to gain contact with the spirits that live in animals, plants and rocks. If you lost something you need only eat a piece of Datura and you would see where to find your possession in a dream. Stramonium was recognized as so powerful that you only used it when other methods failed and even then you made sure you had a good singer whose strong voice could help direct its power!

In fever the co-ordinating ability of the brain is disturbed, so data is not interpreted as before. Fright also brings on this state. If there is no fear, fear becomes part of the picture. As in Aconite the fear is very visible but whereas the Aconite patient's fear is direct and under-standable, the fear of Stramonium is imaginary. The fear comes from the nightmare, or is imagined in the dark. There is a *dread of the dark* because they see ghosts and *imagine all sorts of monsters in the dark*. In particular they *see animals jumping about*. In delirium the *eyes stare*, as in Belladonna, but there is a *cold sweat* as in Aconite, and the mind *raves*. In the nightmare, *the child screams even before it is awake* and *when awake it is as if it is still in the nightmare* and cannot really come to and recognize those around it. They may not even recognize Mum and you may feel you need to waken them up even though apparently they are awake. Very young children in this state may be *stiff as a board*. When older, the patient may have a great *desire to escape* when delirious. A useful keynote of Stramonium is *consciousness in fits*. You cannot describe the above as a fit, but will recognize this strange quality of consciousness whilst yet not in control.

Cognition and perception are distorted.

There is in Stramonium the same excitement of the sensorium that we find in Belladonna, hence the *staring eyes* and the keynote < *looking at glistening objects*. Bright objects cause delirium, spasm and convulsions. Another keynote to do with the changed state of the sensorium is *small objects look large*. The patient may also wake with 'a shrinking look as if frightened at the first object seen'. The cognitive processes of the brain have been disturbed. It is not surprising with their world disorientated that the patient *cannot bear to be alone* and *wants their hand held*. The Navajos said Datura made the mind go round and out in many directions. Things are called by the *wrong name*, or the patient *talks incessantly* or is *struck speechless*. It is << *alcohol* which confuses the brain. Stramonium can be used for the fright alcoholics get when they see things!

ACTIVITY 11 List the different delusions attributed to Belladonna, Hyoscyamus and Stramonium. Search through this section of Kent's Repertory to find more. List also the disturbance of sensorium and disturbances of cognitive faculties for these three remedies.

In Fever

As in Belladonna, blood moves upwards to the head producing a number of symptoms but notably *face hot and red with cold hands and feet*. Stramonium differs from Belladonna in that the heat *is* accompanied by *sweat*. There may be dry, glowing heat all over the body as in Belladonna. With headache the Stramonium patient becomes *incoherent in speech*. The main Strange, Rare and Peculiar symptom is *painlessness* in inflammation where other symptoms would normally suggest pain. Suppressed inflammation goes inwards as *spasm* to the brain and spinal cord. The spasm of Stramonium is as highly marked as in Hyoscyamus. It comes on from *fright* or from *suppressed eruptions* such as measles. The twitching of Stramonium may be only in a single muscle or group of muscles, or it may occur only *in the upper half of the body*. Another difference between Stramonium and Hyoscyamus is that during the convulsions the Stramonium patient remains *conscious*. When deeply disturbed, or when the inflammation in the brain is caused by emotional crises, you may find the patient *prays* or *sings all the time*. In mania they *may talk all the time*, or as *moods swing between joy and sadness* they may *alternately talk or sit speechless and sad*. When the brain is much disturbed it is one of the remedies of madness.

ACTIVITY 12 Note down the symptom picture of Stramonium in the following minor ailments. Pay attention to modalities.

Measles
Sore throat
Fright.

Similar Remedies

Aconite is commonly used in children after fright. Whilst Aconite produces paralysis, Stramonium produces disturbance of consciousness, though both could produce inflammatory illness.

Phosphorus sees monsters in sleep and waking as does Stramonium. Both hate the dark but can find the light too much. Like Stramonium, Phosphorus loses boundaries between one state of consciousness and another.

Opium This patient dwells in dark caverns peopled with black animals as in Stramonium. There is much fear and fright and lack of control.

Tabacum

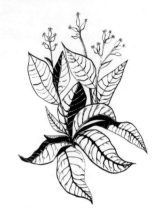

Nicotiana tabacum

Latin name:	Nicotiana tabacum
Common name:	Tobacco
Botanical family:	Solanaceae
Habitat:	It grows in warm, dry climate zones.

Origin

The proving was done by Lembke, Schreter and others from a tincture made from fresh leaves.

Characteristics of the Plant

The plant grows 4–6 feet. The main alkaloid is nicotine from which the vitamin niacin is derived. This same alkaloid is used as an insecticide. It is found in the leaves which are the source of the remedy. The leaves are covered in hairs, some of which secrete a viscid, gummy substance. There is a considerable amount of citric acid also present which is interesting in the context that the vegetable acids antidote the effects of tobacco and of other Solanaceae.

Essence

The remedy has a most powerful effect on the central nervous system, producing spasms or flaccid paralysis. The patient is put out of touch with themselves through nausea and vertigo. J H Clarke mentions several provings in which there is irritability, followed by memory loss. During the out of touch phase one prover experienced vivid imaginings which he only remembered on recovery.

Keynotes and Characteristics

- **Nausea**
    - **> open air**
    - **> uncovering the abdomen**
    - **as if the stomach hanging down**
- **Vomit < movement of any kind**
- **Vertigo on opening the eyes**
    - **< rising**
    - **< looking up**
    - **> open air**
    - **> vomiting**
    - **increases to loss of consciousness**
- **Death-like pallor**
- **Nervous tremor**

- **Debility**

- Weak irregular pulse

- Weak sinking in stomach
- Icy coldness of skin with cold sweat
- Icy coldness from the knees down
- Sensitive to noise and light
- **Loquacity**
- **Apathy**
- Despondency
- **Paranoid**
- **Spasm**

This is the beginning of the state of disassociation of mind and body. Seasickness > in the open air.

It leaves a weakness and inability to concentrate or focus.

Accompanies the nausea and vertigo temporarily.

This is a chronic state which is antidoted temporarily by smoking a cigarette.

May be very deep and chronic. Can attack suddenly.

The next symptoms are found to occur with the debility in acute and chronic states.

As in Stramonium and Belladonna.
Is the overactive mental phase.
Is the equivalent of flaccid paralysis in the mind.
Accompanies many other symptoms.
He feels someone is out to get him.
These are tetanic in the poisonings. Death is caused by paralysis of the respiratory system.
They come with deathly nausea and are often followed by prostration.

• Palpitations from use of tobacco	Smokers often end up with heart problems such as angina pectoris.
• Paroxysms of sneezing last weeks	< lying on the left side.
• **Constriction of muscles of hollow organs**	**Strange, Rare and Peculiar**. What language would the patient use to express this?
• **Cramps in calves**	Develops into severe circulatory symptoms in smokers.
• Renal colic	An example of spasm in vital organs.
• Spasms of anal sphincter	From oral to anal fixation!
• Hiccough	Spasm of the diaphragm.
• Dry, tearing cough > sips of cold water	
• Prolapse ani	This is the relaxed stage.
• Seminal emissions involuntarily at night	
• **Vision < looking at white objects**	Showing oversensitivity of the sensorium.
• **As if looking through a veil**	Now the eyes are slow to focus.
• Blindness through atrophy of the retina or optic nerve	The final stage of withdrawal from the world!
• **Periodicity**	Headaches occur regularly.

ACTIVITY 13   Separate and list the symptoms under the categories:

Strange, Rare and Peculiar
Mental and Emotional
General
Particular.

ACTIVITY 14   List the symptoms of spasm and relaxation.

ACTIVITY 15   List the modalities of Tabacum. Are you aware of any exciting causes? Separate into:

Exciting causes
Aggravations
Ameliorations.

Characteristic Presentation of Symptoms

All acute and chronic phases of the symptom picture are accompanied by *prostration*, *a deathly pallor* and *a cold sweat*. It is thus a remedy of collapse resembling China, Veratrum Album and Camphor. The mode of activity is through the nerves which act upon the muscles to first relax then constrict or tense the muscles. When the drug is used in its crude dose by those with nervous tension, as with the tobacco smoker, it cures this temporarily. When the effects wear off they reach for another cigarette.

In its action it 'lets go.' Thus it appears the opposite of remedies like Nux vomica that tense up. Letting go is a loss of integrity and organization, so *nausea* and *vertigo* represent a separation of consciousness from the body. The nausea may be violent with a death-like pallor and *vomit that brings no relief*. The epigastric area may feel empty and limp. Curiously the *nausea is better when the abdomen is uncovered*. It is also *improved by acid fruit or drink* that starts the next phase, contraction. The nausea comes through *excessive stimulation of the senses*, as in the constant control needed in sea travel to change and accommodate the eyes to the moving landscape.

The vomiting represents the spasm and contraction of the stomach. It is very violent and worse for movement of any kind, so you will see them in a deathly pallor, with eyes closed, clinging to the mast of the boat out in the open air. This is how they will travel.

The relaxation can be seen at its worse in the inveterate tobacco-smoker whose circulation is so affected the *veins relax*. Coldness can then be seen to start at the knees. When disease reaches the heart we see *palpitations*. Then the spasm of *angina pectoris*. Before that stage there will be *cramps in the calves* and the restricted movement of *intermittent claudication*.

Vertigo is another type of relaxation which may plague the long-term smoker, but it is more likely to affect the non-smoker exposed to a quantity of the crude dose. If we note the symptoms Tabacum can be used curatively when vertigo is produced with *nervous exhaustion*. *The vertigo is worse opening the eyes*.

Relaxation then contraction can be seen in many local symptoms of the tobacco smoker. There is a constant need to urinate when the bladder is relaxed, lack of hunger when the stomach is contracted and, in the morning copious catarrh from relaxed mucous membrane and a dry smoker's cough.

ACTIVITY 16 Study the disease patterns of some smokers known to you. Trace the increasing disorder to the vital force. Try to identify the difference between symptoms of relaxation and contraction.

ACTIVITY 17 It is difficult to sort out the symptom picture caused by the long-term use of the drug and the constitutional type that will respond curatively to the remedy Tabacum. The first is a symptom picture showing maintaining causes. To help you identify the second, I would like you to sketch the symptom picture of the following ailments:

Travel sickness on a bus
Cholera
Constipation.

The Neurasthenic Type

This term is not commonly used in medicine today. J T Kent and Sigmund Freud would use it easily to describe the Tabacum type who ranges from the hysterical, fainting patient to the ME sufferer of today, from the Ignatia/Ipecacuanha type to the Camphor/Veratrum type.

The Tabacum patient is sensitive and easily disturbed, producing nausea, vertigo or fainting. They are pale in colour, shake and tremble easily and exhaust quickly. Their pulse may be weak and irregular when they have icy cold skin on the extremities. There is a clamminess from cold sweats.

The senses are so sensitive that exposure to light may bring on a headache and the deathly nausea.

They are introspective, insecure types. Often this gives rise to a state of apathy, or one in which they feel sorry for themselves. So involved in themselves are they, that they cannot take note of others. They are self-centred.

When the cognitive faculties slow down they are confused. At the same time transmission to voluntary muscles slows down so they move more slowly and may be clumsy. When the mind is more prostrated, imbecility may result but first there is loquacity, 'silly talk' as they 'let go'. The patients are so introspective they may appear paranoid, that someone is out to get them. Despondency is the rule when ill.

ACTIVITY 18 Examine the symptoms of ME from a perspective of comparing it with neurasthenia. How does the Tabacum symptom picture fit that of ME?

Similar Remedies

Ipecacuanha is a sensitive type who produces travel sickness after over-stimulation of the pneumogastric nerve, > closing eyes and not relieved by vomiting. It is a remedy of relaxation of mucous membrane producing copious discharge.

Ignatia is a sensitive type who is strongly affected by tobacco. There is a lot of spasm in Ignatia, particularly of the diaphragm and there is emptiness in the epigastric area. Fainting is common.

Camphor has faintness and prostration with a deathly coldness and is > coldness. There is also a great deal of spasm in the remedy. It tends to have more energy than Tabacum to produce distress rather than despondency.

Veratrum album has sudden sinking of strength with coldness and cold sweat. It too is > cold. It has violent spasms often brought on by tobacco-chewing. It is often called the cold Arsenicum.

Dulcamara

Solanum dulcamara

Latin name:	Solanum dulcamara
Common name:	Woody nightshade, bittersweet
Botanical family:	Solanaceae
Habitat:	It grows throughout temperate Europe in damp, shady places.

Origin

Hahnemann proved the remedy prepared from a tincture of the shoots and leaves before the plant flowers.

Characteristics of the Plant

The red berries are poisonous. At first they taste bitter then the action of saliva produces a sweet taste, hence the name bittersweet. The base of the plant is woody, but Gibson says the upper branches '. . . climb and trail restlessly over shrubs and hedgerows by twining around any available support. This urge to keep moving is characteristic also of the Dulcamara patient.'

Essence

Dulcamara affects the mucous membrane and the lymphatic system, also all areas where fluid is absorbed or secreted. The Dulcamara patient has a rheumatic diathesis, < cold, damp weather.

This is a deeper and slower remedy than the four Solanaceae we have studied so far. The active alkaloid is solanin rather than atropine or hyoscyamine. Solanin paralyses nerves and muscles.

Keynotes and Characteristics

• **< cold, damp**	**Exciting cause.**
• **< getting soaked**	**Exciting cause.**
• **< chilling, after overheating**	**Exciting cause.**
• **< suppressed sweat**	**Exciting cause.**
• **Cutting pain at the navel**	During the diarrhoea.
• **Green, slimy stools**	When chilled, after overheating.
• **Sour smell**	Especially with the stool, but also vomit and sweat.
• Yellow, watery stool < damp weather	This patient is very responsive to weather conditions.
• **Restlessness**	With a strong desire to move and > motion.
• **Spasms and twitching**	This precedes the paralysis stage.
• Restless in sleep	Movement prevents stiffness.

• **Excessive urination**	After cold, damp weather.
• **Milky deposit in urine**	After getting soaked.
• **Perspiration on the palms**	
• Offensive sweat over all body	Night and day.
• **Rheumatic dropsy**	< suppressed sweat or eruptions or exposure to cold.
• Tearing pains in limbs	After cold, damp weather.
• **Paralysis from lying on damp grass**	The side lain on is affected.
• One sided paralysis	After exposure to cold, damp weather.
• One sided paralysis with speechlessness	After getting soaked or exposure to cold and damp.
• Dry, red, crusty eruptions	Worse on the head.
• Crusts red rimmed	As in tinea capitis.
• Intense itching, > cold < scratching	This remedy is very similar to Rhus toxicodendron.
• Depressed	When the sluggishness affects the mind.
• Can't concentrate	As above.
• Confused – cannot find the right word	This is a deeper stage to the above. Stiffness affects the mind so it cannot function. This will increase as the state increases.
• Head feels large	Rather than bursting and full as in Belladonna.
• Eyes discharge	Rather than stare.
• Eyes twitch	In cold air.
• Menses suppressed	There is a tendency for discharge to be suppressed by cold, damp weather or by a soaking.

ACTIVITY 19

List the symptoms under the categories:

Strange, Rare and Peculiar
Mental and Emotional
General
Particular.

ACTIVITY 20

List the exciting causes and modalities of Dulcamara. Some aggravations and exciting causes are the same this time. Separate into:

Exciting causes
Aggravations
Ameliorations.

Characteristic Presentation of Symptoms

In the provings the symptoms produced are not inflammatory, or in the blood, as in Belladonna. Dulcamara is a remedy of the mucous membrane and the lymphatic system. It affects the water balance of the body and those areas where fluid is absorbed or secreted. An example of its common usage is given by Kent who saw many cases of watery diarrhoea brought on when the child was rapidly cooled in the evening after a day of intense heat. *Chill after overheating* is a keynote.

In children it is usually the digestive system that reacts. *Cutting pain at the navel* and *green slimy stools* (not unlike Chamomilla) are two keynotes that illustrate the disturbance in the digestive system and also remind us of the violence of Belladonna (i.e. the cutting pains), but they also point to Dulcamara's special action on epithelial (lining) tissue causing it to over-secrete (mucus in this case, hence the slime). The special nature of the gut is worth noting. Greater activity here can greatly reduce the need for activity on the whole, because part of its function is to expel matter. The vital force can therefore acquire a quiet space to allow healing to proceed elsewhere. Greater activity in the gut means vomiting and/or diarrhoea, of course. A baby will often react to excess heat or chill with diarrhoea. When Dulcamara is the remedy the diarrhoea usually contains mucus and is accompanied by colic. It may have a *sour smell* or be *yellow and watery* especially if the weather is *damp*. Another exciting cause of Dulcamara is < *wet weather*. As Lippe and Tyler point out, the diarrhoea, or simply a mucous discharge, may occur when the child has been *wading in cold weather*. This may also lead to a *milky deposit in the urine* which is less common than simply producing *excessive urination*. Another symptom of excessive discharge can be found as *perspiration on the palms*.

In the deeper stage, the mucus is produced in the chest whereas in the more chronic patient, especially the adult, it becomes rheumatism which I often label 'catarrh in the joints' to emphasize the link. Rheumatism most often affects synovial joints which contain a capsule of fluid to lubricate the joint against the wear and tear of movement. It is excess fluid within this capsule that produces swelling in rheumatism. In the Dulcamara patient these joints are often affected, but there is also dropsy which comes after suppressed sweat or suppressed eruptions, or after exposure to cold. The *dropsy* may be part of the chronic symptom picture.

The limbs may show severe reaction to the cold and damp, producing *tearing pains* or paralysis. *Paralysis from lying on damp ground* is a keynote that even the susceptible child may produce, i.e. who is not at the rheumatic stage.

The skin symptoms which are next in importance are like those of Belladonna, i.e. with *dryness* and *redness*. There are *thick, crusty eruptions* especially about the head, often with reddish borders. The *intense itching* is *better for cold*. This is a deeper, more chronic stage than the digestive symptoms.

ACTIVITY 21 Note which symptoms form the symptom picture of Dulcamara in the following ailments. Pay attention to modalities and exciting causes. Try to list symptoms from each of the four categories, Strange, Rare and Peculiar, Mental/Emotional, General and Particular.

Laryngitis
Headache
Cystitis.

Nervous Affections

Dulcamara is also a remedy of spasm like the other Solanaceae, but this is occluded by the strong effect causing paralysis. Two major keynotes are *paralysis after lying on damp ground* and *one-sided paralysis*. If you only think of Dulcamara as a remedy of paralysis, you will miss it when you meet the rheumatic who is restless and on the go, whose *pains are better for movement*. When Dulcamara reaches the paralysis stage in a chronic case, it is very advanced in pathology.

It is not so violent as the other Solanaceae. There is little excitability in the brain. Disturbance of perception is limited to such symptoms as *the head feeling large* due to congestion. Disturbance of cognition is less clear. There is *confusion*, so *they cannot find the right word*. They *cannot concentrate*. *Speech* and *co-ordinating faculties may disappear*. There is little delirium.

Temperamentally there is excitation with impatience and aggression. J H Clarke is clear that there is no anger in the aggression. The irritability comes to resemble more closely the other rheumatic remedies such as Rhus toxicodendron and Bryonia. They are *dissatisfied* and do not know what they want. Later they are *depressed*. Dulcamara's energy compares with Bryonia rather than Belladonna. It is slower and the symptoms are deeper.

ACTIVITY 22 Compare the temperament of Dulcamara with the other rheumatic remedies, Rhus toxicodendron and Bryonia.

Similar Remedies

Rhus toxicodendron shares the exciting causes < cold, damp weather, < soaking, < suppressed eruptions. Both produce a rheumatism that is better for motion.

Chamomilla produces a green, slimy stool when chilled, but they tend to be more vociferous patients, with more inflammation. Both remedies throw away what they asked for.

ACTIVITY 23 Construct a table of comparison as a summary of your work in this lesson. Compare Belladonna, Hyoscyamus, Stramonium, Tabacum and Dulcamara using headings as follows:

Exciting causes
Modalities
Symptoms in fever
Symptoms in delirium
Spasm symptoms
Paralysis symptoms
Effect on mucous membrane
Effect on skin.

 SELF-TEST QUESTIONS

Test your understanding of the lesson with the questions below. All the remedies are Solanaceae. You will find the answers in the Lesson when you review it. (See answer section at the end of book.)

1. Name three remedies which bite and strike out.
2. In which of the Solanaceae is the patient struck speechless with fright?
3. State three factors about the nausea of Tabacum.
4. Which remedy has paralysis after lying on damp grass?
5. When ill, this remedy may pray all the time.
6. In which remedy do red streaks radiate from the breast?
7. Which remedy has a sinking weakness in the stomach when ill?
8. Which remedy drops the jaw?
9. Give four modalities of Tabacum.
10. The cough is excited by a dry spot in the throat. Which remedy?
11. Which two of the Solanaceae will have ailments after fright?
12. This remedy has a death-like pallor and cold sweat with nausea.
13. Name two remedies which laugh in delirium.
14. Which remedy has painless sore throats?
15. Name three exciting causes of Hyoscyamus.
16. Describe the skin of the Tabacum patient.
17. Which of the Solanaceae dreams of fire?
18. This remedy has sour smelling sweat and diarrhoea.
19. In fever, this remedy prattles and picks at the bedclothes.
20. Name two of the Solanaceae with a hot, red face and cold extremities.
21. Which remedy might sneeze for weeks?
22. Which two remedies bore the head into the pillow and move it from side to side?
23. Name three of the fears of Hyoscyamus.
24. Which remedy has spasm on the top half of the body only?
25. After a soaking, which remedy has one-sided paralysis?
26. Which two remedies are aggravated looking at shining objects?
27. Crusty eruptions on the head are red-rimmed in this remedy.
28. Which remedy is conscious in convulsions?
29. Eyes twitch in the cold air in this remedy.
30. Which remedy is so relaxed it has seminal emissions in the night?
31. Which remedies see monsters?

32. Which two symptoms might describe the deceitfulness of Hyoscyamus?
33. Give three symptoms of the nightmares of Stramonium.
34. Give four exciting causes of Dulcamara.
35. In fever, you can see the carotid artery pulsate.
36. In which remedy do small objects appear large?
37. The optic nerve of which remedy is atrophied?
38. Which remedy has cutting pains at the navel, with green, slimy stools?
39. The pupils are dilated, the eyes stare in three remedies.
40. Describe the madness of Hyoscyamus.

Further Studies

Hyoscyamus

1. Describe the Hyoscyamus patient in fever and compare this with the Belladonna and Stramonium patients.
2. When does Hyoscyamus present symptoms similar to Phosphorus, but much more exaggerated?
3. Hyoscyamus and Nux vomica are both very spasmodic remedies. Compare their modalities. How does the constipation of Hyoscyamus resemble that of Nux vomica?
4. Compare the mental side of Lachesis and Hyoscyamus. How might this present in patients today?
5. List six Strange, Rare and Peculiar symptoms of Hyoscyamus.
6. How might you relate Hyoscyamus to a Presbyterian Scottish character? (e.g. *Hatter's Castle* A J Cronin; *The House with the Green Shutters* George Douglas-Brown.)
7. Compare the cough of Hyoscyamus, Drosera and Pulsatilla.
8. Hyoscyamus and Rhus toxicodendron both want to drown themselves. Compare how these two remedies get into such a state.

Stramonium

1. When would you choose Stramonium rather than Aconite for a frightened child? Describe the different symptom picture in detail.
2. Compare the delusions of Stramonium and Opium.
3. Which remedies desire to escape?
4. Compare the religious affections of Stramonium, Hyoscyamus and Lachesis.
5. Which other remedies have painlessness in inflammatory ailments?
6. Study psychosis and neurosis as they might apply to Stramonium and Hyoscyamus.
7. When might you need to differentiate between Stramonium and Phosphorus?

Tabacum

1. Compare the travel sickness of Tabacum, Ignatia, Ipecacuanha, and Cocculus.
2. How do the collapse symptoms of Tabacum resemble those of Camphor and Veratrum album?
3. Describe the heart and circulatory symptoms of Tabacum.
4. Compare the spasm symptoms of Tabacum and Nux vomica.
5. Compare the disturbance of perception and cognition in the Solanaceae.

Dulcamara

1. Describe the symptom picture of Dulcamara in respiratory problems.
2. Which remedies are worse getting soaked? Sketch the resulting symptom pictures.
3. Make a table of comparison of the rheumatic remedies, Dulcamara, Bryonia, Rhus toxicodendron, Rhododendron, Ranunculus bulbosus.
4. Compare the digestive symptoms of Dulcamara, Chamomilla and Colocynthis.
5. Describe the skin symptoms of Dulcamara. Which remedies compare?
6. Which remedies have one-sided paralysis?

Four Irritable Remedies

Arsenicum Album, Apis Mellifica, Rhus Toxicodendron, Hepar Sulphuris Calcareum

Aim: To discover the different aetiology and essence that gives rise to a similar symptom picture of irritability.

Objectives: To demonstrate the similarity in the symptom picture of these four remedies.
To label the similarity and difference in the exciting cause and modalities.
To define the underlying weakness of each constitution.

Headings: INTRODUCTION
ARSENICUM ALBUM: Origin; Characteristic of the Metal; Essence; Keynotes and Characteristics; The Exciting Cause; Over-control; Common Acute Patterns; Similar Remedies
APIS MELLIFICA: Origin; Characteristics of the Bee; Essence; Keynotes and Characteristics; The Exciting Cause; Fluid Balance; Similar Remedies
RHUS TOXICODENDRON: Origin; Essence; Keynotes and Characteristics; The Exciting Cause; The Personality; Similar Remedies
HEPAR SULPHURIS CALCAREUM: Origin; Essence; Keynotes and Characteristics; Sensitivity; Suppuration; Similar Remedies
SELF-TEST QUESTIONS
FURTHER STUDIES

Introduction

Human beings are wonderfully dynamic creatures. If we were simply to list the symptoms and find a remedy that matches, we would frequently fail to cure. To find the best-fit remedy, you need more than a list of symptoms. You must also match the intensity and importance of the symptoms.

I have already drawn your attention to the different value of symptoms in putting them into categories, Strange, Rare and Peculiar, Mental and Emotional, General and Particular. The vital force affects the organism as a whole, but when disturbed it will attempt to localize the disease to the extremities. Nonetheless, the individuality may be most clearly represented in the other three levels. There is thus a distinct hierarchy of symptoms where we must seek the individuality. Individuality is also recognizable in the exciting cause and modalities which may be of paramount importance in some remedies.

In the next four remedies the physical presentation is so similar that we will need to look at constitutional types to differentiate them. We will trace the different weaknesses and the strains and pressures to which they are sensitive, then how this translates into symptoms.

Arsenicum Album

Latin name: Arsenicum album
Common name: Arsenic oxide

Origin

A preparation was prepared from the white oxide by Hahnemann.

Characteristic of the Mineral

This is the first mineral we have studied. It is found as an impurity in many metals. It is added to copper products to increase resistance to erosion and it is added to lead products to improve shape. Mostly it is used as a weedkiller, to preserve wood or clear glass. Since its presence is more abundant than its use, it is one of the main components of toxic waste.

In the chemical periodic table it occurs between antimony and phosphorus. Allied chemicals include bismuth. Thus the homoeopathic remedy, Arsenicum album is related to remedies prepared from these metals.

Essence

There is a very great deal of energy in this remedy. They are great organizers and pioneers. J H Clarke describes Arsenicum 'for the effects of feats or prolonged endurance'. However, when ill, a marked characteristic of almost all Arsenicum cases is *profound prostration*. The energy used is so great the patient is used up.

Keynotes and Characteristics

• **Sudden prostration out of all proportion**	They are prone at the least provocation.
• **Chilly**	This is one of the coldest remedies in the Materia Medica.
• **Burning pains > heat**	**Strange, Rare and Peculiar.** All complaints > heat except headache.
• **Thirst for small quantities**	He continues to take small sips to prevent dryness, but not enough to cool down.
• **Right-sided**	
• **Complaints return annually**	Hence Arsenicum is often indicated in Hay Fever.
• **Itch, dryness, heat**	Refers to skin in general.
• Urticaria after eating shellfish.	This is a major remedy of food poisoning.
• **Restlessness**	Of the mind. At night he/she goes from one bed to another.
• **Anxiety about health**	There is a great insecurity about this remedy.
• **Great fear of death**	The ultimate insecurity – can I extinguish?
• Fear of suffocation	So much so, that in respiratory problems they will not lie down.
• **Despair of recovery**	So does not take the medicine.
• < alone	All fears and anxieties are < alone.
• **Fear of the unknown**	Underlines many symptoms. The Arsenicum patient must be in control.
• **Suicidal**	Would rather take control and commit suicide than wait to die.
• **Ambitious**	Somehow they must prove themselves. In doing, or in being something, they exist.
• **Fastidious**	There is an obsessiveness about the remedy.
• **Well organized**	Thus they keep insecurity, the unknown, at bay.
• **Watery diarrhoea**	At any chill in the stomach or slightest food poisoning.
• **Diarrhoea smells of rotten meat**	You can smell it when you come into the room.

• **Diarrhoea excoriates the anus**	There is much acidity present.
• Duodenal ulcers	There is so much heat and anxiety.
• **Nausea at sight or smell of food**	Arsenicum has a profound effect upon the stomach.
• Stomach sensitive to ice cream	This remedy wants to be warm.
• Watery coryza excoriates the nose where it exits	Similar to the diarrhoea.
• Tears burn the cheeks.	All discharges are acrid.

ACTIVITY 1 Arsenicum is a remedy of great anxiety. List the symptoms above that relate to anxiety.

ACTIVITY 2 Find and list the modalities of Arsenicum. Separate into aggravations and ameliorations.

The Exciting Cause

The Arsenicum symptom picture is triggered by three factors:

- Anxiety
- Chill
- Food poisoning.

Anxiety

These people have terrific strength and perseverance to achieve. They are well co-ordinated, well-organized and well-integrated leaders and pioneers. It is as if they are driven yet, out there on their pinnacle, they are fragile and isolated. They are not separate from the mass because they are always checking they are taking the mass along. They are anxious to get it right and thereby win esteem. *Dread of death*, *of the unknown*, is a threat to the self and of the existence they have given themselves in their grand plan. This may be hidden in the *ambitious, well-organized* business man until his deal goes wrong. He may still maintain a brave face, but it takes so much energy to do this that the strain may show in *duodenal ulcers, high blood pressure* or even cancer. Still, he is *fastidiously correct*, fastidiously dressed and hassles others to maintain his standards. He, himself, may not be into menial tasks. Yet, it is his energy and vision that keeps the whole functioning. When self-esteem is dented, or the energy output is at last exhausted, chaos reigns. Organization crumbles around him/her. The body crumbles too, so a wide range of degenerative diseases now enter. It may be rheumatism, arthritis, cancer, etc. If there is only a set-back, the shock of his infallibility and anxiety may lead to an acute lung disorder, such as bronchitis or pleurisy. The chronic state of this would be asthma. On the mental level they may become *obsessive about small things*. They may continually turn back to check the gas is off. Now they need even more energy to maintain their empire and they are very consciously near chaos. Now it is difficult to hide the anxiety.

Chill

Chill as an exciting cause affects the stomach and lungs most clearly, causing the *watery excoriating discharges* and *the nausea at the sight and smell of food* that have an underlying essence of destructiveness. They are alien to life, breaking up order and reason in the body. On the general level the Arsenicum patient is so chilly. This *lack of heat* is lack of life. I have encountered a situation of stomach disorder piled high with blankets at an outside temperature of 130ºF. What is enough life to this patient? When well, they consume vast quantities of energy; when ill, they consume vast quantities of heat. So much energy is burnt up they need so much more. The flow of life is uneven.

The *pains* of Arsenicum *are burning* denoting inflammation – excessive blood is taken to the part bringing more life and nutrients.

In the skin this imbalance of heat/life dries, creating heat and itch.

The discharges are burning and excoriating, acid could be seen as super abundance of heat/life.

Food Poisoning

Sensitivity to food poisoning illustrates the intolerance of the body to a foreign condition. It is violently and *suddenly debilitated.* Nausea to the sight and smell of food shows the depth of the disorder. Watery, excoriating diarrhoea shows the excessive, internal heat, externalized.

ACTIVITY 3

List as many symptoms of Arsenicum as you can that show *active integration* and as many symptoms as you can that show *broken down integrity of the whole.*

Over-control

Arsenicum symptoms are produced in the body through the action of adrenaline or histamine. Both of these control reactions to the outside. Adrenaline is a hormone that acts on the general level. Histamine acts locally under the skin. Both create heat and activity. Between them they can produce asthma, eczema and a range of allergic reactions.

ACTIVITY 4

Find out the changes that adrenaline and histamine make in the body. Which symptoms of Arsenicum correspond to the effect of adrenaline and histamine?

On the mental level the over-control comes out in obsessiveness, fastidiousness, and in organization. They are intense people. They cannot bear not to know. Their fears are of the unknown. In business, all factors and avenues need to be explored before they will commit themselves. If the way is not clear they will create their own way and use their powerful will and ingenuity to back up their plan. So potent is this need to control that they will commit suicide rather than wait on death! If ill, they will take over and fantasize great illnesses even though they have been told otherwise. Their greatest fear is that they might have cancer (cells out of control) or heart problems (disintegration of the central co-ordinating mechanism).

ACTIVITY 5

When the Arsenicum patient breaks down on the physical level there is much fluid imbalance. Research this and note characteristic conditions and symptoms.

Common Acute Patterns

In Colds

The Arsenicum cold will start on exposure to cold. There is an excoriating, watery discharge from the right nostril. Sometimes the eyes are also affected with acrid lachrymation. This is similar to Euphrasia (eyes < and coryza bland) and Allium cepa (left nostril < and eyes bland). All three remedies occur commonly in the hay fever pattern.

Arsenicum seldom produces coughs. When the cold goes deeper the chest is affected. There may just be dryness and suffocating breath, but the fully developed picture will include burning pains, exhaustion, anxiety, constant sips of water.

In Skin Problems

Arsenicum produces a number of different skin problems. They are very sensitive, reactive people, so the skin is likewise.

Nettlerash may quickly occur when touching plants like scented geranium, or cats. The same may be produced from foods eaten. The Arsenicum patient may produce the rash within seconds of eating spoiled fish, shellfish or meat that is slightly off. Tomatoes and watery vegetables may produce the same. The skin is red, hot, itching with raised weals. The patient does not suffer silently, but needs something done *now*! He/she will go to the best doctors, try the most elaborate procedures, anything that keeps them in control and status.

Arsenicum is also a remedy of chronic skin problems such as eczema. The skin, like that of many other remedies, will be dry, very itchy, red and scaly. When scratched the skin will bleed. There is little here to tell the difference between Arsenicum and any other remedy. To prescribe you must go on the underlying character and aetiology.

Disturbed Digestion

The digestion is very easily disturbed in the Arsenicum patient. The major causes are spoiled food or chilling (ice cream when overheated). The emotional picture can produce disturbance in digestion though. You must question the patient carefully.

The diarrhoea is first produced. It may become excoriating only when the situation is serious. A pungent odour is more common. The awful cadaverous odour appears only in deeper disturbance. There may be colic with burning pains. When the whole symptom picture shifts to cholera or dysentery, the full blown picture will appear, plus constant thirst for cold water which they sip, chilliness and restless anxiety. All is well covered except the head which always likes to be cold – this is especially individualistic about Arsenicum. The nausea does not always come with the diarrhoea. Indeed it may come without it. It may accompany prostration when the patient has over-exhausted himself. It is usually found in the cancer in which the patient is so alien to himself.

Asthma

Arsenicum is commonly an asthma remedy. This comes from two characteristics:

- The sensitivity of the patient
- The annual periodicity.

The dryness is there, plus the constriction in the chest and the aggravation at 1–2 a.m. There is also such fear of suffocating that they will not lie down. There is still little here to distinguish Arsenicum – you must study the character weaknesses to prescribe with confidence. Arsenicum is strongly marked as better when *not* alone.

ACTIVITY 6   List the symptoms which indicate the drying effect of Arsenicum.

Similar Remedies

Lycopodium has the same basic insecurity and need for status. It also has a strong effect on the lungs and digestive system. The modalities and appetite are different. Lycopodium < 4–8 p.m. Arsenicum < 12–2 a.m.

Phosphorus shares the sensitivity and fears of Arsenicum. Both are desirous of company. Both are major lung and digestive remedies. The Phosphorus is a more open, trusting and optimistic character.

Natrum muriaticum like to control to relieve anxiety, like Arsenicum. They are very emotionally vulnerable, but can be much more empathetic with others than Arsenicum.

Aconite is another fear remedy that affects respiration. It also has fear of suffocating and is < midnight. Adrenalin plays a key role in the symptom picture of both.

Apis Mellifica

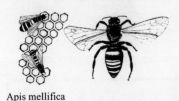

Apis mellifica

Origin

The whole bee was crushed by Constantine Hering to make the tincture for the provings.

Characteristics of the Bee

The honey bee is a social animal. Organization in the hive is around the queen who is the only productive female. Almost all the other bees are infertile females. They are busy continually doing the many jobs about the hive, cleaning the hive, tending the young and organizing food. They have a great ability to communicate with each other by doing a complex dance. They do not like cloudy, rainy weather, or excessive heat – they may get quite aggressive then.

The queen is very jealous. When another queen hatches, if she does not kill it the old queen leaves with many of the hive. Apart from mating at the beginning of her life, this is the only time she leaves the hive. Whilst in the hive, the worker bees do everything for her, even feed her.

When they sting, bees die. All the anger is in one outburst as it were and they pay for it with their lives.

Essence

The bee is an active factor in a well-integrated female system. The remedy has a powerful effect on the fluid balance of the body and on the emotions. On the emotional level disintegration gives rise to a hysterical scattering of energies. On the physical level Apis produces *oedema* on the skin, mucous membrane and the surface of organs. The tissues are so waterlogged, the surface pits when pressed. The skin has a shiny, rosy-red glow. The nerves are affected by pressure, so problems of co-ordination arise.

Keynotes and Characteristics

• **Bright red, shiny swellings**	As in a bee sting.
• **Burning, stinging pains**	It is more severe than an itch.
• **Oedema pits on pressure**	
• **Heat is > cold applications**	As in Belladonna this is as you would expect it. Hypericum swellings and pain are < cold.
• **Thirstless**	Though unexpected in fever this is not surprising with all the oedema around.
• **< touch**	The nerves are already pressured by the fluid.
• **<< heat**	Already there is too much, but also the tissues are so congested they cannot cope with more activity.
• **Right-sided**	
• **Always busy**	Like a bee.
• **Jealous**	Like a queen bee.
• **Suspicious**	Of someone taking over their empire.
• **Fears they will poison her**	The queen is so vulnerable.
• **Head bores into the pillow with a piercing shriek**	Because the cerebro-spinal fluid is congested putting pressure on the brain. This is seen in meningitis.
• **Opisthotonos**	Apis bends the back further than any other remedy.
• Swollen, hot joints, shiny red with burning stinging pains	As in rheumatism and arthritis. They still use bee stings therapeutically in these diseases.
• Swollen right ovary	The ovary is an area of potential, lost or unrealized in the bee.
• **Great debility**	The patient is exhausted.
• **Clumsy**	Nerves are affected.
• **Lack of co-ordination**	Because of the effect on nerves.
• Urine scant and dark coloured	Eventually in oedema the kidneys are affected.
• Involuntary urination with much irritability of parts.	
• Chest oppressed as if the patient would smother.	There is even greater similarity to Arsenicum when we add burning pains as a characteristic.
• Diarrhoea involuntary as if the anus was wide open.	Similar to Phosphorus.

ACTIVITY 7
List the general symptoms of Apis that are similar to Arsenicum. Which general symptoms are different?

ACTIVITY 8   Compare the modalities of Apis and Arsenicum.

The Exciting Cause

Allergy

Like Arsenicum, Apis is a sensitive remedy that is often found in allergies. It may be contact with an obnoxious substance which produces *swollen, red patches* that are so itchy they *sting*. Frequently Apis is the indicated remedy after stings and bites. As in Arsenicum the reaction is very fast. The distinctive symptoms that allow the choice of Apis are:

- redness is *bright red and shiny*
- *swelling* is so great the limb may double in size or the *skin pits on pressure*
- heat is *better for cold applications*
- *pains burn and sting.*

These symptoms appear on mucous membrane as in the throat when an allergen such as mercury is swallowed (i.e. some tinned fish). The soft tissue at the back of the throat swells considerably and may even affect breathing. Apis was used frequently in the past as a remedy of diphtheria. Some allergy situations are so severe the whole body swells and the situation may be fatal if the mucous membrane lining the respiratory system is involved. When Apis is indicated the situation is much relieved in 5–10 minutes. In one patient, the soft tissue of the eye blistered out and vision was obscured after handling a cat. 15 minutes after Apis 6, one pill, she was able to cycle off into the London traffic nonplussed.

Emotional/ Hormonal

The mental and emotional symptoms of Apis take centre stage, as in Arsenicum. There is a great deal of *insecurity*. This is a bit more *hysterical* in Apis. She gets *jealous*. She is *suspicious* of others and is more sly to Arsenicum's subtleness. She is a busy bee, usually quite content if let be, but a *restlessness* arises if she is not given her due. *What caused all this?*

She is *fussy, fidgety* and *hard to please*. What do we mean when we say someone is a queen bee? They are in control and all revolves around them. They make the choices, often not considering others' needs at all. Are they so needy? They demand so much that it is not surprising the others cannot fulfil their needs. She is conscious of what she has and what she has not, and what others have, so suspicion and jealousy arise. She becomes so *anxious* and *excitable* that hysteria is the next step, or paranoia, that they are out to get her – *she fears they will poison her*, will spoil her chances.

There are places where this would be regarded as typical female behaviour! – the harem, the chorus line, the corps de ballet, the opera company. The flighty, artistic temperament here is not often put down to hormones as it may be elsewhere. The *tearful, depressive moods* that lead to *indifference* describe many premenstrual women, especially when we add *bloating* and *fluid retention*. Even the *clumsiness* and *lack of co-ordination*, which come with PMS, describe the effect of Apis on nerves.

ACTIVITY 9   Relate the symptoms of Apis to what you know of PMS and Menopause.

Fluid Balance

Apis affects the mucous membrane and serous membrane. First it engorges tissue with fluid then it dries up tissue. It can be recognized as the appropriate remedy in pleurisy or pneumonias, or in meningitis. It was a favourite of Kent and Tyler in meningitis when the cerebro-spinal fluid was so increased that *opisthotonos* resulted, arching the back so severely the patient's *head bored back into the pillow*, and the notorious *cri célèbre* was sounded. This was a *piercing shriek*. This cry is also sounded by the child before urination when suffering from cystitis. In this case, the mucous membrane is so dry the *urine burns severely* as it passes down the ureter. The child knows it will be painful so hence the shriek. Dryness of the cornea, dryness and rawness of the genitalia or throat is less commonly covered by Apis – Cantharis may be a better remedy or even Arsenicum – but Apis may occur.

Malfunction of the kidneys, leading to *retention of urine* and *bloating of the extremities* may require Apis if the rest of its symptom picture agrees. The patho-physiology of this situation may be altered levels of aldosterone controlling the fluid balance. This also accounts for the very bloated cases of high blood pressure (HBP) that respond to Apis.

The immune response discussed above may be seen in the auto-immune disease, rheumatoid arthritis. The characteristic symptoms of this disease very much resemble the characteristic Apis symptom picture:

- swollen joints
- red and shiny
- with severe stitching, stinging, burning pains.

Also a high proportion of the sufferers from this disease are females. In all of these situations of fluid retention, Apis is characteristically *thirstless* and << *heat*. Understandably there is a sensitivity to touch or pressure.

ACTIVITY 10   Describe the symptom picture of the sore throat of the Apis patient. Pay particular attention to exciting cause and modalities.

ACTIVITY 11   Read up on anaphylactic shock. Why do you think Apis would be a good remedy for this? Note any keynotes and characteristics of Apis that might apply.

Similar Remedies

Belladonna has the swollen red parts, but is not shiny, and stitches, throbs and pulsates, rather than stings. Both are remedies of cerebral congestion but in Belladonna action is through the blood and heat whilst in Apis the cerebro-spinal fluid is affected. Both < heat and > cold.

Hypericum affects the nerves and has the red swelling with pains shooting along the nerves. Once again it will throb rather than sting. It has the same numbness and paralysis as Apis but is not as affected by the hormone cycle as Apis. Hypericum is < cold.
Hypericum is used for bee stings.

Cantharis has swelling of mucous membrane and stinging, burning pains. Both have a strong effect on the kidneys and on fluid loss or retention. Cantharis is more burning than stinging.

Urtica urens has the burning, stinging pains of Apis, where skin and mucous membrane are affected by overheating or inflammation. The breasts and genital organs are strongly affected by burning, stinging and swelling. Both have a strong effect on the kidneys. Urtica urens has a uric acid diathesis – Apis has simple oedema.

Natrum muriaticum strongly affects the water balance in the body and the nerves and also is strongly affected by change in the hormone cycle in the female. Both have oedema, clumsiness and lack of co-ordination. Both are < before menses.

Rhus Toxicodendron

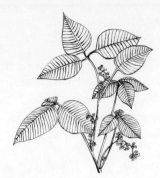

Rhus toxicodendron

Latin name:	Rhus toxicodendron
Common name:	Poison ivy
Botanical family:	Anacardiaceae
Habitat:	Found in woods throughout North America.

Origin

A tincture is prepared from the leaves freshly gathered at sunset before the plant flowers. Hahnemann did the first proving.

Essence

This remedy is so sensitive *irritability* describes its symptom picture. The limbs need to move, the mind is anxious if it has space. There is stagnant flow especially in cold, damp situations, so toxins build up and there is irritability. Anything that encourages flow ameliorates – heat, motion, massage.

Keynotes and Characteristics

• **Irritability**	This applies in all disturbances. Mostly it is physical.
• < **rest**	Irritability keeps them on the move.
• < **1st movement** > **continued movement**	This keynote applies to all levels of physical disturbance.
• < **cold, damp**	It sinks into the bones to stiffen limbs.
• < before storms	They are more sluggish, so more irritable.
• Parts lain on become sore	As in Arnica.
• > heat	Which increases circulation.
• > rubbing	Because flow is stimulated.
• **Dreams of great exertion**	Wakes up exhausted.
• **Restless at night**	Mostly limbs but also very anxious and apprehensive.
• < **chilled after overheating**	There is a lot of flow in heating, then it is suddenly shut down.
• < **suppressed sweat**	How do you suppress sweat but by chilling.
• < **after being soaked**	Once again this creates chill.
• **Fear of poisoning**	The tissues are full of lactic acid which causes an autotoxic situation. May apply to rheumatism or flu.
• **Itching, red rash**	Occurs in response to the release of histamine.
• < hairy parts	**Strange, Rare and Peculiar**.
• < uncovering	Chilled again.
• **Red spot with pus**	As in chickenpox or smallpox.
• Spots come together when scratched.	
• Vesicles along the tract of nerve	This is a major remedy of shingles.
• Burning, itching, scaly eczema	On a chronic level when there is too much acidity in the body. Diet helps.
• Cracked tongue except for red triangle at tip	This comes with a much disturbed digestive system.
• Cough as if would tear something out of the chest	Shows the violence of the reaction.

ACTIVITY 12 Look up the rubric *irritability* in the Repertory. List the modalities that apply to Rhus toxicodendron.

ACTIVITY 13   Find out about the chemical changes that take place in a muscle during exertion.

The Exciting Cause

This is a remedy of acid reactive constitutions, hence the essence is *irritability*.

Under the skin, excess heat or allergies produce histamine release, so there is *intense itch* and *heat*. Great *red blotches* appear which *join together when scratched*. The skin may break to form a *crusty, moist eruption*. The *hairy parts are especially favoured by eruption*. If only the skin could be cooled inside relief would come. In fact the *itch* is much *worse when the patient uncovers*. This skin condition is common in the summer *after eating acid fruits*, such as strawberries and tomatoes.

The same symptom picture may be present in those who overindulge in alcohol. The alcohol increases the acidity and heat in the system. This time the irritability may be more widespread, so the mental and emotional realm is affected. The Rhus toxicodendron patient is renowned for his/her *volatile temper*.

In acute illness such as chickenpox, where the spots are red with yellow heads, the irritability is seen as an intense itch which burns.

Rhus toxicodendron is a useful remedy in first aid situations such as sprains, or in overuse of muscles, because of its strong effect on connective tissue. What is happening here? The overuse, or sprain, creates lactic acid in the tissues. This causes them to tire, then to heat up. *The parts stiffen* and congest quickly. You know if this happens that it is best to keep the part moving so nothing can settle, that *heat and massage improve the situation*. The body has already provided a lot of heat. There is too much activity here yet, although it is temporarily > cold it is ultimately > *heat*. In this semi-rheumatic state we see the *aggravation from cold*. There is a static situation developing here, so anything that increases flow benefits the patient whilst what slows down flow further disturbs the patient. Thus the part is improved by heat, massage and movement and is aggravated by initial movement, cold and rest. In the susceptible type, the situation is brought on by *chilling after overheating*, by *soaking*, or *cold, damp weather*. The really sensitive will feel the barometric pressure drop, and the chill come over as a storm approaches. These types will be particularly sensitive at the time of year when the weather changes, especially to cold.

In the chronic rheumatic, the synovial joints are singled out. There is swelling and heat, locally. Whilst the patient may be uncomfortable when too hot, they are generally chilly types. Since the pain builds up with stagnation, they are constantly on the move. Even at night they are restless because *parts lain on become sore and stiff*, even *numb*. It can be quite a painful ordeal for them to move. This is the type who might *dream of great exertion* and wake up exhausted because, indeed, they have been on the move all night.

ACTIVITY 14   Explain how digging the garden, or moving furniture, might bring on a Rhus toxicodendron symptom picture. What keynotes might apply here?

The Personality

The Rhus toxicodendron is an irritable person, often stereotyped as a crotchety old colonel. It is easy to see how the acid, irritable type might evolve from the physical type. However, many create this type by overindulgence in acid-forming foods, or by a lifestyle that puts stress on connective tissues. Still others, with an inherited rheumatic diathesis may succumb when living for years in a cold, damp climate.

The Rhus toxicodendron person is worn out, but this implies that there was a great deal of energy in the first place – remember their dreams of great exertion. They are conscientious, industrious types, but the strain is too much, so they become irritable when anything gets in the way. Like Nux vomica they have a volatile temper and need to be active. There is a lot of hostility and blaming of others, so they steadily become more isolated. They may even become paranoid that others are out to get them particularly to poison them. As the metabolism slows down they become confused or forgetful. At first they struggle to keep thoughts together. Eventually they just sink under it all. Life is a struggle to them and their cup runneth over. When they cannot cope they drown themselves, literally and metaphorically, in their sorrows. In their body, the tissues drown when they become oedematous. Physically they may end up with congestive heart disease when the centre is overwhelmed and drowned.

ACTIVITY 15 Read up on the symptoms of rheumatic fever. Why do you think Rhus toxicodendron would be a good remedy for this? Note any keynotes and characteristics that might apply.

ACTIVITY 16 What are the symptoms of congestive heart disease? How might these apply to the Rhus toxicodendron patient? Note any keynotes and characteristics that might apply.

Similar Remedies

Arnica shares the same effect on muscles and tendons. Both are common in sprains and strains, where the part is < first movement, > continued movement, > rubbing, > heat. Arnica is better indicated where there is bruising. Rhus toxicodendron can be used where the skin is broken without producing erysipelas.

Ruta is difficult to tell apart from Rhus toxicodendron in muscle and tendon problems. Both are < rest, and < first movement, and > continued movement. The rheumatism of both is < in cold, damp weather, > heat and rubbing. Ruta desires cold drinks, whereas Rhus toxicodendron does not. Ruta takes the disease, constitutionally, into the digestive and pelvic organs, where there is bruising and lack of tone. Rhus toxicodendron goes deeper to affect heart and circulation.

Dulcamara like Rhus toxicodendron is a remedy < for a soaking. This brings on the aching muscles and even paralysis. Both are < before a storm and have a rheumatic diathesis that is < chilling after overheating. Dulcamara in the last situation will often produce diarrhoea. Rhus toxicodendron is more irritable than Dulcamara.

Hepar Sulphuris Calcareum

Impure mixture of sulphur and calcium carbonicum.

Origin

It is prepared from 'finely powdered oyster shells and quite pure flowers of sulphur kept for 10 minutes at white heat'.

Essence

Hepar sulphuris calcareum patients are very sensitive. They are easily disturbed but are so profoundly disturbed recuperation is slow. There is the irritability of the Sulphur and the depth of the Calcareum in the Hepar sulphuris calcareum symptom picture.

Keynotes and Characteristics

- **< slightest draught of air**
- **< slightest touch of clothing**
- **Chilly**

- **< cold dry winds**
- So sensitive – faint with pain
- **Irritable**
- Volatile temper

Exciting cause.
On affected parts.
They could wear a fur coat in the middle of summer.
Cold brings on many minor ailments.
This reminds of Chamomilla.
Become angry and abusive.
They do not suffer silently.

• **Impulsive**	As in Nux vomica.
• **Overwhelming desire to kill**	Even people they like.
• Capricious	Restlessness on the mental level.
• Nothing pleases	They can be insolent if they do not get their own way.
• Everything disturbs	
• **Quarrelsome**	It can be difficult to differentiate this remedy from Nux vomica.
• Desire constant change	When irritable they move on.
• **Haste**	In speech, eating and drinking.
• Dreams of fire	The system is over-reactive.
• Dreams of danger, of guns and sickness	There is much violence in the remedy.
• **Everything festers and suppurates**	Recuperation is so slow.
• Boils	Illustrate the toxic state of the patient.
• **Discharges smell of old cheese**	They smell sour.
• Splinter-like, stitching pains	Arising from irritability of parts touching.
• Desires highly-seasoned foods	As well as being over-stimulated they need more stimulation.
• Desires strong tastes such as acids	

ACTIVITY 17   List the symptoms above that correspond to irritability.

ACTIVITY 18   List the modalities of Hepar sulphuris calcareum. Separate aggravations from ameliorations.

Sensitivity

The Hepar sulphuris patient is *very sensitive*. The *slightest draught of air* may bring on a cold or even croup. The tonsils or the ear may flare up rapidly after exposure. This patient is so sensitive to the cold that they appear always well wrapped up, even wearing a fur coat in summer. This is the type who harangues you to keep the door closed because the draught chills them. You may find them wrapped up in scarfs, stalking the house to seek out the draughts, muttering irritably all the while.

As well as the discharge being *sour*, the patient is 'sour' of disposition. *Nothing pleases* them. They settle to nothing, but *continually change irritably*. Like the Chamomilla patient they are *capricious*, constantly changing their mind. The Chamomilla patient is vexed and thwarted, whereas the Hepar sulphuris patient is simply irritable. Any stimulus will disturb them. It is as if they go out of their way to find things to quarrel over. Their *temper is volatile*. The remedy closely resembles Nux vomica in its need for activity, but there is lack of direction in the activity of the Hepar sulphuris patient. You could associate this with fire which consumes everything, often spitting and spluttering. The Hepar sulphuris patient *dreams of fire*. Their *dreams of danger*, guns, accidents and sickness give an idea of the instability of this remedy and of the suddenness with which they disintegrate. The *haste* is to be seen on the mental and emotional level in the speed with which they speak, eat and drink.

On the physical level, sensitivity can be seen in their reaction to pain. They faint. The *sensation of a stick in the throat* is an interesting keynote. There is, of course, no stick in the throat. As the mucous membrane starts to dry it is very sensitive. Where parts touch there is severe pain as if a splinter were present. The Hepar sulphuris patient is generally *sensitive to touch*.

ACTIVITY 19   Draw a sketch in words of how you would expect the Hepar sulphuris patient to behave after rising in the morning. Use as many general, and mental and emotional symptoms as you can.

ACTIVITY 20   Explain how the appetite of the Hepar sulphuris patient illustrates the need for activity.

Suppuration

Irritability in Arsenicum, Apis and Rhus toxicodendron produces a histamine reaction with irritation on the skin. This also occurs in the Hepar sulphuris patient where it can be recognized by the sensitivity to the cool air touching the skin. There is a similarity to the Rhus toxicodendron skin which itches when taken out from under the bedclothes. The Hepar sulphuris patient's skin quickly goes further to chap or crack. It dries as in the Arsenicum patient then it easily exudes moisture, so cold sores are common, but it also quickly suppurates so impetigo is a possibility, as in Rhus toxicodendron. The difference is often one of degree, so you must watch carefully for the modalities and the underlying trends.

In Hepar sulphuris the skin heals poorly. Boils and abscesses are common. Any discretion of diet may produce boils – as do indiscretions of temper! Abscesses form on wounds, or where parts are slow to heal. These are full of yellow pus which smells foetid. They are very sensitive to touch and cold air. These modalities now distinguish Hepar sulphuris from Silicea and Phytolacca.

All discharges are foul. They are described as sour or smelling of old cheese. There is much catarrh with inflammation of the tonsils and glands. The sensitivity is shown when the stick pain is worse, extending to the ears when yawning. The leucorrhoea is foul-smelling with sensitive labia.

Hepar sulphuris is most useful as a croup remedy, when the dry stage has passed and catarrhal discharge is copious. The paroxysms of cough are then recognizable as Hepar sulphuris because they are brought on by the *slightest* breath of cold air.

ACTIVITY 21   Describe the symptom picture of the following in detail, using the general characteristics of the remedy and keynotes, modalities and exciting causes:

Sore ear
Sore throat
Headache.

Similar Remedies

Nux vomica is also a very irritable remedy with a volatile temper. Both need activity and have a degree of violence or suddenness. They both crave stimulating foods and are < cold dryness. Nux vomica has more direction. It also affects the digestive system and the nerves whereas the action of Hepar sulphuris is more visible on the skin.

Bryonia Both remedies are very sensitive to touch. Both produce copious discharge at one phase which dries, so the mucous membrane has stitching, sticking pains. Bryonia is very much worse motion on the physical and mental/emotional level. Hepar sulphuris needs to move all the time.

Rhus toxicodendron has the irritability of Hepar sulphuris but is more physical in its restlessness.

Silicea has the same degree of suppuration and poor ability to heal. Although very sensitive the Silicea patient is less volatile. Silicea is a meek remedy.

ACTIVITY 22   Make a table of comparison for Arsenicum, Apis mellifica, Rhus toxicodendron, and Hepar sulphuris showing the following:

Effect of heat
Effect of cold
Skin symptoms
Weakness of lymph system
Exciting causes
Modalities.

?   *SELF-TEST QUESTIONS*

Find your answers in the text and then compare with the answers in the answer section.

1. Which remedy fears poisoning?
2. Which remedy wants to kill?
3. Which remedy has a thirst for small quantities?
4. Which remedy has such a fear of death they kill themselves?
5. Which remedy has nausea at the sight and smell of food?
6. Which remedy is < first movement and > continued motion?
7. Which remedy has shiny, red swellings?
8. Which remedy is < for the slightest touch of clothing?
9. Which remedy dreams of
    a.   great exertion?
    b.   fire?
10. Which remedy desires constant change?
11. What are the modalities of Rhus toxicodendron?
12. What does the diarrhoea of Arsenicum smell like?
13. Which remedy is jealous?
14. Name two remedies that suffer when chilled after overheating.
15. What characterizes the pains of Hepar sulphuris?
16. What are the modalities of Hepar sulphuris?
17. What distinguishes the pains of Arsenicum?
18. Of what is the Apis patient afraid?
19. Where in particular do you see the red, itchy rash of Rhus toxicodendron?
20. What do the discharges of Hepar sulphuris smell of?
21. What are the modalities of Arsenicum?
22. Give an example of the busyness of Apis.
23. How is acid metabolism expressed in a Rhus toxicodendron patient?
24. Give an example of Arsenicum's fastidiousness.
25. Describe the pains of the Apis patient.
26. State three exciting causes of Arsenicum.
27. What is peculiar about the oedema of Apis?
28. What effect do strawberries have on Rhus toxicodendron patients?
29. What distinguishes the cold of Arsenicum?
30. How does Apis affect the nerves? Give two characteristic symptoms.

Further Studies

Arsenicum

1. If Arsenicum is the homoeopathic adrenalin, compare the action of both physiologically.
2. Compare Arsenicum, Lycopodium and Phosphorus in stomach disorders.
3. Compare Arsenicum and Ipecacuanha in asthma.
4. Describe the eczema of the Arsenicum patient.
5. Draw a table to differentiate between Nux vomica, Arsenicum and Sulphur.
6. Catarrh, worse in the evening on lying down. How many remedies have this symptom and how do you differentiate between them?
7. Name the remedies of marked periodicity and differentiate between them.
8. What is a herpetic eruption? Which are the main remedies that have these?
9. Compare the fastidiousness of Arsenicum, Nux vomica and Sulphur.
10. When, and where, would the Arsenicum patient develop ulcers?

Apis Mellifica

1. What is the difference between a bee sting and a wasp sting?
2. How would an Apis patient present with high blood pressure?
3. Compare the effect of Apis, Cantharis and Urtica urens on the fluid balance of the organism.
4. What symptoms would relate Apis to Natrum muriaticum and Natrum sulphuricum as an acute?
5. How could Apis be of use in congestive heart disease?
6. Study the effect of Apis on the nerve system. Which remedies does it compare with?
7. How does Apis compare with other remedies of diphtheria?
8. Describe the symptom picture of an Apis child with meningitis.
9. How might Apis be a useful remedy in poliomyelitis?
10. How does aldosterone affect the kidneys? Relate this to the Apis picture.

Rhus Toxicodendron

1. Describe the backache of Rhus toxicodendron.
2. How does the rheumatic diathesis affect the head?
3. Discuss the modalities of Rhus toxicodendron in relationship to the rheumatic diathesis.
4. Read up on Rheumatism in a modern pathology textbook.
5. What is rheumatic paralysis? How does it present in the Rhus toxicodendron patient?
6. Compare:
   Rhus toxicodendron and Sulphur in skin problems
   Rhus toxicodendron with Bryonia, Gelsemium and Nux vomica in flu.
7. Compare Rhus toxicodendron and Hepar sulphuris calcareum.
8. Compare the acute picture of Rhus toxicodendron with that of a Calcarea carbonicum patient and/or a Natrum muriaticum patient.
9. Discuss the use of Rhus toxicodendron in childhood diseases. Read Dorothy Shepherd *Homoeopathy in Epidemic Diseases.*
10. Name those remedies that are worse getting soaked and distinguish between them.

Hepar Sulphuris Calcareum

1. Select *one* word to describe the essence of Hepar sulphuris calcareum, then find up to ten symptoms to illustrate this.
2. Compare Hepar sulphuris calcareum with Aconite and Spongia in croup.
3. Name two remedies that are as chilly as Hepar sulphuris calcareum. Differentiate between *one* of these.
4. Compare Hepar sulphuris calcareum and Sulphur skin problems.
5. Compare Hepar sulphuris calcareum and Silicea and differentiate between them.
6. When would Hepar sulphuris calcareum be of use in a first aid situation? Describe its symptoms.
7. When would you choose Hepar sulphuris calcareum rather than Mercurius in a digestive problem?
8. What are the similarities between Hepar sulphuris calcareum, Nux vomica and Rhus toxicodendron?
9. Which symptoms of Hepar sulphuris calcareum resemble those of Lachesis?
10. How do the urinary symptoms of Hepar sulphuris calcareum resemble those of Causticum?

Three Remedies of Suppressed Anger

Nux Vomica, Ignatia, Staphysagria

Aim: To explain how *one* powerful, exciting cause can produce different symptom pictures.

Objectives: To identify the symptoms that arise from suppressed anger in the symptom picture of Nux vomica, Ignatia and Staphysagria.

To differentiate between the symptom pictures of Nux vomica, Ignatia and Staphysagria.

To describe how the symptoms arise from the essence of each of these remedies.

Headings: INTRODUCTION

NUX VOMICA: Origin; Essence; Keynotes and Characteristics; Over-stimulation; Out of Harmony; Tension; Anger; Similar Remedies

IGNATIA: Origin; Essence; Keynotes and Characteristics; Worse Emotional Distress; Overwhelmed; A Romantic Idealist; Sensitive; Similar Remedies

STAPHYSAGRIA: Origin; Essence; Keynotes and Characteristics; Passionate; Situations of Suppressed Emotion; Physical Effects of Frustration; Similar Remedies.

SELF-TEST QUESTIONS

FURTHER STUDIES

Introduction

Emotions have a special place as stimulants. Some people act strongly to emotions, whilst others are calmer and cooler. Is there anyone who cannot be provoked eventually to anger? We are all different and we each have our trigger factors and our threshold of reaction. Think of the different types around you? What kind of person sits on their anger, or swallows it? Nux vomica sits on anger, so ends up with piles, or pains in the rectum! Ignatia swallows anger, so has choking throat problems! Staphysagria holds it like a red hot coal, that tortures them, and causes burning pains, searing, lacerating pains!

Why do we suppress anger? In some cultures it is not acceptable to express anger. In other cultures the Nux vomica may have no problem. Yet it is still ugly, giving rise to contorted grimaces that identify the Nux vomica patient immediately. Depending on the level of sophistication, the Nux vomica may punch you, twist your ear off threateningly, shout at you more or less crudely, or lash out with vicious words. They are active people, so stifled from outward action anger will turn internally to destroy them, or may end in depression, which is another kind of destruction.

Ignatia is more sensitive of others. It is not external constraints that determine the expression of anger, but the degree to which they allow themselves to feel the anger. It may come out as in any other remedy, or it may go deeper to affect their breathing, with great sighs. This contrary remedy easily turns anger into its opposite – grief, sorrow, pity. They can be so empathetic to the other, they lose self, or become depressed at the lack of self.

Staphysagria is offended in anger. If one is shocked, it is because the world is so different from what one expects. Does the expression of shock depend on culture, or sensitivity? Rather it depends on the degree to which the shock is objectionable. Then the symptom picture will depend on the degree of knowledge of self, to bounce back, or side-step the objection. It is a personal response. Thus Staphysagria can mimic either of the above remedies.

Let us now look in more detail at the symptom picture.

Nux Vomica

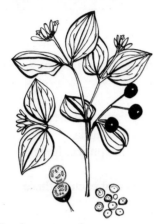

Strychnos nux vomica

Latin name:	Nux vomica officinarum
Common name:	Poison nut
Botanical family:	Loganiaceae
Habitat:	A native of the East Indies it is found on the Colomandel and Malabar coasts

Origin

The proving was done by Hahnemann, the tincture being prepared from the seeds.

Essence

The main active ingredient is strychnine which affects the nervous system, to produce *tension*, first overexciting with spasms, then exhausting or paralysing. It may work on single nerves, particularly the digestive system, or it works on the general and mental/emotional level. There is great sensitivity of the sense organs.

Keynotes and Characteristics

• **Impulsiveness**	Everything happens suddenly.
• **Impatient**	Need everything to happen immediately.
• **Spasm**	Is present in most symptom pictures.
• **Quarrelsome**	So irritated can pick fights.
• **Dissatisfaction**	Nothing contents, the remedy is out of harmony with reality.
• **Fastidious**	These patients are perfectionists, they have their own ideas of what is right.
• **Fault-finding and critical**	Of others and self.
• **Desires stimulation**	Applies to food, consciousness, life style, etc.
• < cold, dry wind	**Exciting cause.**
• **Chilly**	But rapidly overheats when covered.
• < slightest noise	It makes them very aggressive.
• < music	Especially if it is in a different rhythm.
• **Anxiety**	There is tension holding everything together precariously.
• Sleepless at night, sleepy in day	Their sleep patterns are out of order.
• **Reversed peristalsis**	The more they try to push out the stool/vomit, the more difficult it is.
• 'If only I could vomit . . .'	
• Vomits bile	Because the liver is over-stimulated.
• Water brash	Acid rises with reversed peristalsis.
• Bitter eructations	Contain bile.
• **Desire alcohol**	Has the same role as the remedy – stimulates then depresses.
• **Desire highly seasoned foods**	Because they are stimulating.
• < overeating	These are gourmets. They overindulge.
• < rich foods	Which bung up the liver.
• Desire fats	**Strange**, **Rare** and **Peculiar**, it is one of the very few remedies that desire fatty foods.
• Constant, ineffective urge to stool	The more they try the less they appear to pass.
• As if part of the stool remains behind	It waits on the next wave to pass on.
• Jerking limbs	Especially at night when they relax.

72

- Tetanic Spasms
- < **Touch**   This can start the spasm off again.

ACTIVITY 1   Pick out those symptoms of over-stimulation. Which symptoms refer to the exhausted stage?

ACTIVITY 2   Go through the Anxiety rubric in Kent's Repertory and list all those in which Nux vomica appears.

ACTIVITY 3   List those rubrics in the *Mind* section of Kent's Repertory that correspond to fastidious and fault-finding.

Over-stimulation

This remedy may be called the remedy of our age. It's essence is *over-stimulation* yet it craves *more stimulation*.

The nut (Lt. nux) contains a great deal of strychnine which causes *spasm* of a tonic nature. Nux vomica is a great remedy of the nerves. People who need Nux vomica are *restless* but this manifests as a great surge of energy outwards and onwards. The Nux vomica patient is a 'doer'. In harmony with their surroundings they may become great achievers and sound pillars of society. The nut, once the skin is removed, is composed of a finely interwoven structure that looks like the girders of an edifice – so the Nux patient seeks structure and the correct way of doing things. This leads them to become *perfectionists*, strict organizers who do things by the book or crusading defenders of the faith. In health the Nux vomica patient is *zealous* expending enormous quantities of energy. All is well if the flow is unimpeded but two factors stop the flow:

1. Obstacles in the patient's way
2. When the patient simply runs out of energy.

Out of Harmony

The 'obstacles' produce some of our classic stereotypes of Nux vomica patients who may sometimes be seen as 'brawn' rather than 'brains'. Dam a stream and its energy is increased so it may force away the dam or force a way round it. Thus in the textbooks we find classic concepts of Nux vomica behaviour include *impulsive* which may be expressed as *outbursts of anger* – the patient lashes out or '*throws the baby in the fire*'. They cannot bear to be kept waiting as this is inactivity. The restlessness now becomes *impatience*. They may get annoyed or *complain* in a queue. They may even become *abusive* or bad-tempered if kept waiting on a meal. At traffic lights, the clutch is held ready to leap off, or the engine is revved up like a growl that cannot otherwise be expressed in human society. They may *swear* or curse, or look critically around them. Robert Burns puts it into just a few lines in his description of Tam O'Shanter's waiting wife 'gathering her brows like a gathering storm, nursing her wrath to keep it warm'. This patient has a remarkable face, with deep lines sucked down from the brows into the top of the nose – a wee bit more than liver lines – and frequently a lop-sided mouth full of half-chewed daggers as yet unthrown. *A scowling face.*

ACTIVITY 4   Give some examples of your own that might fit the Nux vomica situation.

Tension

The obstacles produce a great deal of tension but there is also *tension* as a state of being. The young executive may be so full of get-up-and-go tension, that high blood pressure is produced

73

as the adrenaline keeps the patient at the ready. Tension develops along the shoulders with the continual tension and control exerted sitting at a desk writing, or driving a car, or simply carrying the weight of the world on his shoulders as Nux is inclined to do. This Nux vomica patient is very *conscientious* and takes responsibility on himself. This last may be seen in the way the head sinks into the shoulders as if avoiding the weight above. Indeed the keynotes of the Nux vomica headache are *pain on the vertex* and *as if a weight pressed down on the vertex*. The pace of life of this workaholic may be so great that he can do nothing but work so he finds that come night-time he cannot switch off his mind to sleep. The mind works on or he wakes in the night worrying about problems and cannot sleep until exhausted at daylight. In the Materia Medica we find this symptom as *sleepy by day, sleepless at night*.

The tension releases adrenaline which alters the fat balance in the body releasing energy for use. Of course the type of energy this process catered for originally was physical energy but today the poor Nux vomica patient is chained to his car or his desk. The unused energy eventually becomes fatty tissue lining arteries leading to arterial sclerosis, *ischaemias*, angina and *fatty degeneration* of various organs, particularly the heart. The heart of course is the final pathology in this egotist. *High blood pressure* and *apoplexy* are plagues on the way. Before this the body will protect itself with *exhaustion* so the patient is more and more worn down. Go to any bar in the business sector and you will recognize the Nux vomica patient. To keep himself together he will reach for *stimulants* – coffee to keep his mind active and tobacco to give his restless hands something to do, alcohol to relieve the tension. Being well into the structure of society he is not usually on sub-culture drugs such as marijuana, but in some cultures you may find him on cocaine which replaces coffee as a stimulant. Of course the result of stimulants is to wear the nerves down further.

Before exhaustion sets in there is a state of *nervous overactivity* which is spasm. *Parts may twitch and jerk* as when excessive coffee is used. The nerves may be so taut the patient *startles easily* or reacts to more stimulation with *irritability*. The sense organs are overactive but the Nux vomica patient is so *sensitive to noise*, especially slight noise, that they find themselves straining to hear even against their will and this loses more energy. They strain to hear because the individual parts are still overworking even when the brain says no. Rhythmic noise may bring violence because the Nux vomica patient is *out of harmony* and has lost his own rhythm. This is his sore spot because all the above activity is a search for harmony. Nux is very sensitive to what is harmonious and 'right'. External rhythm captures the weakened nervous system imposing a structure in its beat – the Nux patient does not have the energy at this stage to throw off the intrusion. The energy needed is squandered in *irritability* (like a fibrillation of the heart muscle) and *complaining*, or it is repelled by one violent impulse which the originator of the noise may not appreciate. On the mental level the equivalent of this is *quarrelsome* or *< contradiction*, both *keynotes* of Nux vomica.

ACTIVITY 5 After some research make notes on the effects of strychnine. Differentiate between chronic, tonic and tetanic spasm.

Anger

The anger is antisocial so it is taken within, but it is still energy so the system must speed up in consequence to expel this enormous wave to the edge of the pond. It is usually the digestive system of Nux that bears the brunt of this. First, secretion increases, so there are more digestive juices leading to *acidity – heartburn*, vomiting, bile, colic, indigestion. Some excessive secretion of course leads to *ulceration*. As spasm affects the muscle of the gut there is first increased movement along the gut, then overactivity produces *reversed peristalsis*, i.e. *constipation* where the stool is in little bits or *sheep dung stools*. Hiatus hernia rises from the violent spasm of the stomach pushing material back up the oesophagus – *projectile vomiting* is often produced by the Nux vomica patient at this stage. One keynote symptom easily recognizable, and very common, is *nausea* but unable to be sick – '*if only I could be sick*'.

As with the stool the more the patient tries the less possible it becomes to pass anything – each effort creates more spasm pushing the material in the opposite direction. Nux vomica is useful in travel sickness often caused by tiredness or over-stimulation and the patient is better if he can sleep.

On a deeper level, or after chronic exposure, the liver is affected. It is congested by excess stimulants and toxins, especially alcohol which the Nux vomica patient craves. These are very active people. If they cannot throw out the anger into activity, they must become active in themselves. Thus they eat more, indulging themselves in *rich foods*. Eventually this abuses the liver so it becomes *congested*. A common result of this is a *bilious headache* – as if a weight pressing down on the vertex, plus nausea, 'if only I could be sick', << noise and a feeling *as if poisoned*. This poisoned feeling is a sign that everything is out of harmony. Nux vomica is a frequently indicated migraine remedy, especially when the patient is stressed and irritable, suppressing anger.

In today's world Nux is often produced as a symptom picture because *stimulation* is a key factor in our culture, yet we live at such a sedentary pace there is no outlet for our activity, rather it wears down the nerves. The tensions produced in us and the emotions we repress respond to Nux vomica but note that after it is administered 'things' move outwards with considerable force – feelings, faeces, vomit, etc.

ACTIVITY 6 Outline the symptom picture of a Nux vomica patient's headache. Pay attention to the exciting cause and modalities. Do the same to show the symptom picture of a Nux vomica patient with indigestion.

ACTIVITY 7 Using either Allen or Von Lippe, take note of the symptoms in black type. List those of the digestive system that do not appear in this lesson. List those of the nervous system that do not appear in this lesson. Divide these symptoms into those belonging to the central nervous system (voluntary) and those of the autonomic nervous system.

ACTIVITY 8 Find out about the food cravings and aversions of the Nux vomica patient.

Similar Remedies

Sulphur resembles Nux vomica more than any other remedy. Indeed, it is called the 'chronic of Nux', i.e. it may be needed when the Nux symptom picture moves deeper.

It is a remedy of excessive heat and over-stimulation. Like Nux, it has a strong effect on the digestive system. Sulphur is also an egotist who can be fastidiously correct, and can force his will with a violent temper.

Ignatia

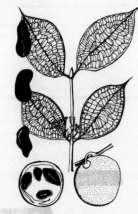

Strychnos ignatia bergius

Latin name:	Ignatia amara
Common name:	St Ignatius's bean
Botanical family:	Loganiaceae
Habitat:	It is a climbing shrub found in the Philippines.

Origin

Hahnemann proved the remedy from a tincture prepared from the seeds.

Essence

This remedy contains even more strychnine than Nux vomica. It is a contrary remedy. Here impulsiveness is because of hysteria or instability. This patient is so scattered there is no direction. They are *overwhelmed*.

Keynotes and Characteristics

• Globus hystericus	A lump in the throat!
• **Grief**	This is too big to swallow.
• Silent grief	They cannot express what is within.
• **< disappointed love**	Even decades later. They are romantics – they live in a dream of love.
• Fall in love with inappropriate people.	It is a fantasy.
• Sighing respiration	Deep spasm of the diaphragm.
• **Fickle**	Today we might call this scattered.
• Contradictory	They go from one pole to the other in instability.
• Laughs when should cry	A horrifying result of shock.
• Moods alternate	They are easily influenced.
• **Introspective**	A lot of time is spent in musing.
• **Thinking makes it so**	They will have any symptom that is mentioned to them.
• Internal trembling	This is the 'scattered' body.
• **Symptoms same hour daily or annually**	They remember the event and it recurs!
• **< tobacco**	There is a very strong reaction to this.
• Fear of robbers at night	This is a fear of loss, that something will be taken from her.
• Paradoxical	You expect the opposite.
• > indigestible foods	i.e. when digestion is upset they will happily eat tomato sauce.
• **Emptiness at the pit of stomach not relieved by eating**	**Strange, Rare and Peculiar**. It is the nerve that is affected.
• **Hiccoughs**	A form of spasm.
• Yawns spasmodically.	The diaphragm draws more air in.
• Convulsive twitches	The nerves are overstimulated.
• Tonic spasms	As in Nux vomica.
• Jerks on going to sleep	They hold so much in that there is much activity when they let go.
• Pains in small spots	**Strange, Rare and Peculiar** symptom that applies to many patients.
• Throat pains > swallowing	**Strange, Rare** and **Peculiar**.

ACTIVITY 9 List all the symptoms of Spasm to be found in the keynotes and characteristics.

ACTIVITY 10 Note all the paradoxical symptoms you can find.

ACTIVITY 11 Find associated rubrics in the *Mind* section of Kent's Repertory for 'overwhelmed', 'introspective'.

Worse Emotional Distress

The Ignatia state most commonly arises after emotional shock. Hence the keynotes include *< grief* and *< disappointed love.*

In the schoolgirl, or boy, loss of the first love causes *anguish* and distress. The first love is the most *romantic* of all love affairs. The blow seems to shatter the patient and surges of emotion well up to swamp all rational thought. The storm expresses itself as a *restlessness* which prevents quiet thought – *thoughts dwell* on the loved one, blocking out all else. He/she cannot sleep, cannot concentrate on anything else, cannot eat. Usually there is a great amount of tears and loud sobs which cause the chest to heave violently. Later *deep sighing* illustrates the spasm in the diaphragm. Strong spasm in the throat may make crying painful as the copious flow of fluid needs to be swallowed and it is as if there were a lump in the throat – *globus hystericus*. The remedy may also be used when the meeting with a loved one produces a light-headedness, a *flutter in the stomach* and a *very dry mouth* that makes speech difficult.

Overwhelmed

In grief the patient may be so beside herself that she is temporarily out of her mind so she *laughs when the matter is really serious*. Or she may behave as above. The globus hystericus is very common when overcome by emotion and is recognized in the common phrase 'it brought a lump to my throat'. So at the graveside the Ignatia patient can be seen literally choking on her tears. But the grief of the Ignatia patient may also be so great that she is *overwhelmed* – she cannot express the grief because she cannot encompass its reality. She may be stunned and have no feelings because they are locked within – it is as if the door shut tight with a jerk and she does not know how to open it. Of course this is an extreme form of *silent grief* or delayed reaction and perhaps rare. Ignatia is a remedy for extreme reaction to shock. The most extreme reaction is *paralysis* after grief as when the patient is struck dumb or is deaf or blind when the shock of what he/she heard or saw is too great. Such paralysis may continue for a lifetime if not released by a remedy such as Ignatia, or another strong emotion.

ACTIVITY 12   I am sure you have seen people in grief or after disappointed love. Write up some notes on how you remember their symptom picture.

A Romantic Idealist

The Ignatia patient is essentially an *idealist* who is brought down to earth with a thud by outside events. The romanticism comes across in their choice of lover who is never down-to-earth or boy-next-door. They reach for the unattainable and when hurt either disintegrate or reach further for universal love or ideals that cannot hurt them. They become nuns, or crusaders for lost causes, or live all their life true to the romantic ideal of the unobtainable love, often of the young man who died in the trenches. They are the heroines of Greek tragedies. Little upsets produce dramas in which they *faint with excitement* or take a *fit if contradicted*, or jerk and twitch with frustration. Reason does not reach them when the mind is not down on earth. The arrival of menstruation creates greater instability and many states are aggravated by then. Notably, the Greek word for the womb has the same root as *hysteria*.

Sensitive

Ignatia patients are extremely sensitive people, very *sensitive to criticism* and *easily exhausted* by their work on behalf of others. They easily tend to *introspection* which leads to the keynote <*thinking about things*. In thinking of things they lose sense of reality (*proportion*) because they are buried in the mind away from reality and the strength of emotional reaction prevents the reason from balancing the situation. In depression they become *confused* and do not know the way ahead or are afraid least they do the wrong thing or in case they have neglected their duty. At this stage the keynote *contrary* becomes evident. The *moods change rapidly* as if there were no substance to them. They are *easily offended* and then may react outrageously, or unpredictably.

One of the common first aid uses of the remedy will be in travel sickness which demonstrates the sensitivity and the keynote *thinking makes it so*. The sickness arises in particular because of *sensitivity to tobacco smoke*. Yet once they are disturbed they will smell tobacco smoke even when it is not there and their anger may be directed to a phantom smoker somewhere at the back of the bus. Basically their nerves are too sensitive to take the stimulation of travel.

ACTIVITY 13   Outline the symptom picture of the Ignatia patient's headache. Pay attention to the exciting cause and modalities.

Similar Remedies

Natrum muriaticum is most similar to Ignatia. It is often required when the symptoms go deeper so is called the 'chronic' of Ignatia.

They are vulnerable types who are easily offended. They may feel separate from reality or retreat from it when grieved or disappointed in love. Like Ignatia, there is a degree of polarity.

Staphysagria

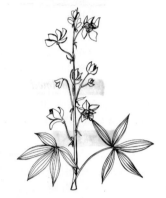

Delphinium staphysagria

Latin name:	Delphinium staphysagria
Common name:	Stavesacre
Botanical family:	Ranunculaceae
Habitat:	It grows in Mediterranean climates

Origin

The remedy was proved by Hahnemann from a tincture prepared from the seeds.

Essence

The remedy excites the nervous system then paralyses it. There are no boundaries. It is a remedy of over-excess. Reaction is *over the top*.

Keynotes and Characteristics

• **< suppressed anger**	**Exciting cause**.
• **< wounded pride**	**Exciting cause**.
• **< sexual excess**	**Exciting cause**.
• **Indignation**	Takes offence easily and broods on it.
• Trembles	Like Ignatia but not only internally.
• Grinds teeth	It is as if they desire to get their teeth into it but can only go through the motions.
• **mind dwells on sex**	They seek a deep peace!
• < masturbation	Some might say quite an indignity to the body!
• **Violent outbursts of passion**	They want to reach out. There is much frustration.
• Violent itching	This remedy gives rise to a lot of irritation.
• Crawling, as from insects, especially genitalia	
• Itching on the margin of lids	On the edges.
• Burning, prickling sensation	A bit more than an itch, you may find it in wounds or in cystitis.
• Crumbling, black teeth	
• > breakfast	This is something they can get their teeth into to ground them.
• Ravenous appetite for days before fever starts	**Strange, Rare and Peculiar**
• As if stomach hanging down and flabby	**Strange, Rare and Peculiar**
• **Desires tobacco**	This is one way of telling the difference between this remedy and Ignatia.
• As if a drop of urine rolled along the ureter	This is seen in cystitis.
• After urination, urging as if bladder not empty	There is much irritation and rawness.
• Burning when not urinating	This will enable you to separate this remedy from Cantharis.
• One-sided paralysis from anger	

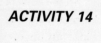 **ACTIVITY 14**   Using the *Mind* section of Kent's repertory, find associated words to *indignation*.

ACTIVITY 15 This remedy can be described as *over the top*. Which symptoms would you pick out to illustrate this?

ACTIVITY 16 Which keynote or characteristic symptoms show an effect on the nerves?

Passionate

The Staphysagria patient embraces a situation fully. In the healthy patient there is a joy and a lust for life. Alas few people and situations can match such a *passion*. Culture often does not allow it either. So the poor Staphysagria patient has to keep herself on a tight rein.

Staphysagria patients when they take the passion within are still volatile, hence they *over-react* to situations. They take *offence* at the slightest hint but the reaction is so strong, they are bowled over – *outraged*. When this is internalized it becomes *anguish*. It is unbearable.

This is such a potent remedy of suppressed anger because these people are *torn apart inside*. Their distress may be so great they cannot hold it. Very deep diseases may arise in the tissues if the anger does not get out.

Thus the remedy is useful for patients who are confined and restricted in expression in some situations, where they are deprived of action.

ACTIVITY 17 What other remedies which you have studied are listed in Kent's Repertory under 'ailments from anger'?

ACTIVITY 18 Go through the *Mind* section and list all those rubrics which mention Nux vomica, Ignatia and Staphysagria.

Situations of Suppressed Emotion

Staphysagria arises out of clear situations that might repay study. It is called variously the spinster remedy, the mother-in-law remedy, the civil servant remedy, the rape case remedy. In each of these situations the patient is *helpless to change the situation* and can simply cry with *frustration* or rage aimlessly at cruel fate. The potential of the individual is subordinated in each case.

The spinster in Kent's day had to sit and wait for a man to take notice of her. Whilst some may have coped, others became *indignant* which might mean discontented, hard to please, nagging. Needless to say the emptiness of some marriages might similarly have lead to a Staphysagria situation.

The mother-in-law may fit into this category – her own life devoid of joy, deprived of a role now the children have left the nest, a helpless soul who is imposed into a situation which others find themselves helpless to alter. Frustration arises on both sides. Such phrases as '*a pain in the neck*' and '*gets under the skin*' describe the reactions of the combatants. An itching restlessness, an impulse to do something – a bit similar to Nux vomica. But Nux vomica does something, is decisive; the sensitivity of Staphysagria holds back. (Compare with Hyoscyamus which goes into madness.) Thus Staphysagria goes into pathology or *depression*.

The civil servant is defined by the role he or she performs and cannot act individually. The rule book sets up a structure to enable fairness to all, but many individual deviations are genuine and heart-breaking to a sensitive person. The sensitive official is disturbed but his hands are tied. The situation is much worse if the client is angry and shows his/her frustration. What can the official do? Rage inside in frustration!

What can the rape victim do, or the victim of a mugging or robbery? Such people have been *violated*. After the event there is no one to say sorry, to be angry with. All protestation is in vain and the hands of the clock move on regardless. *After operations*, especially involving epidurals or lumbar punctures which affect the nerves, Staphysagria is well indicated for the resultant indignation of the body. In operations especially, the cut is across the natural lines of the body and is an intrusion or violation. Cuts which require Staphysagria are not satisfied that Hypericum heals the nerves, there is still the outrage to be soothed. So it is often said in the books on first aid to use Staphysagria when Hypericum does not relieve pain or after razor-type cuts. Episiotomy is another medical situation that responds well to Staphysagria.

Head lice or fleas produce another interesting condition. Their presence causes intense irritability and frustration, expressed as an itch at body level. The fleas or lice are intruders who violate the individual's space. They may even induce helpless anger. A most interesting example of this concerned a cat who developed fleas after castration. For a year nothing seemed to have any effect until the homoeopath added the flea condition to that of repressed sexuality and the fact the creature had an epidural for the operation – Staphysagria was given. The fleas almost dropped off minutes later – a simple combing removed them, but for a whole week afterwards this over-affectionate little cat would not permit any handling at all and was especially sensitive on the lower spine where he had had the epidural injection. Seven years later the fleas have still not returned. This case shows not only the Law of Cure, but the strong effect of Staphysagria on subjects who have been sexually frustrated especially those who continually think of such matters!

Physical Effects of Frustration

Conditions produced by indignation and suppressed anger in the Staphysagria patient include *styes* and *tarsal tumours* of the eyelids and cystitis as the remedy affects the mucous membrane with rawness and irritation – most notably it is useful for *'honeymoon cystitis'* – and thus the keynote *burning when not urinating*.

They tend to *crunch their teeth* in frustration, so producing problems in that area. The teeth turn *black, crumble and decay* at the edges. There may be a considerable amount of *tension in the jaw*. It often comes up as a remedy of toothache which is very sensitive to the slightest touch but fine when a firm touch such as in chewing is applied. Toothache is also worse from exposure to cold.

On a deeper organ level, *eczema* is a chronic condition produced by frustration. In the Staphysagria patient there is *violent itching*, worse at any offence or insult. They will scratch this passionately and with no temperance. To prescribe the remedy, you must go back to trace the cause. Once you have this clearly, Staphysagria will cure remarkably.

ACTIVITY 19 Describe the symptoms of a throat problem that might respond to Staphysagria as a remedy. Note the individualizing symptoms, the exciting cause and the modalities.

Similar Remedies

Pulsatilla is the chronic of Staphysagria. It is more easy to see the Pulsatilla patient produce a Staphysagria acute when her simple trusting nature is violated.

The mother-in-law could easily be a Pulsatilla who has lost her role and is so demanding and voracious that she is a pain in the neck. Or, in her deep need to be loved she is vulnerable to insult and rejection.

 SELF-TEST QUESTIONS

Which remedies suit the following situations? Look for characteristic patterns and keynotes. Check your answers in the answer section at the end of the book.

1. After hearing bad news, the patient withdraws and wishes to be left alone. She is weak and trembling and messages to the muscles are so confused she lacks co-ordination.
2. The patient has numbness of parts and is, at first, unable to move on rising from a patch of dew-laden grass.

3. Since an operation which involved an epidural, the patient is very depressed.
4. Since hearing her lover ran off with someone else, speech has been incoherent and the patient is sleepless and very excitable.
5. Her car sickness is accompanied by a profuse cold sweat and violent vomit as soon as she tries to move.
6. Very violent, spasmodic contractions during labour cause the patient to faint. She is worse from heat and worse from cold air.
7. The patient prattles continually during a high fever and cannot bear to be alone in the dark.
8. Cystitis has persisted since she was found out to be on the bus without a ticket by the conductor. The burning pain in the urethra is present when she is not urinating.
9. He is a chilly person who finds the heat of the bed unbearable as it causes burning pains in his swollen feet and ankles.
10. A severe throbbing headache on the right side is accompanied by a hot head and a flushed face, < touch, noise and light, especially light, and is < lying down.
11. Very severe neuralgic pain from a torn tendon causes the patient to be exhausted.
12. He has eyes like balls of fire after straining them all day at close work without his glasses.
13. His headache is heavy and feels as if there is boiling water in the brain. Objects seen appear yellow. The pain is < looking at bright things and < the sound of running water.
14. The patient is hot and irritable and yet sensitive to the slightest draught and coughs as soon as any part of the body is uncovered.
15. Drinks little often, eats seldom but much.
16. The diarrhoea resulting from anger is hot and smells of rotten eggs.
17. The menses disappeared after a fright.
18. An urticaria type eruption appeared after the patient was long exposed to cold, just before the menses started. This eruption burns after it is scratched.
19. The parts lain on feel cold and bruised, especially after lying on the left side or when the weather is cold and damp.
20. She finds her husband trembling all over after his boss told him off for going home five minutes early. After all he was in at work 15 minutes early this morning.

Further Studies

Nux Vomica
1. When would you use Nux vomica in a first aid situation?
2. Describe the Nux vomica headache. How does it compare to other remedies? Repertorize the symptoms.
3. Describe how the Nux vomica teacher would behave in a classroom crisis.
4. When would the Nux vomica present as 'The Irish Remedy'? Do you think this is a fair description of the symptom picture?
5. What symptom picture does the Nux vomica patient present when the anger is suppressed?
6. What ailments does the Nux vomica patient suffer under stress?
7. Explain how Nux vomica affects the nervous system.

Ignatia
1. Give *six* symptoms that illustrate the contrariness of Ignatia.
2. Describe the love-sick teenager who needs a dose of Ignatia – compare with Antimonium crudum and Pulsatilla.
3. Compare the rape victims who need Ignatia and Staphysagria.
4. Ignatia and Nux vomica are both spasmodic remedies. Compare them.
5. Describe the behaviour of the grief-stricken Ignatia patient at the side of the grave.
6. Compare the excitement of Ignatia and Phosphorus.
7. Compare the modalities of Ignatia and Natrum muriaticum.
8. Compare Ignatia with other remedies that are worse for fright, e.g. Aconite and Causticum.
9. Compare the religious affliction of Ignatia, Lachesis, Hyoscyamus and Pulsatilla.
10. Compare the throat symptoms of Ignatia and Lachesis.

Staphysagria
1. How might you confuse this remedy with Nux vomica?
2. When might the Pulsatilla patient need Staphysagria?
3. When might you use Staphysagria in a first aid situation?
4. Describe the sore throat of Staphysagria.
5. Differentiate between the Staphysagria child and the Chamomilla child.
6. Describe the Staphysagria spinster.

Different Levels of Response to the Exciting Cause

Euphrasia, Bryonia, Gelsemium, Baptisia

Aim: To illustrate how the same exciting cause can produce different levels of response and different symptom pictures.

Objectives: To be able to identify different levels of response.
To be able to identify individuality in similar symptom pictures.
To relate the characteristic weakness of a remedy to the symptoms produced.

Headings: INTRODUCTION
EUPHRASIA: Origin: Essence; Keynotes and Characteristics; The Scrofulous Constitution; Eye Injuries; Case
BRYONIA: Origin; Essence; Keynotes and Characteristics; Congestion; Different Levels of Disturbance
GELSEMIUM: Origin; Essence; Keynotes and Characteristics; Different Levels of Disturbance; Excitability Becomes Prostration
BAPTISIA: Origin; Essence; Keynotes and Characteristics; Different Levels of Disorder
SELF-TEST QUESTIONS (REVISION)
FURTHER STUDIES

Introduction

All four remedies are common in colds and flus. In bringing them together it is not my intention to present you with 'cold remedies' because any constitutional remedy may be appropriate in an acute episode of disease. Rather I want to introduce you to the different levels of activity of which remedies are capable.

In many of the little books on minor ailments, with which you may be familiar, there are short snippets on symptom pictures that contain perhaps half-a-dozen keynotes and characteristics. Not all the symptoms are present in a case, so we need to look deeper to find the role and position of any symptom in the disturbance. In later years of study you will find there is even more depth to the study of remedies.

Some remedies will go deeper than others. When a cold first starts the symptoms are minor. In relatively healthy individuals it may remain so.

One group of remedies will cover the type of cold which produces minor symptoms of sneezing, runny nose and fever. Another group will indicate a deeper disturbance when throat pain and catarrh arise. Yet another group will represent the type of cold that develops into the chest, or even involves the kidneys. Yet another group may produce flu.

Thus the Aconite patient will start to sneeze almost immediately on exposure to intense cold. Within a few hours a fever may develop which responds well to a hot bath and a milky drink and bed. By morning all is well.

The Euphrasia patient's eyes may start to water shortly after exposure, then the nose may run copiously and the sneezing start. This patient may be well next day or the throat may start to produce copious catarrh.

The Bryonia patient seldom sneezes right away. He takes a little longer to develop the symptoms and they are deeper. The tonsils may be congested or the throat and/or the chest may be involved, first with copious catarrh then a painful dryness.

The Gelsemium patient does not often localize the disturbance but starts to shiver on a run up to a flu. A few days after exposure the limbs are heavy, the eyes are heavy and the patient is exhausted, chilly and dopey.

In the lesson we will look at this in more detail. As well as the symptom picture characteristic of the remedy, we will see why the patient susceptible to this remedy is predisposed to catch cold and we will study the conditions under which this happens.

Euphrasia

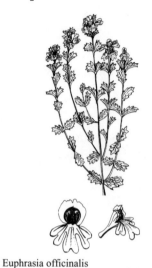

Euphrasia officinalis

Latin name:	Euphrasia officinalis
Common name:	Eyebright
Botanical family:	Rhinanthaceae
Habitat:	Throughout Europe and North America. It grows in meadows and verges in town and country.

Origin

Hahnemann proved the remedy using a preparation of the whole plant.

Essence

The remedy works on scrofulous, catarrhal constitutions localizing markedly in the eyes.

Keynotes and Characteristics

- **Profuse lachrymation** — Occurs in almost any complaint.
- **Acrid lachrymation**
- Redness and swelling of the eyes — Caused by acrid tears.
- Burning sensation in the eyes — Caused by acrid tears.
- Photo-sensitive eyes — The eyes are a weak organ in the Euphrasia patient.
- **Copious fluid discharge from nose** — Which is bland.
- Violent cough — Arising from a tickle in the throat < exposure to warmth.
- Hawk catarrh in morning — Indeed so much catarrh, gag till vomit.
- **Catarrh flows in night lying down** — This is **Strange, Rare and Peculiar**, so distinguishes the remedy from many others.
- **> lying down** — This is a general symptom which applies to the patient in many different ailments. Most patients are > rest, but scrofulous (catarrhal) patients are more blocked up on lying down. This symptom can then be very significant.
- Frequent yawning, walking in open air — They need not have a cold.
- **Chilliness** — As a cold deepens the general level is more disturbed.
- Heat descends the body — Found in the fever. This is **Strange, Rare and Peculiar** as the majority of remedies have ascending heat.
- Sweat on the front of the body only — Particularly about the chest. Where there is congestion in the chest it may be more difficult to spot this symptom as unusual. Perspiration on the front only. Other remedies will produce sweat on the localized part, i.e. the chest in this case.
- Pressing pain beneath the sternum — When congestion is concentrated in the trachea.
- Eyes agglutinated in the morning — This is a deeper disturbance on the local level.

84

• Dimness of vision	Usually this is the chronic disturbance manifesting locally.
• As though a hair hung over the eye	This is also the chronic level and is **Strange, Rare and Peculiar**.
• As if sand in the eye	As above. It is more common where there is liver disturbance (Sepia also has this symptom under the same conditions).
• **Menses very short**	Last only one day, or even just one hour.
• Amenorrhoea with catarrh in the eyes	The last two symptoms are both signs of chronic disturbance.

ACTIVITY 1

Assign the symptoms above to one of the four categories:

Strange, Rare and Peculiar
Mental and Emotional
General
Particular.

Two of the symptoms might be described as common in circumstances. Which are these?

ACTIVITY 2

Which symptoms may be described as sensations? Which symptoms may indicate pathology. What is the possible underlying pathology? *Study the latter in a pathology textbook so you understand the relationship to the symptom.*

The Scrofulous Constitution

This phrase occurs commonly in some homoeopathic textbooks. Strictly speaking it refers to a patient with a family history of tuberculosis, who has a personal medical history of catarrhal problems. The term is used more loosely to refer to patients whose constitution produces catarrhal problems whenever there is a breakdown in health.

If you look at the list of keynotes and characteristics of Euphrasia, you will see that it has a strong effect on mucous membrane, lubricating tissue, so copious mucus is produced.

Now we have the overall pattern, what is different – individualistic, in the Euphrasia patient? First, *the eyes are strongly affected*. Sulphur shares this affinity with Euphrasia but in Euphrasia *the discharge is acrid*. It contrasts with Allium cepa which has a discharge from eyes and nose, but has the acrid discharge from the nose and bland from the eyes. The discharge of Euphrasia is *worse in the morning* and *on entering warm places*. Indeed the exciting cause is *exposure to warm winds*. In the textbooks you will see this described as 'a warm south wind'. If you translate that into today's world, you may find the Euphrasia condition in the shop assistant who has to stand under the overhead convection heater that blasts out warm air. The centrally heated office or school will often produce a Euphrasia condition. Pulsatilla produces catarrhal conditions in similar situations, but the discharge is always bland and the Pulsatilla patient is worse lying down when the catarrh cannot flow. Euphrasia is > *lying down*. This is most unusual and therefore an important symptom when found in a patient.

As the cold progresses, it reaches deeper into the respiratory system. A violent cough may arise from *a tickle in the throat* (Phosphorus). As the mucus thickens the patient may start to *hawk it up in the mornings*. It is so copious he/she may *gag until they vomit* (Bryonia, Ipecacuanha, Drosera). This is common in whooping cough where this remedy is further distinguished by copious lachrymation and a *cough only in the daytime* because the patient is better lying down.

Should the Euphrasia patient develop a headache with the cold, there will be *a bursting sensation* or *a bruised feeling* as the sinuses fill with catarrh. At night little itching pains may start all over. The eyes will feel bruised and may be *photophobic*. Opposite to the discharge state, the head and eyes are better for open air. As the cold deepens further, *the eyes may feel as if there is sand in them* (Sepia). The general symptom of *chilliness* will appear. This may be accompanied by two Strange, Rare and Peculiar symptoms: *heat descending the body* (more commonly it ascends, as in flushes), and *sweat on the front of the body only*, particularly about the chest. Congestion may then be concentrated in the trachea giving rise to a *pressing pain beneath the sternum*. This deepening situation is a little less common but may be present in whooping cough or in measles before the spots appear. It is interesting to note that measles also has an affinity for the eyes. In the Euphrasia case there would be excessive lachrymation and fluent coryza.

Usually in a scrofulous constitution the lungs are affected more markedly. In Euphrasia the remedy is able to localize through the minor organ of the eyes and would only go into the lungs if this drain were blocked, e.g. with allopathic drugs. The chronic situation in the eyes will produce thicker catarrh which will *stick the eyelids together* in the morning. There may be frequent blepharitis. Vision may be affected so the patient *continually closes the eyes* and presses them to clear the vision. Spots and vesicles may appear on the cornea and the acidity may give rise to ulcers there. Throughout this the eyes will appear red-rimmed and will smart.

ACTIVITY 3 Compare the catarrhal state in at least two other remedies, paying attention to:

The nature of the catarrh
The areas affected in each remedy
The distinguishing features in each remedy.

Of the remedies you have studied you could use Bryonia and Cantharis.

ACTIVITY 4 You cannot imagine the different types of catarrh. Use the repertory to explore this, looking up *catarrh, discharge, coryza,* under the sections for nose, throat, expectoration.

Eye Injuries

Two factors make Euphrasia a useful remedy in injury to the eye. The first of these is of course its affinity for the eye. The other factor is *the bruised sensation* Euphrasia produces. What happens when a part is injured? – It bruises of course. Thus Euphrasia may be found in other injuries where there is bruising.

When the eyes are injured they *frequently water. Photophobia* also occurs frequently, and *smarting* is not uncommon. In injury, the stitching pain, which flits on and off is accompanied with much restlessness.

In severe injury, there is a sensation *as if a hair hangs over the eye*. The patient is continually trying to sweep this away.

In more serious injury, catarrh can follow or accompany inflammation. In a prolonged situation sight can be affected *as if there is a film covering the cornea*.

ACTIVITY 5 Compare Euphrasia with Arnica, Ledum and Symphytum in eye injury. Look at the symptoms each produces and look for individual differences.

Case

During a flu the patient is so chilly he cannot get warm in bed. During the day there is a lot of heat giving rise to a red face but it is as if the heat descends, although the hands are cold. Perspiration is worse at night, on the chest, where there arises a most offensive odour. In the morning the cough starts as the expectoration flows more profusely. There is a lot of gagging to clear this and as he does this, the eyes start to water so the crusty deposit that sticks them together becomes a gummy mess.

After all this activity the patient receives much comfort and relief from lying down again.

ACTIVITY 6		In the case above, pick out the characteristic symptoms of Euphrasia.

ACTIVITY 7		Pick out the modalities of Euphrasia from the text, separating aggravations from ameliorations.

Bryonia

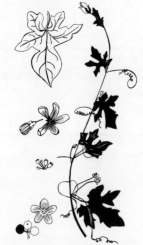

Bryonia alba

Latin name: Bryonia alba
Common name: White bryony, wild hops
Botanical family: Cucurbitaceae
Habitat: A climbing plant that grows in hedgerows in Europe. Gibson says it creeps quietly and unobtrusively, often hidden by other foliage

Origin

The remedy was first prepared by Hahnemann from the milky juice extracted from the root, taken before the plant flowered.

Essence

The Bryonia plant is a climber, with specialized tendrils with which to hold on. Thus it is very sensitive to touch and movement. It seeks stability. In the mental realm this is experienced as *insecurity*. The patient is very conservative in outlook. On the physical level, congestion arises from lack of movement and 'holding on'.

Keynotes and Characteristics

• **Slow onset**	Bryonia is a slow mover.
• **< cold damp**	It grows in damp hedgerows.
• Affects epithelial lining tissue of serous and mucous membranes.	These are the damp places in the body.
• **Copious white catarrh**	In the early stages of illness. This is like the milky juice that can be pressed from the roots of the plant.
• **Thirst – great quantities**	Because so dry. This patient drinks by the glassful in the dry state.
• **< slightest movement**	Because the tissues are so dry – the lubrication is gone so there are stitching pains.
• Child dislikes to be carried	
• **Lies on the painful side**	To prevent movement of the dry, unlubricated part.
• Grasps painful part to stop it moving	This may be especially seen in the cough.
• **Sticking stitching pains**	Arise out of dryness of epithelial tissue.
• Cannot breathe deep enough	
• **< heat**	The patient is so congested. Heat increases congestion and movement.
• **Touchy**	There is great irritability of tissue and the mind.
• **Fear of poverty**	This might be considered a drying up of resources and nurture. It epitomizes the *insecurity* of the remedy.
• **Cries to be taken home in delirium**	Both this, and the next symptom show insecurity.
• **Talks anxiously about business when ill**	

- Sensation of fullness and stuffiness

  Because of congestion and dryness. These will be found in any affected part.

- Bursting headache

  Congestive, often associated with slow-functioning liver, so toxins build up in the blood. This is a remedy of migraine that would once have been called a bilious headache.

- Vomits bile
- **Dry, hard stool, looks burnt**

  The intestines are so dry. This gives rise to constipation.

- Constipation when abroad

  This is a new situation, incurring insecurity.

- Vicarious menstruation

  The part is congested and feels full, but there is a drying up of flow which comes out elsewhere, especially as nose-bleeds.

- **Stone hard breasts**

  It has a great effect on the glands of the body. The breasts are especially affected before the menses.

- **< before menses**

  Congestion increases at this time as the liver tries to expel oestrogen. The slow liver then has more work to do and is overcome.

- **< 9 p.m.–3 a.m.**

ACTIVITY 8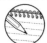

Label each of the above symptoms with the category of symptom to which it belongs:

Strange, Rare and Peculiar
Mental and Emotional
General
Particular.

Congestion

Bryonia's field of action is epithelial tissue such as mucous and serous membrane. Slowly it builds up a congestion so tissue has a *dark red, purplish hue* as it becomes engorged. At first, *copious discharge* is produced as the tissue is irritated. Later it dries, producing the typical *stitching pains on movement* and *aggravation to heat*.

Congestion occurs wherever there is epithelial lining tissue. It is most common in the respiratory system but is also found in tonsils, the intestines and appendix. Bryonia works especially on epithelial tissue which secretes. Hence its first action is to produce excessive mucus and its second action is to dry this up. Bryonia also has a strong effect on the glands which are the gateway to the lymphatic system, as in the tonsils and adenoids, or have a more specialized secretory function as in breasts, ovaries and testes.

In the last it can be seen to be markedly *right-sided*. The glands respond on the epithelial lining tissue with much swelling, engorged with fluids. If visible they have a purplish hue, many have stitching pains or *feel as if they will burst*. They are markedly > *for any firm pressure* that stops movements – this is notable in appendicitis which is usually diagnosed by 'rebound tenderness'.

At a deeper level the Bryonia rheumatism is concentrated in the synovial joints which are usually well lubricated. In the first instance the synovial fluid builds up giving rise to *swellings*. The Bryonia rheumatic is *very touchy* in temperament and worse for any heat or movement.

Different Levels of Disturbance

This remedy is deeper than Euphrasia, Aconite, Belladonna or Chamomilla. Onset is slow as the congestion takes time to build up. During that time, the patient will gradually feel more debilitated. The vital force has been afflicted but has not yet shown a reaction – there are no real prescribing symptoms, though a good homoeopath will already have noted the slow onset and the exciting cause. The exciting cause may be a soaking (i.e. < *cold and wet*), *anger*, or *chagrin*. The patient is affected according to his/her vitality. The healthy may simply produce catarrh from the nose for a few days. If it is worse he/she may get a little stuffed up and dry, finding it a little difficult to breathe. He/she will desire drinks and may be a trifle hot and bothered. It is possible a stuffy head cold will develop in which the dryness, thirst and irritability are a little more marked. A *bursting headache* may develop, *aggravated on stooping*, or *in a stuffy warm room*.

Instead of the head, the disturbance in the Bryonia patient may centre in the tonsils, or the minor organ of the ear. The *right-sidedness* will be evident. The usual symptoms will be present, of *fullness, throbbing* or *bursting pains < heat*. At the throbbing, full state, there may be *copious catarrh*, but as this dries up the pain will change to *stitching* and there will be *an attempt to hold the part to prevent movement*.

As the disease progresses at the acute level, or without precursor in the less vital or the aged, bronchitis may result, with a characteristic *hard cough* that first brings up copious expectorations. In a further stage, the cough may still be there because the dryness creates *irritability*, but now there will be the *stitching pain on each spasm*. The heat will cause the patient to struggle for breath and *drink copiously*. The temperament will be irritable and *anxious regarding their work and business*. In pneumonia or pleurisy the symptoms will be more marked because they are more serious. Here you will find the patient *lying on the painful side* to prevent movement of any kind. There will be so much *dryness* each breath will be drawn in with difficulty. You will find the patient more *touchy* and more distressed. Now you might see the symptoms *< 9 p.m.–3 a.m, fear of poverty*, or *desire to go home*. You must look at this patient with the dull red face and realise he/she is expressing a need to be cosseted and safe.

In another patient the disease may not go deeply into the respiratory system but may strike out on the general level as flu. Here there will be a slow build-up. The congestion will gather in the muscles producing aching. When the symptoms come out there will be *much heat especially around the head* – the flow of blood is again to the head. The head may throb or feel full to bursting. The copious catarrh may rapidly pass to dryness of right tonsil. There will be much thirst. The patient will be *dopey* but will *arouse angrily if disturbed*.

Notice how the keynote and characteristic symptoms repeat themselves and how each new symptom represents a deepening of a trend already there?

Bryonia has a strong effect on the liver and digestive system, so the same story can be unfolded through diarrhoea and dysentery to typhoid, with a minor localization in appendicitis and a deepening on a more chronic level to constipation because of dryness in the gut. This last symptom produces a characteristic *hard, dry stool* that may look *burnt*. The constipation may become an acute problem when the patient is faced with insecurity, e.g. *when abroad*, off to boarding school for the first time, or with a *financial worry* hanging over him/her.

Bryonia has a profound effect on the reproductive system because testes, ovaries and breasts are glands. This is noticeable in the female also because of the added burden to the congested, slow liver, of regularly disposing of oestrogen. The Bryonia female is much *< before menstruation*. As congestion builds up *the breasts are tender*, sore to touch and may need held to stop them bobbing up and down in some situations. Irritability increases as the period approaches. The *abdomen may distend and feel full*. The patient slows down, becoming more sluggish. *Constipation* is often present. *Bursting, bilious headaches* may occur. The menses start slowly with dark coloured blood, often clotted. On some rare occasions, it may even be *black and stringy*, or the system so congested the body has to relieve the pressure elsewhere as in *nosebleeds*.

The movement up to the head, bursting headaches and nosebleeds may be present when this remedy is of use in high blood pressure. These people are irritable, anxious about their security and well-being, sluggish, congested and *easily overheated. Anxiety* and stress is the key here. On a chronic level the Bryonia patient is more likely to have chronic bronchitis or emphysema especially if they have lived in *damp surroundings or climate*. This patient may develop rheumatism and end up with congestive heart disease. Throughout all this, the characteristic symptoms and modalities will be present.

ACTIVITY 9 Describe the Bryonia headache in detail, noting which parts of the characteristic symptom picture are best represented.

ACTIVITY 10
Go through each entry in the Repertory under 'expectoration' and list those under which Bryonia appears.

ACTIVITY 11
Go through each entry in the Repertory under 'cough' and list those under which Bryonia occurs.

ACTIVITY 12
Go through each entry in the Repertory under 'stool' and list those under which Bryonia occurs.

ACTIVITY 13
List the modalities of Bryonia. Separate into aggravations and ameliorations. How do these illustrate the character of dryness and congestion?

Gelsemium

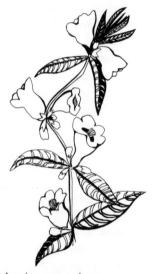

Gelsemium sempervivens

Latin name:	Gelsemium sempervivens
Common name:	Yellow jasmine
Botanical family:	Loganiaceae
Habitat:	It is a native of Southern Europe, USA, Carolina, Tennessee, etc. where the climate is warm and winters cold

Origin

It was proved separately by Douglass and Hale from a tincture of the bark.

Essence

Gelsemium is similar to Bryonia in its speed of onset. After exposure to cold, damp conditions, the patient may take several days to develop the symptoms. It attacks the nervous system, especially motor nerves, causing first, overexcitement, trembling, then weakness, fatigue and even paralysis.

Keynotes and Characteristics

• **Trembling**	This occurs in voluntary and involuntary muscles.
• **Tremble so much – want to be held to stop the trembling**	This may be seen after grief or bad news.
• **Heaviness – (limbs) described as leaden**	It especially refers to the eyes which they cannot keep open. It is often caused by venous congestion.
• **Relaxation and prostration**	Of muscles and nerves. Want to lie down.
• **Apathy and indifference**	As the heaviness reaches consciousness. The cerebro-spinal fluid becomes congested.
• Want to be left alone	Because they have no energy with which to respond.
• **Numbness**	e.g. of the tongue.
• **Lack of co-ordination**	Occurs as the nerves are disturbed in their action.
• Cannot grasp thoughts	As above, though in the brain, nerves are disturbed in their action.

• **Answer slowly**	Because nerves are affected.
• **Shivers up and down the spine**	The spine is very sensitive as it is the channel of all the nerves. Sensations arise when nerves are affected, e.g. by congestion of fluid.
• **A sensation of coldness up and down the spine**	This is a common sensation in colds.
• **As if the heart would stop beating if they ceased to move**	A **Strange, Rare and Peculiar** symptom which relates to action on the inhibitory cardiac fibre (See Neatby & Stonham).
• **Thirstlessness**	In fever, because congested.
• Headache > urinating	Is a particular symptom that illustrates the congestion and fluid imbalance.
• **Yellow**	Of thickly coated tongue; of skin in jaundice; of discharges. Gelsemium is a remedy of malaria and jaundice.
• Sensation of emptiness in the epigastrium	This is an affectation and weakening of the nerves.
• < **bad news**	All the **exciting causes** that follow affect the
• < **disappointment**	nervous system as shock. They excite, tremble,
• < **fright**	then paralyse.
• < **anticipation**	
• Paralysis	This is the final stage of the nervous system. Note it is primarily the motor nerves that are attacked.
• Diarrhoea	Appears after exciting causes such as anticipation or fright. In the first instance the nervous system is excited and diarrhoea is the result of this.
• **Vertigo**	Dizzy with blurred vision as the disturbance affects higher nerve functions.
• Fear of falling	As well as higher nerve functions affected there is a lack of co-ordination.
• **Never been well since flu**	The nervous system is a deep level of disturbance and is less capable of recovery so a patient may have *never been well since* an acute ailment such as flu.

ACTIVITY 14 Put each of the above symptoms into the categories:

Strange, Rare and Peculiar
Mental and Emotional
General
Particular.

ACTIVITY 15 List the modalities of Gelsemium (as opposed to the exciting causes).

ACTIVITY 16 Using an anatomy and physiology textbook, review the functions of motor and sensory nerves.

Different Levels of Disturbance

This remedy affects deeply and strangely, because the exciting cause is a shock to the nervous system. In the first instance there is overexcitability then weakness.

Where the constitution has been established it is not impossible that the Gelsemium patient will react to *cold, damp* episode with a *runny nose* and *sneezing*. A strange, rare and peculiar sensation might then be ... *as if hot water were running from the nose*. The same sensitive constitution will produce similar symptoms in the summer because of sensitivity to the sun's heat. The predisposition for such reaction is a weakened nervous system and, because the nervous system affects the totality of the patient, it is not always easy to tell the difference between local and general disturbance. The exciting cause of *shock* is almost always behind the illness, even if a flu.

On the acute level shock may produce *diarrhoea, hysterical lack of co-ordination, paralysis* or *apoplexy*. Diarrhoea may come suddenly as a result of *fright. Bad news* may produce *trembling* and weak knees. They may be *incoherent in speech*, unable to co-ordinate muscles to perform simple tasks, the tea cup may rattle severely as they attempt to pick it up, or they may become so dizzy and light-headed, *vision is blurred*. Such symptoms may last minutes, hours or days. If more deeply disturbed a functioning part may be *paralysed*, e.g. they can no longer speak or are struck deaf after a shock (see Aconite). The same symptoms may appear in *anticipation* of an event, a driving test, exam, or stage appearance. Influenza is a general disturbance on the acute level. There may be general *chill* then trembling of extremities. As the patient is more affected the *limbs become heavy*, they cannot keep the eyes open. There may then only be a runny nose, then dryness with exhaustion, better after one or two days in bed. If the situation goes deeper the spine will be involved. First chill and *shivering*, then stranger sensations, as if *coldness is running up and down the spine*, as if there is *cold water trickling down the spine*. The *prostration* is now increased. The patient may be hot and sticky. If even more deeply disturbed there is *apathy* and *indifference*. They *want to be left alone* – there is no energy for communication. It is difficult to co-ordinate thoughts. As the fever rises the head becomes more affected. There is *thirstlessness*, the full *headache may be better urinating* or the cerebro-spinal fluid may be so congested there is *vertigo* and *dizziness* coming from the occiput, with an inability to focus the eyes. The same scenario of symptoms may be produced by dysentery or malaria. In the last the *sticky sweat* may be more prominent, the time modality *2–3 a.m.* may be present, and the *yellow colouring* may be more evident.

The chronic state is produced when the patient has never fully recovered from the above. It may mean he/she is more prone to produce flu, digestive disorders or bouts of malaria. The person may be *melancholic, slow of thought* and even *suicidal* at times. Digestive disturbances may include chronic *loose yellow stool, thickly coated yellow tongue, emptiness around the epigastric area* and dull headaches as if there were a *band around the head* or a dull ache extending into the shoulders.

When the paralysis occurs on a chronic level it is usually after a particularly traumatic exciting cause.

ACTIVITY 17   When might you see the 'all-goneness' over the chest area rather than the epigastrium?

Excitability becomes Prostration

Every homoeopathic remedy has two actions, the first action is opposite to the second. It is common to see only the second action stressed in the symptom picture, as above, but in a remedy like Gelsemium it is important to study the whole remedy because we may not want to wait until the full symptom picture develops to prescribe the remedy.

The excitability of Gelsemium may be seen in the child whose nervous system is strongly stimulated by events. Trembling with excitement, heart thuds, he/she may even become giddy with joy but the over-stimulation may overload the system so prostration is a result. Which mother can then explain the apathy?

The old person may deteriorate considerably after flu. It takes a great deal of energy to produce an acute disorder, so afterwards the weak patient may seem to slump further. If we recognize this we need not take the state as advancing senility.

The same symptom picture may be seen in the exam student who has crammed his/her head full of facts. There is so much over-stimulation that confusion results leading to a paralysis of action because the brain cannot sort out the right connection between themes or organize ideas and thoughts. It is the same in stage fright, where the actor simply freezes.

If we look at a drunk person, we will see a similar incoherence of speech and lack of co-ordination following the over-stimulation of alcohol.

In some disorders such as multiple sclerosis the same overexcitability of nerves precedes the weak state. The motor nerves are attacked. There is lack of co-ordination and blurred or even double vision. Here the situation extends to paralysis of the motor nerves. In many such cases you will find mental/emotional shock at the beginning of the disease.

ACTIVITY 18   Describe in detail the nervous state of an old person who may not have recovered from flu.

Baptisia

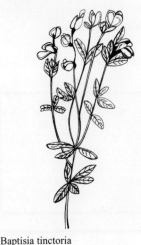

Baptisia tinctoria

Latin name:	Baptisia tinctoria
Common name:	Wild indigo
Botanical family:	Leguminosae
Habitat:	The plant is a native of the southern part of North America.

Origin

The preparation of the remedy comes from the root of the plant. Allen lists twelve provers, but no systematic provings. Neatby and Stonham complain that most knowledge of the remedy is from clinical experience.

Essence

The remedy produces severe, acute disorders with great rapidity of onset. It is claimed that the Baptisia patient produces the typhoid state faster than any other remedy. Action is through the blood. As in septicaemia, or states produced by zymotic fevers, there is rapid mental prostration, better described as besotted than delirious.

Keynotes and Characteristics

• **Besotted**	This mental state is most marked. The patient is confused.
• **Drowsy**	Most of the time is spent in sleep.
• **Rapid prostration**	The patient is suddenly very ill.
• Dull red face	Often bloated as in chronic drunkards.
• **Fall back to sleep halfway through a sentence**	There is no energy to stay awake.
• Mutter in delirium	This is part of the confusion of consciousness.
• **Feel bruised and sore all over especially parts lain on**	There are many endotoxins in the system.
• **The bed feels too hard**	As above.
• Chilly in the daytime only	It may not be too easy to distinguish this symptom. The patient may not notice because he/she is confused.
• Burning heat on the face	Gives rise to the dull red colouring.
• **Sense of duality**	We do not feel ourselves when ill. Here the patient is conscious of a self and of feeling decidedly different.
• One limb speaks to another	The next three symptoms occur in the confused state when priorities change somewhat.

- One part is in contact with another
- Parts feel scattered about the bed
- Eyeball sore when moved — As in the limbs, it is the muscles that are sore.
- Patient can only swallow liquids — Because the mucous membrane is so bloated.
- **Painless ulcers** — **Strange, Rare and Peculiar**.
- Phagedenic ulcers — Join together to eat at the surface.
- **Offensive discharge** — There is so much toxin to exude, all discharges smell.
- Dry tongue with brown streak down middle — Strange, Rare and Peculiar, but present only in the deepest state.
- Bitter taste in mouth — The digestive system is much disturbed in Baptisia.
- < after 2 a.m. — A modality when the digestive system is deeply disturbed.
- < after first waking — Because more confused.
- **< fog and damp** — **Exciting cause**.
- **< sewers, swamps and inhaling foul vapours** — Where one is exposed to zymotic fevers.
- < night watching — **Exciting cause**. The healthy person is exhausted.
- < Bad news — There is a blow to the nervous system.

ACTIVITY 19

List the above keynotes and characteristics under the categories:

Strange, Rare and Peculiar
Mental and Emotional
General
Particular.

ACTIVITY 20

List all the symptoms of sensation.

ACTIVITY 21

Using the Repertory find out about other types of ulcers. Look under 'ulcer' in the following sections:

Skin
Throat
Abdomen
Stomach
Extremities.

ACTIVITY 22

What kind of smells are associated with discharge? Use the Repertory to look under 'discharge', 'leucorrhoea', 'coryza', 'catarrh', in the sections on:

Skin
Throat
Nose
Genitalia.

Different Levels of Disorder

The Baptisia patient succumbs deeply and quickly on the general level. There is little localization and this is not the kind of state that can be perpetuated long enough to reach the chronic level.

There may be a build-up of toxins in *the limbs so they ache and feel heavy*. This may be noticeable in a flu that resembles Bryonia or Gelsemium. The ache is stronger than the heaviness. Baptisia resembles Arnica in flu. The *parts feel bruised*, the *bed feels hard*. Unlike any of these remedies the mind of Baptisia is quickly overcome. At first he/she may only appear tired and *drowsy*, can't keep their eyes open. They may try to find the energy to talk but will *sink back rapidly* into the pillows. As the poisoning proceeds the heat will gather giving the *face a dusky hue* or even a *purple, bloated appearance*. If they mutter in delirium it will be about the sore parts. As the mind becomes more *besotted*, the conversation will become stranger. This is when the *sense of duality* is most pronounced so that *parts talk to one another*. It may be more notable in the morning when the patient is dopey and *confused after sleep*. With a purple, bloated face the Baptisia patient will resemble the Lachesis patient after sleep.

The flu may follow *exposure to foggy, damp weather*. The Baptisia may arise in the child who has fallen into the polluted river. When it is of use in diphtheria, the disease is most malignant, as in Lachesis. Baptisia has a strong effect on the throat. *Septic tonsils* or quinsies may call for Baptisia.

The throat is *engorged* and purple. *Ulcers eat into the tonsils* or back of the throat but they are *painless*. The patient's *breath is foetid*. When the homoeopath sees such an advanced case, we do not despair, especially where the onset is rapid. No matter how low the prostration, the vital force has the ability to match in energy a strong-acting remedy that will quickly restore equilibrium.

ACTIVITY 24 List the modalities of Baptisia. Separate into aggravations and ameliorations.

ACTIVITY 25 Describe the symptom picture of a Baptisia patient with a quinsy in the throat.

ACTIVITY 26 Compare the Baptisia and Arnica patients in flu.

? **SELF-TEST QUESTIONS**

Answers can be found in the answer section.

1. Find the remedy below. It may be *any* of those you have studied. Remember to look for characteristic symptoms and keynotes.
   a. Swollen tonsils with a purplish hue and patient drinks small amounts constantly. The patient is exhausted but relatively pain-free. Breath is foul.
   b. The patient has a very painful sore throat which is bright red and dry, < on the right side. As it worsens pain shoots up to the right ear.
   c. The tonsils are greatly swollen especially on the right side. There is much dryness and an inclination to drink plenty of water although each swallow increases the pain and the patient grasps the throat to ease the motion of the swallow.
   d. The tongue is numb and feels so thick he/she can hardly speak.

  e. There is a dry hoarse cough on expiration since the exposure to the cold outside yesterday.

  f. The burning pains in the throat started after exposure to cold, wet conditions. The patient is very tired and worn by these pains. She sips water continuously.

  g. Copious amounts of mucus are dislodged in the morning. During the day coughing to bring up mucus also brings tears to the eyes.

  h. The patient has a dry bark and sharp little pains in the throat after experiencing severe cold conditions yesterday. She shouts at the children irritably when the door is left open as it causes draught.

  i. The rash on the hands is red and swollen. The itch is so awful it stings. The patient jerks about restlessly, casting venomous glances at the cat whom she blames.

  j. Sour smelling diarrhoea during teething problems. Much crying occurs as soon as the child is put down in the cot.

  k. The voice is quite hoarse after four hours' carol-singing. At first there is no sound at all but the croak gets a bit distinctive as he goes on. It is better too with warm drinks.

2. Compare the modalities of Bryonia, Gelsemium and Baptisia.
3. In what way does Gelsemium resemble Aconite?
4. Belladonna, like Baptisia, works through the blood. Compare the developmental stages of the two.
5. Bryonia is often labelled a 'sycotic' remedy. This means overproduction, overreaction, or over-function. Give at least six symptoms of Bryonia that you feel would verify this label.
6. Compare Aconite, Euphrasia and Arsenicum. How are they similar?
7. How does the mental disturbance of Baptisia compare with that of Stramonium and Hyoscyamus?
8. Compare Bryonia and Dulcamara.
9. Show how Gelsemium, Ignatia and Staphysagria differ in how they receive bad news.
10. Create a table of comparison to show which symptoms all the remedies you have studied so far will produce in a cold or flu.

Further Studies

Euphrasia
1. Compare the cold symptoms of Euphrasia, Allium cepa and Arsenicum.
2. How does Euphrasia resemble Pulsatilla. In what type of disease do they overlap?
3. Relate the scrofulous symptoms of Euphrasia to Tuberculinum.

Bryonia
1. Why is Bryonia a useful remedy in appendicitis?
2. When might Bryonia be useful in a patient suffering from PMT?
3. Describe the rheumatic state of the Bryonia patient and compare it to that of Rhus toxicodendron.
4. Describe how the cold of the Bryonia patient progresses down into the chest.
5. How does Bryonia resemble Pulsatilla?
6. Describe a stereotype of the Bryonia constitutional type and give reasons for your choice.
7. What symptoms relate Bryonia to Sepia as its acute equivalent?
8. Describe the menstrual symptoms of Bryonia and relate these to the essence of the remedy.
9. What miasm most relates to Bryonia?

Gelsemium
1. Gelsemium has two symptom pictures, one of hyperactivity and one of sluggishness. Describe each of these and discuss progression from one to the other.
2. Give three keynotes of Gelsemium.
3. Distinguish between Gelsemium, Aconite and Apis in retention of urine.
4. Describe the headache of the Gelsemium patient.
5. Describe how the Gelsemium patient behaves after hearing bad news.

Baptisia

1. Describe the sore throat of Baptisia.
2. Compare the symptom picture of Baptisia and Lachesis.
3. How would you first become aware of the Baptisia flu and how would you then differentiate it from other remedies?
4. How would you make use of Baptisia on a trip to India? Give details as to how you would identify the remedy.
5. Compare the tongue of the Baptisia patient to that of the Bryonia patient.
6. In the event of a nuclear holocaust how might Baptisia be of use?
7. Compare Baptisia to Apis, Bryonia, Gelsemium and Rhus toxicodendron.

Three Major Polycrests

Lycopodium, Sulphur, Calcarea Carbonica

Aim: To illustrate the character of the essence present on all levels of the remedy's action.

Objectives: To identify the essence of the remedy in all its symptoms.
To label the variety of expressions of one essence.

Headings: INTRODUCTION
LYCOPODIUM: Origin; Characteristics of the Plant; Essence; Keynotes and Characteristics; Modalities; Inertia; The Personality; Digestive Disturbances; Respiratory Disturbances; Similar Remedies
SULPHUR: Origin; Characteristics of the Mineral; Essence; Keynotes and Characteristics; Modalities; Unstable Heating Mechanism; The Personality; Respiratory Disturbances; Similar Remedies
CALCAREA CARBONICA: Origin; Characteristics of the Mineral; Essence; Keynotes and Characteristics; Modalities; A Slow Metabolism; The Head is a Focus; The Lymphatic System; Similar Remedies
SELF-TEST QUESTIONS
FURTHER STUDIES

Introduction

When we study polycrests, you must be aware of the great breadth of their action. Before, we could speak of the characteristic presentation of the symptoms and could draw up characteristic general symptoms, modalities and exciting causes that ran through each presentation of the remedy in minor ailments. This field is too narrow when speaking of a polycrest. Although the essence remains the same, only a few of the enormous range of symptoms are found in any one patient. Although the essential inner nature, motivation and weakness are the same, the variety of personalities is as wide as human nature. Each one shows a different shade of the same colour. The note C repeated in a different octave has an essential quality that does not change, but the note in each octave is different. Now we must seek more deeply into the symptoms before us to find the underlying quality of the patient. Although each symptom will contain this quality, it may only be visible when placed in a group of concomitant symptoms.

Lycopodium

Latin name:	Lycopodium clavatum
Common name:	Club moss, Wolf's claw
Botanical family:	Lycopodiaceae
Habitat:	It grows on dry heaths and pastures throughout Europe and North America.

Origin

Hahnemann proved the remedy after triturating the spores.

Characteristics of the Plant

The plant is one of the primitive mosses. This is one of the first plants to evolve leaves which

99

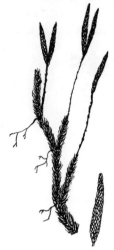

Lycopodium clavatum

are arranged like scales on either side of the stem. In the human, Lycopodium affects all the paired organs arranged on either side of the trunk. There is no direct anatomical connection between these organs, so no reason in allopathic terms why one remedy should affect them all.

In the Carboniferous Era, two types of Lycopodium, Lepidodendron and Sigillaria, grew into a tall tree of over 90 feet. These arborescent club mosses did not survive the Permian ice ages. They represent in the Lycopodium type a potential of greatness which underlines many symptoms. The Lycopodium person is often conscious of potential greatness which is, as yet, unveiled to the masses!

Essence

Inertia explains the expression of the Lycopodium symptoms. They never quite made it. They have a dread that they might not reach the grade.

Keynotes and Characteristics

• Thin, spare with a sallow complexion	Digestion is poor.
• Wrinkled forehead	Even children look wrinkled and old.
• **Angular shape**	This is seen particularly in the head.
• Emaciate from the neck down	So have a thin, scrawny neck and angular head and large buttocks.
• Mind is better developed than body	They live through their mental faculties.
• Hair grey in spots	The hair symptom is a common occurrence.
• Baldness in spots or widow's peak	Once again, it is easy to find this symptom in both sexes.
• Hair greys or balds early in life	As above.
• **Anticipatory fears**	They may not be able to hold together to perform.
• **Fear of failure**	They may not talk of this but it underlines many of their inhibitions.
• **Fear of the future**	This leads to anxiety and anticipatory fears.
• **Inferiority complex**	But know they are superior.
• **Dictators**	At home only, although it could apply in the office where the man is chief over the typists or in the army, where officers rule insubordinates.
• **Cowardice**	Outside the home. They will even lie to save face.
• **Fear being on their own, but hate crowds**	Company is fine in the next room!
• Dislike company but dread solitude	
• **Avoid responsibility**	In all fields. It often means they do not marry.
• **Traditionalist**	This protects them from holding their own opinions.
• **Arrogant**	Domineering dictators or traditionalists.
• **Dread least they forget**	Before the lecture they will make copious notes.
• **Contrary symptoms**	One of the few remedies that have this.
• Hate to be contradicted but full of contradictions	There is one rule for themselves and another for others.
• Hungry but full after a few mouthfuls	They cannot explain why.
• One foot hot, the other cold	Usually the right foot is hot.
• **< kept waiting for food**	They may become very nasty.
• **< fasting**	Headaches and all sorts of symptoms occur.
• **< onions**	Makes them more flatulent.
• **Craves sweets**	Adds to uric acid diathesis.
• **Flatulent – even after a few mouthfuls**	This is one of the most flatulent remedies in the Materia Medica.
• **Tympanic abdomen**	Because of flatulence.
• < Pressure of clothes	Because of flatulence.

• **Emptiness in stomach not relieved by eating**	So they will eat a full meal immediately after another.
• Duodenal ulcers	They are anxious speedy types.
• **Constipation**	Because of inactivity of the gut.
• **< 4–8 p.m.**	This general symptom often shows in the digestive system.
• **Lack of vital heat**	No visible stamina, easily tired out.
• **Numbness in spots**	**Strange, Rare and Peculiar**.
• **Symptoms move from right to left**	There is a marked sidedness in the remedy.
• **Impotence**	From shrunken or relaxed genitalia.
• **Brick red, sandy deposit in urine**	They have a uric acid diathesis.
• **Gout**	Is an end result of the above uric acid diathesis.
• **Kidney stones**	Is an end result of uric acid diathesis.
• Burning pains > heat	As in Arsenicum.
• Fan-like motion of the alae-nasi	When very ill. Also has sooty deposits here.

Modalities

< 4–8 p.m.	> **warm drinks and food**
< **pressure of clothes**	> **eructations**
< **fasting**	> **micturition**
< **eating**	> after midnight
< **milk**	
< **onions**	
< **windy weather**	

 ACTIVITY 1 List the symptoms above that illustrate the contrariness of the remedy.

 ACTIVITY 2 List the symptoms above which are associated with an inferiority complex.

 ACTIVITY 3 List the symptoms above that reflect *inertia*.

Inertia

This is one of the remedies that most clearly demonstrates the 'magic' of the homoeopathic potentization process. In past times Lycopodium was used universally by pharmacists to coat pills as it was seen to be inert. The essence of this psoric remedy is *inertia* and, of course, in the potentized form it is capable of revitalizing an essentially inert constitution.

Inertia in Lycopodium is seen on all different levels.

One role of the blood is to distribute heat evenly throughout the body. The chilliness or *lack of vital heat* in the Lycopodium patient is an indication of the under-functioning of the circulatory system whilst *constipation*, as it manifests in the Lycopodium patient, is an indication of under-function of the liver which does not secrete enough bile to stimulate the gut. A secondary effect of the liver's under-functioning is *flatulence* or fermentation in the gut with the very great *distension* and *tympanic abdomen* of Lycopodium, very sensitive to the pressure of clothes, and, of course, these are the symptoms we see in the patient when he/she first comes along to the clinic. The Lycopodium patient is one of the windiest in the Materia Medica – an honour shared by Argentum nitricum, Carbo vegetalis and China officialis – and is the archetypal pot-bellied adult. Luther, in the play of that name, by John Osborne, is a typical Lycopodium type – he sits on the toilet throughout the play trying to move his bowels, yet thinking, thinking, thinking, all the time in an abstract way. Of course, not all Lycopodium patients are as disturbed as this, though their intellectual pursuits do tend towards constipation.

Most Lycopodium patients are thinkers, or at least actively seek a rational explanation of life. There is little inertia here and indeed this may discount our theory as most of the activity of the Lycopodium is in the mind which is very active. The work of Rudolf Steiner's anthroposophical medicine is of great interest here, as he understands the mind to be the death pole which balances the metabolic (life) pole which is the digestive system. Whilst one assimilates, the other analyses. By 'mind' Steiner means rational thought which he sees beginning to develop around the 7th or 8th year of the child's life. To think rationally one has to hold (or kill) thoughts in order to analyse, or compare. In Steiner education, the child who develops the death pole too early is the young child taking things apart to see how they work, rather than colouring in pictures or using his/her imagination. Such a child is often found to have a small head, in the same proportion to the body as found in the average adult. This description could easily fit the average Lycopodium child who has a small angular head, in great contrast to the Calcarea carbonica child who has a large head and great difficulty with rational thought.

One more point of interest regarding Steiner's concept, is that the situation is recommended to be remedied by administering sweet-tasting foods to encourage the imagination-dream faculties, whereas the under-developed rational faculties of the Calcarea carbonica child are reputed to respond to salty foods. To the homoeopath the most interesting point here is that the Lycopodium patient *craves sugar and sweets* – nature gives us always the direction we should take.

The inertia in the Lycopodium mind is the continual *fear of failure*, the *lack of confidence* which is camouflaged by *arrogance*. The Lycopodium patient works very hard to be sure of his/her performance, mentally, but is dogged by the fear that his/her memory will let them down. There is a considerable anxiety which brings typical lines to the brow and may cause him/her to freeze during the performance, but is much more likely to be transmuted into excessive activity of the bowel, i.e. diarrhoea and/or flatulence before the show or test. The Lycopodium patient is also likely to totally opt out of the performance, unconsciously by becoming physically ill!

ACTIVITY 4 Outline the symptom picture of a Lycopodium type about to sit their driving test.

The Personality

The causative factors in Lycopodium lie mainly in the personality. In a few words we can label them as *sensitive intellectuals with an inferiority complex*. They are motivated by a constant anxiety that they are not good enough. It is size they are concerned with, so they are sensitive to their status and they may show great versatility to be on the winning side. One thinks of politicians! It may be that they will hide feelings or will be very well-read intellectuals who quote or drop names to show how well-connected they are. Their thoughts, or opinions, may be defended with considerable arrogance. At home they may be *dictators* or *traditionalists*.

They are traditionalists because they need to know the ropes – *anything new threatens them* because they have to learn anew, so the mind's ability and their status is challenged. Aggravations will often appear when they are away from home, e.g. *constipation away from home*. They may even have a marked aversion for Chinese or Indian food – any of that foreign stuff! The dictator is especially evident at home if they are male, because there is a traditional stereotype of the patriarch. As bosses, this may show in benevolent paternalism. In both of these stereotypes there is a concept of superiority and that the traditional status is unquestioned and unchallenged. The Lycopodium patient feels safe with this. In other types he/she may be the dictator at home simply because he/she has created a situation in which she is tolerated and will get away with bad graces that would never be shown outside the home because of *cowardice*.

The nervous intellectual lecturers who finds it difficult to talk in anything but concepts and ideals may need Lycopodium. Though recognized as brilliant by others, some tolerance is needed of his foibles, and is given because it is accepted that genius is flawed.

He may be isolated or part of a group of trendies. There is an arrogance even in such a group which sets itself above the others. The young executive may be more socialized and part of society than the nervous lecturer. He has accepted an obvious social structure and ascribed status. He will also live on his nerves and on adrenaline and may end up with serious digestive dysfunction, especially duodenal ulcers, perhaps even Crohn's disease or diabetes. A very acid metabolism will create rheumatism, gout or stones in the kidneys. If the lungs are affected bronchitis may result, or even TB. In Kent's Materia Medica we will find the TB type is *emaciated from the neck down*, has *profuse night sweats* and a hard cough.

The contradiction which is part of the Lycopodium picture is found in these TB types. Many of the contradictory symptoms are also keynotes of the remedy.

ACTIVITY 5

This is a common stereotype, so study a few at a bus stop, in a cafe, etc. Make a few notes.

Digestive Disturbances

There are a great variety of these in the Lycopodium type:

- As he rushes his food he will *often burp*.
- Because he chooses sugary foods, there is much fermentation in the gut, so it *rumbles* a lot, can be grossly disturbed, so he *must loosen his belt* and he passes a lot of *noisy flatus*. She wears *loose clothes*.
- A constant worrier, his stomach *over-secretes acid*. His stomach churns as he wrestles with problems at work. The *burning pain in the epigastrium* is *ameliorated by heat*. There are so many possibilities he can see, but he either cannot make up his mind, or *does not want the responsibility* for the outcome. The pain gives him an excuse for poor functioning. He gets *impatient* and *angry if he has to wait for his food*. He lives on his nerves. He is decidedly < *between 4–8 p.m.* The constitutional type is *thin and cold*. He/she may find it difficult to eat in company. She may feel *full after only a few mouthfuls* then hungry again when out of the restaurant and in the theatre. It is at this level that *one foot may be hot whilst the other is cold*. It is this patient who will *react strongly to onions*.
- *Away from home*, the Lycopodium type may have *constipation*. They hold themselves together strongly in the new environment. On stage, before a lecture, or an examination, *anxiety* may be so great they cannot hold themselves, so run to the toilet often with *a loose bowel*.

ACTIVITY 6

How does the essence, inertia, appear as an underlying factor in the digestive symptoms above?

ACTIVITY 7

Explain how shellfish disturb the digestion of the Lycopodium patient.

Respiratory Disturbances

Colds are frequent in the emaciated type who lacks vital heat. These may stick at the throat as a raw, tight feeling that causes them to *swallow constantly* – just as in nervous situations the Adam's Apple is seen to bob up and down. In fact they have a *feeling of a ball rising up to stick in the throat. Warm drinks ease the situation*.

Colds rapidly develop into the chest. At first the *cough is dry and tickling*. It can become deep and hollow. Breathing is difficult because of the dryness and the chilly sensation of the air. They want to breathe deeply but the *chest is tight and burning*. When the discharge comes it is greeny-yellow and tastes salty, smells foul. The situation can become quite serious in some patients. Pneumonia may develop. The older, weaker patients may have *hydrothorax*. TB is not uncommon in the Lycopodium type, even today, because the remedy tends to form *abscesses* and *cysts*.

The respiratory system is weakened by grief and shock. This may refer to disappointments, or failures they have faced. As insecure persons the chest may be weakened when they have no support or love over a long period.

ACTIVITY 8

Inferiority is found in the personality and in the insufficiency of parts. List the symptoms that fit in here. Look through the *Mind* section of Kent's repertory. Which rubrics would fit 'inferiority'?

Similar Remedies

Arsenicum is also a remedy of the insecure executive who develops ulcers, gastric this time, with burning pains > heat. Arsenicum is fearful for its existence and status. It does not have the cowardice of Lycopodium though. The essence is different. Arsenicum likes control and is an organizer.

Phosphorus is a fearful remedy with many digestive and respiratory problems which have ulceration and heat. When very down they can also feel sorry for themselves and are a bit of a hypochondriac, like Lycopodium. In health, they are more optimistic and full of themselves, and more social. Here again the essence is different though the symptoms may be the same. *Diffusion* rather than *inertia*.

Natrum muriaticum has a similar essence to Lycopodium. Natrum muriaticum is so vulnerable, emotionally, she builds a barrier and erects a persona out front to hide behind. This is like the status of Lycopodium. Both are defensive. Natrum muriaticum is more optimistic than Lycopodium and thinks always of others, or good causes to support.

Sulphur

Origin

The remedy was prepared by Hahnemann from a trituration of flowers of sulphur.

Characteristics of the Mineral

The mineral occurs naturally in the effluence of volcanoes as 'flowers of sulphur'. It occurs in combination with hydrogen as hydrogen sulphide, which gives the typical rotten egg smell.

The element is found in many proteins, so as a remedy it touches every organ of the body in its action. In Victorian times it was frequently used as an emetic in brimstone and treacle.

Essence

This is a remedy of *centrifugal action* which parallels the primitive action of the *vital force* to throw the symptoms outwards. As in the volcano it is heat that moves outward, often violently.

Keynotes and Characteristics

- **Lazy** — They use their intellect to skive.
- Layabouts, but loaf with style — As in Samuel Johnson
- **Lack energy, so catnap at every opportunity** — But not > after sleep
- **Daydream** — i.e. of winning the pools.
- **Self-centred** — Mean, vain and hypercritical of others.
- Noisy, talkative — Full of life, boisterous.
- **Inquisitive** — They want to know. Poke their noses into others' business.

• **Indulge in philosophical obscurities and abstractions**	Dropouts and hippies, or the sloop-shouldered philosopher of tradition.
• Absent-minded philosophers	They are so lost in their researches and theories, everyday things are unimportant.
• Eccentrics and extroverts	They are sure of themselves.
• **Enthusiastic over causes but do nothing**	Overactivity of the mind costs no energy!
• **Everyday objects seem beautiful**	They are collectors of 'junk'.
• They hate to wash	Children who are tousled tykes.
• **Untidy**	But they know where everything is to be found.
• Leans rather than stands, sits rather than leans	They won't expend energy.
• Redness of orifices	This is marked in emaciated types or in acute cases.
• **Offensive body odours**	Whilst they are offended by others' smells, they do not notice their own.
• **Imagines nasty smells**	Imagines smoke, or gas, for example.
• **Unstable heating mechanism**	Like the volcano.
• Sudden hot flushes	Heat to the head also represents their volatile temper.
• Hot hands and face, cold feet	The heating mechanism is unbalanced.
• Burning feet at night, stick out of bed	This is a common symptom in Sulphur patients.
• **< heat**	It fatigues them.
• Burning pains on vertex	This is the typical headache.
• **Burning, itching, smarting skin**	This is Hahnemann's major anti-psoric.
• **Sudden weakness in epigastrium**	There is an energy imbalance behind the heat imbalance.
• Need to nibble food constantly	As above.
• **Ravenous appetite**	The metabolism is very fast.
• **Better after eating**	Perhaps they are earthed.
• **Hunger 11 a.m.**	**Strange, Rare and Peculiar**.
• Hunger vanishes at the sight of food	A little similar to Lycopodium.
• **< fasting**	Headaches develop.
• **Crave spicy, highly-seasoned food**	Needs stimulation.
• **Crave alcohol and stimulants**	As above.
• **Stool drives out of bed 5 a.m.**	A most urgent call though often a small amount.
• **Stool smells of rotten eggs**	Arnica also has this symptom.
• **Stool burns**	So the orifice is red and sore.
• **Wakes 3 a.m. and can't sleep until morning**	Many of the TB remedies have 3 a.m. aggravation.
• Dreams of falling	

Modalities

< standing	> open air
< after sleep	> motion
< **bathing**	> lying on right side
< **heat**	
< wearing wool	
< atmospheric changes	

ACTIVITY 9   List those symptoms that show the imbalanced heating mechanism of Sulphur.

ACTIVITY 10   Which symptoms show the Sulphur patient's need for stimulation?

ACTIVITY 11   List those symptoms associated with *self-centredness*. Look through the rubrics in the *Mind* section of the Repertory. Which are associated with self-centredness?

Unstable Heating Mechanism

The most notable symptoms of Sulphur are those of its *skin* which well illustrate the trends and characteristic modalities – itchy eruptions:

< heat
< bathing.

Like a volcano, it has an unstable heating mechanism and the skin erupts easily – heat spots are a good example which also indicate the acidity of the body (or fire in the system). Heat spots especially follow acid foods such as strawberries, rhubarb or tomatoes. Or it may be that in hot weather the acid builds up under the skin so they easily come out in *red, raised itchy weals if touched*, especially by *metal* or *wool*. The itch may also arise from a debilitated liver as a result of their craving for *highly seasoned food, fats*, and *alcohol* which are all difficult to digest. Alcoholism may start innocently from the Sulphur patient's *craving for stimulating foods*. They are sensuous individuals who like to indulge themselves. Their craving for highly seasoned foods builds up heat in the gut which may produce another keynote symptom *diarrhoea at 5 a.m. which drives them out of bed*! The skin and the digestive system are closely linked, as the digestive system is the inner tube whilst the skin is, of course, the outer tube. Skin problems such as eczema can be considerably improved if attention is paid to diet or to correcting the digestive disorders. Note that the eczemas of Sulphur are *very dry* and itchy, as well as ≪ *heat and bathing*.

The mucous membrane, the inner tube, is very much affected by Sulphur. It may itch and become raw and sore because *discharges excoriate*. This may be seen in the sore, raw nose that occurs with a cold, or the sore, raw throat of laryngitis, or even in cystitis (sore raw parts). The keynote symptom is the *redness of all orifices* caused by the excoriating discharge. In hay fever or cold, the Sulphur patient has red-rimmed eyes, red nostrils, and in constitutional types we see thin, red lips.

As expected with heat, there is a *copious flow of sweat* which, of course, is part of the movement outwards. The Sulphur patient often *smells strongly* and although he/she can put up with his own smell, he is very sensitive to that of others – this is also a keynote. After heat, *bathing is the prime exciting cause* of the Sulphur patient. He will avoid washing irrespective of smell, or will '*spot wash*' – wash only the dirty bits! The most common stereotype of Sulphur is that of an unkempt individual who cares little for his appearance – unshaved, unwashed, hair uncombed, clothes crumpled or unironed, a chap who slouches, *does not stand if he can lean or sit, will not sit if he can lie down*. The stereotypes allocated to the remedy include the hippy, the down and out, the ragged-tailed philosopher, the dreamer of dreams, the layabout who loafs with style, the intellectual who uses his intellect to skive work!

The unstable heating mechanism of Sulphur means the patient overheats easily. This is why he or she avoids work, but it is physical heat that he especially avoids. The energy of the Sulphur patient *moves upwards to the head*. This reminds us of the intellectual pursuits of Dr Faustus or the absent-minded scientist type and of Lycopodium. Physically the heat in the healthy individual is thrown to the periphery, so a common keynote is *burning on the soles of the feet*. This is obvious if the patient is on his/her feet too much, especially in hot weather, or in bed at night when they lie horizontally. At night they *overheat*, becoming *restless* (remember Sulphur is also the chronic of Aconite) and throws the clothes off. The last is very noticeable in children.

There is much *burning pain*, especially noticeable in the abdomen in digestive disorders. There are surges of heat upwards which is most noticeable in menopause or in the overweight Sulphur patient, but the overweight Sulphur patient is not too common because by their very nature they tend to burn off calories which is why they often *crave fatty foods*. The surges of heat upwards may be seen to connect with yet another keynote symptom – burning on the vertex.

Over-acidity, too much fire, eventually leads to rheumatism which is distinctive in the Sulphur patient by its characteristic < heat. The rheumatism of the Sulphur patient occurs in the summer, in the hot, dry weather!!!

ACTIVITY 12 Hahnemann links Sulphur closely to suppressed skin problems, especially scabies. Find out the pattern of symptoms produced in scabies, urticaria, erysipelas, dermatitis and eczema.

The Personality

On the level of personality, fire is equated with *ego* and whether or not you accept such a correspondence, the marked characteristics of the Sulphur person concern the ego. We have already said they are very *egocentric, self-indulgent* individuals. In truth the Sulphur patient is so involved in his own interests, he finds it difficult to form relationships with others. He finds it difficult to allow space for others. He may bear no ill will for others. He would rather finish his project and does not understand his wife's complaints. In this type of Sulphur patient, the wife may well feel like a servant(!) or if this aspect is greatly exaggerated, this type of Sulphur will never find time to marry at all. He will have a housekeeper or a very, very untidy house. The *opinions of others mean nothing to him*, unless it is a contribution to his project, but even here he may not be able to hear others. He is totally self-indulgent and oblivious to the feelings of others. In another type, nearer to the Calcarea carbonica this time, he may be so easy going and so little affected by outside events that he is described as *easy-going* or *casual*. The hippy-type may fit well here.

Borland writes an interesting account of the Sulphur child whose egotism may come out as *bullying*, or domineering. This can be easily explained by his character which is forceful and will not allow space for others!

They are eccentrics and extroverts who can stand on their own feet. History owes a great deal to them.

On the mental plane, the above theme is represented as *irritability*. The Sulphur patient has a *quick temper* and has very little time for others. They are very egocentric patients who dislike being diverted from their own interests. It may be well worth remembering that this remedy is the chronic (deeper version) of Nux vomica!

ACTIVITY 13 Describe in detail the bedroom of your Sulphur son or daughter.

Respiratory Disturbances

The Sulphur patient is often poorly nourished because they do not look after themselves. This type will *easily catch a cold*. There is an *excoriating, watery discharge that burns* the nose and *causes redness*. The eyes too are red-rimmed as they water a bit.

The centrifugal action of Sulphur is excellent at keeping the disturbance out at the extremities. On the rare occasions when the Sulphur patient has a sore throat the mucous membrane is red and swollen. Once again, as in Lycopodium, there is a *dry tightness*, so there may be the *sensation of a ball rising when they swallow*. Irritation takes the form of a *hair in the throat*. This may even feel *like a splinter*. Too many remedies resemble this picture, so you must look at the essence that permeates all levels to get an accurate prescription.

When the cold of the Sulphur patient goes deeper it will usually go straight into the chest. There may be a violent cough because of irritation. There will be dryness and tightness in the chest. If bad, this may be described as a *constricting band* and burning pains. Breathing will be difficult because of the dryness, so they will *feel suffocated* and want the window open. In chronic cases there will be a weakness in the chest so they will have difficulty bringing up mucus which gathers. Rattling sounds can be heard with the stethoscope. Without going into the full essence there is little here to individualize Sulphur as the remedy. The only distinctive symptom might be the modality < 11 a.m. In case taking, you must take time to find the individuality.

When individualizing the Sulphur remedy in a respiratory problem you might have several clues:

- Follow the development pattern of the remedy. Were the red-rimmed orifices, especially the eyes, there in the beginning? These might still be there even although the chest is the active zone.
- You may see the disturbed heating mechanism. How are heat and cold distributed? How does the patient react to heat and cold? What do the general symptoms and the history show?
- What is the personality type of the patient? How are they handling this illness and what does that tell you about them? The essential nature of the patient is always in front of you.

ACTIVITY 14 A polycrest cures many illnesses when you prescribe on the essential nature. Sketch a symptom picture of a Sulphur child with earache. How do the symptoms present? Describe how the child behaves.

Similar Remedies

Nux vomica shares with Sulphur the need for stimulation. This is seen in the digestive symptoms and in the personality. Whilst Sulphur is self-indulgent, Nux vomica has a direction and a purpose.

Rhus toxicodendron has the irritability and fire of Sulphur which is seen in skin irritation and the temper. As in the Nux vomica, they are less self-indulgent. They are also more physically active than the Sulphur.

Phosphorus patients are also egotistical day dreamers with grand ideas. Phosphorus diffuses its energy, so seldom achieves anything. Sulphur patients are achievers when they rise from their lethargy – the only problem is their goals may not coincide with those of society.

Tuberculinum is a romantic dreamer who also needs continual change and new challenges. It has a profound effect on the skin, lymphatic system and lungs. In the Tuberculinum patient the heating mechanism may have broken down completely, so they are lacking in fire. It is a cold remedy, sensitive to more cold.

Calcarea Carbonica

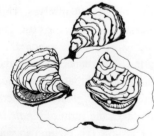

Common oyster

Latin names: Calcarea carbonica
Calcium carbonicum
Calcarea ostrearum
Calcarea carbonicum ostrearum

Origin

Hahnemann did a proving from a trituration of the middle layers of an oyster shell. Koch prepared his proving from a trituration of Calcium carbonate precipitated from the action of hydrochloric acid on chalk.

Characteristics of the Mineral

Calcium plays a very important role in the evolution of life. Before the Calcium age sponges are the main animal fossils found. Plants were unlimited in size. After Calcium enters the life cycle, animals and plants have regulation size. Skeletons appear, first as protective shells, later as internalized back bones.

Calcium brings protection and rigidity to life through its presence in bones. It regulates the speed of metabolism through its action on the thyroid gland where it balances iodine. It also affects the enervation to muscles and as such has a profound effect upon the heart.

We will also see the characteristics of the oyster in the symptom picture of the remedy. These types shyly retreat into their shell, have a large head and a wet handshake. There is a greater preponderance of white muscle tissue, so they have little stamina.

Essence

This is a remedy of *unrealized potential*. Shyness and anxiety keep them from free interaction. They are content, but slow to assimilate.

Keynotes and Characteristics

• Defective assimilation	So they tend to be *fair, fat and forty*.
• Imperfect ossification	So they are late to walk and have problems teething. Fontanelles are slow to close.
• **Bloated appearance**	Like the oyster!
• **Damp, cold, boneless handshake**	Like a damp cod!
• **Lethargic and slow**	Metabolism is slow.
• **Large head, pot belly**	In children.
• **Knotty glands**	These are the gates of the lymphatic system.
• **Clumsy in movement**	Unusual in children.
• **Easily strain muscles and ligaments**	Because muscles are weak.
• **Hate being observed**	They do not like to be exposed.
• **Hate being laughed at**	They are very sensitive.
• **Poor concentration**	Plodders. They will pause when asked a question.
• **Lack initiative**	Or originality. They are content.
• **Sit playing with fingers**	Little energy and actually they are content.
• **Easily frightened**	The oyster is defenceless if not hidden in its shell.
• Fear that something will happen	They are not too quick to react so dislike sudden demands.
• Fear will lose their reason and others will see their confusion	They are so slow they lose thoughts so lose the sense of things.
• Brood over little things of no importance	
• **Thoughts vanish**	Simply no energy to keep a hold of them.
• Repeat themselves over and over	This is the bit they have got hold of.
• **< cold, damp**	Vital energy is already low.
• **Chilly**	This is a sign of low vitality.
• Sweats in cold rooms	Remedy of the lymphatic system.
• Feet cold sweat, as if wet stockings	Circulation is very sluggish. There is little resistance to flow of fluids.
• **Offensive foot sweat**	Smells of cheese.
• Soles raw from perspiration	Which excoriates.
• **Easily tired**	Flabby, relaxed tissue.
• **< ascending**	Because it needs more energy.
• **< heat**	Because the circulatory system is slow to adapt.
• **Right sided**	General symptom.
• **Menses early and profuse**	There is a relaxation of tissue.
• **Breasts painful and swollen before menses**	
• **Feel > constipation**	Because metabolism is slow, it gives them time to take nutrients from their food.
• **Crave salt or sweets**	
• **Crave indigestible things**	Like chalk, coal, white rags (contains starch).
• **Averse milk**	Even babies reject milk. It is too much like lymph which is already disordered.
• **Aggravated milk**	Especially the skin, as in eczema.
• **Desire farinaceous food**	Which is slow to release carbohydrates. They are < for anything that heats them up too quickly.

- **Curvature of bones**   A bit less common today.
- **Rickets**   As above.
- **Kidney and gallstones**   Because of sluggish metabolism.
- Warts on fingers, verrucas on feet   When indicated nothing happens for one month then they suddenly disappear.
- Uterine fibroids   Which tend to calcify.

Modalities

< **exertion**   > dry climate
< **cold, raw air**   > after breakfast
< **ascending**   > lying on painful side
< **dentition**
< **milk**

ACTIVITY 15   List the symptoms that show lack of assimilation. Split these into mental and physical symptoms.

ACTIVITY 16   List those symptoms that indicate a slow metabolism. Many of these will be the same as those in Activity 15.

ACTIVITY 17   Explain the modalities in terms of lack of assimilation and slow metabolism.

A Slow Metabolism

It is one of the remedies we call fair, fat and forty. Behind this lies the slow metabolism of the Calcarea carbonica patient, so he/she is a *poor assimilator of food*. The speed of movement of food through the gut is slow to give the patient time to take nutrients from the food. The Calcarea carbonica patient is one of the few that has *no urge to defecate* and can go for days happily. They are protected in their poor ability to accumulate energy by copious reserves in the form of fatty layers and in their slow rate of metabolism. The wise body even prefers foods such as potatoes that provide starch for slow release energy in the body.

The bones are slow to harden. *Curvature of the spine* and *rickets* were common in Calcarea carbonica children in previous times. Nowadays we still see that the *teething is late* and often a problem. This applies to permanent as well as deciduous teeth. Growth requires a lot of energy. Interestingly, the Calcarea carbonica child may be smaller than normal but shoots up quickly after the remedy is given or after puberty which is often delayed.

The body is underdeveloped in that it appears *childlike*. The *bloated, swollen shape* appears plastic. Sexuality is often underdeveloped. They are not motivated. The male often has breasts like the female. The remedy occurs frequently in cases of undescended testes. It is interesting to note that the oyster is known to change sex. Almost all oysters start off male and become female later in life as they mature.

The body is underdeveloped in other ways. Digestion is poor. The body is slow to absorb food and slow to use it at cell level. The slow metabolic rate can be seen in the child with its *large head* and *large belly*. The *fontanelles are slow to close*. Steiner will tell us that the energy has note yet descended entirely to the metabolic pole and the death pole has not yet given form to the head. Certainly the Calcarea carbonica patient throughout life has *problems holding thoughts* in his head – so much so, that some *fear they are losing their minds*, or cannot fit into normal social situations, because they cannot grasp the conversation quick enough to take part in the repartee.

The child's use of energy is most interesting – like the oyster it sits there, a little blob, waiting patiently on all coming to him, or develops the most amazing, ingenious forms of non-verbal communication. This adorable, smiling little blob appears inactive and indeed he is *very slow to walk and talk*. He appears *lazy* but inside he is slowly assimilating and when he does talk it is a sentence he utters, not single words. He astounds his parents. Later in class he will frustrate his teachers who will call him thick, lazy or an idiot but, given time, and with patience, he will usually show intelligence and though slow to grasp new subjects will not forget once he has done so. He knows he is slow and depending on his upbringing may show a great deal of *anxiety* regarding lessons, or will develop a *stubborn* time-delaying attitude that may frustrate adults, or he will pursue new subjects alone and quietly at his own pace taking great delight in his acquisition of knowledge. The stubbornness of the Calcarea carbonica patient is a protective device to slow things down to his pace. If pushed beyond this pace, we see one of the few times the Calcarea carbonica patient gets angry. It takes a lot to make them angry. They have to be pushed and pushed. Normally they are very easy going and casual ... They do not have energy to spare so they take the easy route.

ACTIVITY 18 Describe the menstrual symptoms of the Calcarea carbonica woman in detail. How does this show a sluggish metabolism?

The Head is a Focus

The head is unusually large in the Calcarea carbonica patient. The oyster is only a head. Some oysters and oyster larvae have one foot, but in the case of the larvae this disappears as they age and set on to the rocks. Everything takes place in the 'head' of the oyster.

In the patient, *blood moves to the head.* Eruptions such as *cradle cap* are common and cover only the head. The adult *sweats at night, only on the head*, or predominantly on the head. I have seen children with enormous heads and tiny, cold, blue underdeveloped feet.

The head of the adult remains active though in a dream world, whilst the body is underdeveloped. They can have very fine minds with deep, intuitive insights. The analytical mind of Lycopodium is not present here.

Ultimately, all activity is in the head. The child sits and watches, taking all in, then it astounds those around by getting up to walk as if it had always walked, or it speaks in sentences when before it did not even say 'mama'. Communication in the Calcarea carbonica child is primitive. It is amazing how much they communicate with no language. It is also amazing how this big head just sits there, taking all in, whilst everyone else acts as his/her hands and legs, bringing to it precisely what it wanted.

The Lymphatic System

This is the primitive great sea of the body in which all cells and organs dwell. In many species it predates the evolution of a blood circulating system. In many molluscs there is no red blood.

The glands are the gateways to the lymph system, often acting to secrete lymph. It is a primitive system without a pump like the heart. It works by osmosis and the action of muscles massaging flow. Yet it comes back to the chest, to the lungs, where it can exit.

It is not surprising to find a primitive remedy like Calcarea carbonica has a specific affinity for the glands of the body and their secretion. The Calcarea carbonica patient is often bothered with tonsillitis in youth. Characteristically the *tonsils become hard* especially on the right side. *Catarrh tastes and smells sour.*

The same symptoms apply to the mammary glands, especially before menstruation. The right swells and may harden. These glands are specialized lymph tissue to secrete milk, one of the main constituents of which is, of course, Calcium. Remember the link between milk and sourness! In the female mastitis, knotty breasts and problems breast-feeding may all be cured by Calcarea carbonica.

From day to day it is the activity of the sweat glands that we notice most. The patient cannot take sudden changes in temperature which require metabolic adjustment. He/she sweats very easily in heat, or after activity, or in the cold there is *clammy sweat.* The sweat smells distinctively sour. The Calcarea carbonica patient has a *chalky, dough-like complexion*, with damp skin. The *hands are like wet cods* to take and hold, whilst the feet feel as if the patient has on wet socks (which smell offensive to the bystander!).

The Calcarea carbonica patient is *easily chilled* and yet cannot take too much heat. He *easily takes cold*, which affects the tonsils and other glands around the throat. These glands harden and copious catarrh resembling thick, white milk occurs. If the condition is very serious, or suppressed, the mesenteric glands can be affected, often giving rise to sore tummies that may be associated with school phobia – anxiety about school may certainly give rise to such a situation.

ACTIVITY 19   Research on the role of Calcium in physiological processes.

ACTIVITY 20   Calcarea carbonica, Lycopodium and Sulphur are distinguished because one is cold in spots, another hot in spots, and yet another is numb in spots. Which is which? Give reasons for your answer.

Similar Remedies

Silica most resembles Calcarea carbonica for its shapelessness, slow metabolism and powerful effect on the glands. Both are stubborn and shy and lacking in adventure.

Baryta carbonicum is slow and simple like Calcarea carbonica. The remedy also has a strong effect on glands. It does not have the wet sweats, though it has the smelly feet. Both remedies are shy and hide behind the furniture. Both hate to be laughed at.

Alumina has a slow metabolism that prefers slow release carbohydrates. It has such bad constipation it has to be manually removed. As the Alumina symptom picture develops, the mind slows down and it is difficult to connect thoughts.

ACTIVITY 21   Create a table of comparison for Lycopodium, Sulphur and Calcarea carbonica using the following headings:

Essence
Modalities
Appearance
Heat and cold
Appetite
Rectal symptoms
Skin
Strange, Rare and Peculiar
Personality.

   SELF-TEST QUESTIONS

Answers can be found in the answer section.

1. Which remedy is very worried about their lecture lest they forget what they will say?
2. Describe the eczema of the Calcarea carbonica patient.
3. Which remedy has an all-gone sensation in the stomach before meals?
4. Which remedy answers questions slowly and is irritable if you notice?
5. What is peculiar about the appetite of the Sulphur patient?
6. Which remedy has a burning pain in the epigastric area > hot water bottle?
7. What is strongly affected in the hay fever or cold of Sulphur?

8. In this remedy the hard swollen tonsils are on the right side. The patient is hot and sweaty.
9. She prefers hot drinks with chocolate biscuits.
10. What adjective describes the sweat, taste and vomit of Calcarea carbonica?
11. Describe the skin of the Sulphur patient in an allergic condition.
12. Describe the abdominal symptoms of the Lycopodium patient after eating onions.
13. These children dread washing.
14. Describe the menstrual symptoms of the Calcarea carbonica patient.
15. These people like to go hill walking in a group because they don't need to speak to anyone.
16. This remedy has constipation so bad he/she has to dig it out manually.
17. Which remedy 'comes down to earth to devour his elevenses'?
18. What are the modalities of Lycopodium?
19. Which remedy tires easily especially going uphill?
20. Describe the Sulphur child in bed at night.
21. Describe the sore throat of the Lycopodium patient.
22. How are the bones affected in the Calcarea carbonica child?
23. Why do some Lycopodium patients never worry?
24. Which remedy is immune to its own nasty smells but imagines others?
25. How would you describe the smell of the Sulphur patient's stools?
26. Which remedy has alopecia or greyness in spots?
27. In which remedy is the right breast sore and hard before menses?
28. Which remedy has skin burns and smarts < heat of the bed?
29. Describe the head of the Lycopodium child.
30. Which remedy might you consider for an undescended right testicle?

Further Studies

Lycopodium

1. Kent says the Lycopodium mind is more developed than the body. He sees the Lycopodium body as emaciated. Does this still hold as true today?
2. How would you recognize the Lycopodium patient in a game of poker?
3. Describe and explain the constipation of Lycopodium.
4. When would you use Lycopodium in renal colic?
5. Compare the modalities of Lycopodium with those of Calcarea carbonica and Sulphur.
6. Compare and contrast Lycopodium, Arsenicum and Phosphorus in chest problems.
7. Lycopodium dreads to be alone, but is happy if the other person is in the room next door. Give two examples your patient may use to illustrate this.

Sulphur

1. How does the symptom picture of Sulphur resemble a volcano?
2. Describe how the Sulphur patient presents in a cold. What other remedies might you have to consider with similar symptoms?
3. Sulphur is a major TB remedy. Describe how you would distinguish it in such a disease.
4. How does the self-centred Sulphur patient resemble the Phosphorus patient?
5. Why does the Sulphur child become a bully?
6. Describe the symptoms of the Sulphur patient with skin problems. What other remedies might you have to consider?
7. How might you use Sulphur in a case of allergies?
8. Explain the modalities of the Sulphur patient.
9. Why is Sulphur Hahnemann's most common anti-psoric remedy?

Calcarea Carbonica

1. Delineate the role of calcium in function of the heart. Relate this to the symptom picture of heart disease. How could Calcarea carbonica help?
2. Compare the laziness of Calcarea carbonica and Sulphur.
3. State *seven* prominent characteristics of the Calcarea carbonica metabolism that may form black-letter type symptoms.
4. Delineate the disease process from Calcarea carbonica through Lycopodium to Sulphur and back to Calcarea carbonica, noting clearly the transition points between each remedy picture.

5. Compare Calcarea carbonica and Mercurius. How could you confuse these two?
6. Belladonna and Pulsatilla may apply to an acute condition in the Calcarea carbonica patient. Give an example for each, paying attention to detail in the symptom picture.
7. Differentiate clearly between the Calcarea carbonica and Silicea child in terms of appearance, symptom picture and behavioural patterns.
8. Describe the Calcarea picture in a menopausal woman.
9. Which symptoms does the Calcarea carbonica patient present in kidney disease?
10. Calcium and Phosphorus balance each other in some aspects of metabolism. Describe the similarities between the remedies Phosphorus and Calcarea carbonica. At what stage may they be confused?

Three 'Women's' Remedies

Pulsatilla, Natrum Muriaticum, Sepia

Aim: To demonstrate how three different essences can yet give rise to a similar symptom picture.

Objectives: To identify the essence of the remedy in all its symptoms.
To describe how the symptoms arise from the essence of each remedy.
To distinguish the difference in the aetiology of each remedy.

Headings: INTRODUCTION
PULSATILLA: Origin; Characteristics of the Plant; Essence; Keynotes and Characteristics; Modalities; Meek and Mild; The Need for Structure; Sensitive; The Lymphatic System; Right-sided; The Reproductive System; Similar Remedies
NATRUM MURIATICUM: Origin; Characteristics of the Salt; Essence; Keynotes and Characteristics; Modalities; The Point of Change; The Personality; The Effect of Emotional Trauma; Similar Remedies
SEPIA: Origin; Characteristics of the Creature; Essence; Keynotes and Characteristics; Modalities; Too Busy; From Irritability to Indifference; The Physical Response; Similar Remedies
SELF-TEST QUESTIONS
FURTHER STUDIES

Introduction

These three remedies are very common polycrests, which are often found to apply to women. All are remedies with strong emotions, which deeply affect the female reproductive cycle or are affected by it. They are also remedies that produce a characteristic symptom picture at points of change in the reproductive cycle – puberty, menstruation/ovulation, pregnancy, menopause. Each one is also a personality type that has problems relating to others, so we will look in depth for the first time into the psychology of a remedy.

Essentially we will portray stereotypes. You must learn to take the essence out of these stereotypes to apply them to other patients or situations. Do not judge patients. We are all surviving. Try to understand the problem that needed to be solved and think on why the patient chose that solution. What possibilities were available to them? What were the results of the choice? How did the organism adapt on each level of symptoms? Which parts are put under greater strain by this adaptation and how are these parts affected according to the essential nature of the being?

Pulsatilla

Latin name: Pulsatilla nigricans
Common name: The wind flower, meadow anemone, pasque flower
Botanical family: Ranunculaceae
Habitat: It grows on chalk downs throughout Europe.

Origin

Hahnemann proved the remedy from a tincture of the whole plant.

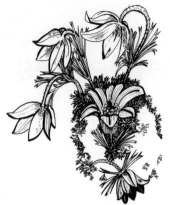

Pulsatilla nigricans

Characteristics of the Plant

The plant flowers in the autumn and spring, a time of change when most Pulsatilla patients visit the clinic with ailments. The plant flowers more in the spring – the patient is especially < change of weather to warm. The plant waves and bends in the wind. The patient is changeable but loves the open air. The purple flower reminds us of venous congestion. The plant bruises easily as does the patient. Whilst the odour given off by the plant when bruised causes fainting fits and headaches, handling the plant causes a dermatitis. All of these symptoms are marked in the Pulsatilla type of patient.

Essence

The remedy is bland and yielding. *Changeable* describes the personality and the symptoms. Pulsatilla is aggravated at times of change, it desires change and is ameliorated by motion.

Keynotes and Characteristics

• **Easily persuaded**	They like to please. Take the easiest course.
• **Mild and tearful**	This is the stereotype of the pretty, blond-haired little girl.
• **Childlike**	They are so naive and trusting.
• **Changeable moods**	Dependent on others, so change as the company does. They are also needy people who react when their expectations are not met.
• **Sulky, moody**	They need a lot of attention.
• **Whine**	They may not suffer silently.
• **Easily offended**	They are sensitive and easily slighted.
• **Sympathetic**	Often weep when you tell your problems to them.
• **Cuddly, affectionate**	You may want to protect them.
• **Shy**	They may need coaxed out of their shell – coy.
• **Desire company**	They need others to define their self and give it structure.
• **Aversion to the opposite sex**	May think sex is sinful. They are so shy and indeterminate they fear they will lose their stability.
• **Religious**	This gives them structure and a channel for their emotions.
• Jealousy	Because need so much themselves.
• **Romantics**	They fantasize and think emotionally.
• **Indecisive**	She sees too many options to choose one.
• **Fear of dogs**	This symptom is often marked.
• Delusions of a naked man in bed with them	They fantasize about their sexual needs.
• Weird dreams	Often of animals.
• **Sleep on abdomen**	This is remarkably common in Pulsatilla patients.
• Sensation of wind blowing through the parts	**Strange, Rare and Peculiar**.
• **Crave fresh air**	This symptom is marked. They sleep with the window open.
• **< becoming heated**	i.e. going into a warm room in summer. **Exciting cause**.
• **Anaemic**	They simply cannot absorb iron. Crude iron poisons them.
• **Low blood pressure**	Gives rise to fainting.
• **Syncope**	Rising from a chair.
• **Vertigo looking upwards**	They are not very well-earthed people.
• **Varicose veins**	Especially after pregnancy.

• **Haemorrhoids**	One form of varicose veins.
• **Right-sided**	This is seen in many symptoms.
• **Right → left**	As in Lycopodium.
• **Copious, bland, green catarrh**	In glandular affections.
• **Mucous membrane dries**	This comes with the thirstlessness.
• **Thirstless**	They are so dry you do not expect this so it is **Strange, Rare and Peculiar**.
• **Desire things they cannot digest, butter, cream, ice-cream, sour, refreshing things**	They eat for emotional comfort.
• **Averse pork, fats**	They have no ability to absorb rich foods.
• **Stool continually changes**	There is so much variety.
• **Menstrual flow changes**	As above.
• **Pains wander**	From one place to another.
• **Throbbing pains**	Because of venous congestion.
• **Pulsation or all-gone sensation in the epigastric area**	
• **Delayed menarche**	Sometimes until 17 years of age.
• **< before menses**	A classic PMS remedy with bloating, tears, headache, sore breasts and irritability.
• **Getting the feet wet**	**Exciting cause**. This brings on colds, cystitis, tonsillitis.
• **Involuntary urination on coughing**	Because the sphincters are lax.

Modalities

< in warm room   > continued or gentle motion
< stuffy atmosphere   > open air
< rich food, pork   > cold applications
< puberty
< menstruation, especially < before menses
< tobacco

ACTIVITY 1   List those symptoms associated with lax tissue. Divide them into general and particular symptoms.

ACTIVITY 2   List those symptoms that show < change and those that show > change. Label the type of symptom, e.g. Strange, Rare and Peculiar.

Meek and Mild

Pulsatilla belongs to the anemone family and like other plants in that group has a delicate flower and a flexible stalk. People who need Pulsatilla are very *adaptable* and *desire to please*, to be accepted and loved. They need to be part of things – problems arise when they are isolated, or have no role in life.

The flower bends to accommodate the wind. The patient is *mild and yielding*. To many this is the archetypal female – passive, obedient and subservient. In classic textbooks the Pulsatilla patient is described as *blond and blue-eyed*. Now, the majority of Scandinavians are blond and blue-eyed – not all are mild and accommodating! The majority of Asians are dark-skinned and dark-haired, with brown eyes, but you still find some patients amongst them that respond to Pulsatilla. The colouring refers to the *laxity of tissue* within the body. Dark coloured people usually have more rigid fibre within the body.

The yielding Pulsatilla is *easily moved to tears* because he/she is so *sympathetic*. In some cultures, e.g. the Scottish (!), the male may only show this in extreme cases, or perhaps when in his cups.

The Need for Structure

The essence of the remedy is *changeability*. She is *worse for any change* because it increases her instability. Too much flexibility leads to *indecision* which is a character much noted in the Pulsatilla patient under stress. The character is formless like water and seeks a shape from its surroundings.

Stress is often about conflict, opening up different paths. The Pulsatilla patient finds choice difficult to deal with, and hence the crisis times are often strongly marked as those times in life when they have to make choices or take initiative.

If the child has a secure upbringing, with clear support and structure, he/she will be charming and versatile, but if there is a lot of change and instability in childhood he/she will be anxious and may crave structure without. This may be the institutionalized person who goes from one institute to another throughout life. It may be the jail, the army, the civil service or the person who turns to *religion* of a strict or sectarian nature. She will form close cliques or special friends, will belong to sub-cultures, social or antisocial, or will come from a close family, or will be *homesick*, or lost, separated from familiar surroundings. In the family role, she will be happy but when the family grow up and leave home, she will be lost and all sorts of physical problems will arise when really she is *lonely*. When you see her as a patient, you will get all her woes and groans and she will *cling* to you so you may have difficulty ending the interview.

Major keynotes that arise from this character structure are:

- Desire for company
- << alone or isolated.

Exciting causes include:

- Disappointed love
- Grief
- Silent grief.

Sensitive

Perhaps the most important keynote after *desires company* is *irresolute*. She is fearful of offending anyone, so does not know which way to turn. When really run down, she may be wishy-washy, because there is *no confidence* to take a clear direction. Pulsatilla patients lack confidence and cannot stand out from a crowd. This could be described as *shyness* or even *bashfulness*. In another context this sensitivity may become the keynote *easily offended*. In the body this becomes *easily bruised*. She is frightened she will be hurt. The coy Pulsatilla maid is *fearful of men*. She *blushes easily* ... even if 'she' is male.

She has a wealth of emotions that can lead to turmoil in an unstable situation. Her sympathetic self is easily overcome, so tears result (the keynote *weeps easily*), or determination (Pulsatillas are *stubborn* too – remember every worm turns!). They fluctuate between moods rapidly, so the child is renowned for its *sulks*. The mature woman may be described as moody, irritable and depressed, especially *before menses*.

The Pulsatilla child is *demanding*, *peevish* and *clings to mum*. This does not sound very sensitive. Why should it do this? Of course there are times when all children behave like this, especially when they are ill so you must see this trait as exaggerated in the Pulsatilla type. He/she is insecure. They need a lot of cuddling and affection but still that is not enough. Mum often gets a bit fed up, so the child starts to take attention. It is a sad situation because enough is not enough, they want even more and often alienate others.

ACTIVITY 3 Describe the Pulsatilla child's first day at school.

ACTIVITY 4 Describe how Grandma behaves when the children forget to give her a Christmas present.

The Lymphatic System

On the physical level, Pulsatilla affects the lymph system, the mucous membrane, smooth muscles (e.g. of veins, especially the portal vein), the reproductive system, and the fluid balance of the body. It acts on the last through the slackness of the veins that offer no resistance to fluid transfer, so *oedema* of the extremities is common in later life.

At the more acute end, the Pulsatilla patient is *prone to colds* and *swollen glands*, often the cervical and submaxillary in today's patient. There is *copious catarrh* of a yellowish colour, or *greenish* if the situation is more severe. The Pulsatilla cold is most likely to go to the head which becomes congested and throbs especially *above the right eye*. As the sinuses are involved, the throbbing may be along the tops of the cheeks. In the throat it is noticeable that the glands are swollen on the *right side*. Pulsatilla is characteristically a *right-sided remedy* that may progress to the left side in more severe cases. The copious catarrh eventually dries but although the pain is worse then, the patient is *thirstless*. This may be one of the few distinguishing symptoms that enables you to tell the difference between Pulsatilla and Bryonia which also has the copious mucus and swollen glands which may progress to the head as a congestive headache. Both remedies are very much *worse for damp weather*. Pulsatilla has the keynote *worse after getting the feet wet*. Both are worse when they become heated but Pulsatilla is more specific here, in that it strongly *desires fresh air* and since it is uncomfortable when the mucous membrane becomes dry, can be seen to be markedly worse in *central heating* or on *going into warm environments*. Being so sensitive, the Pulsatilla colds are seen directly related to the change of weather and hence the keynote *worse change of weather*, or *change of temperature*. Many sinus problems in central heating, or which start with warm weather, or after vigorous use of decongestants respond well to Pulsatilla as an acute remedy.

As the disease process deepens, particularly in the older person, or after the family has left home, or after menopause, rheumatism often appears. The constitution is sluggish and was allowed to stagnate, so a marked modality is *better continual movement*. The condition begins when the weather changes or is worse when the wet weather arrives. It may come on suddenly when the feet are soaked in a rainstorm whilst walking home, or it may appear after the menopause or when the mental problems of grief or isolation begin. The keynote is that the aches *move from joint to joint*, i.e. *wandering pains*. After the nightly rest, the symptoms are worse, as they get going again in the morning. The catarrh also fits into this pattern when it is much thicker in the morning because it has been allowed to collect and stagnate overnight.

ACTIVITY 5

Describe the symptoms of the Pulsatilla patient with:

Tonsillitis
Sinusitis.

Use the appropriate keynotes and characteristics.

Right-sided

Pulsatilla is a very *one-sided* remedy. The majority of affections appear on the *right side* but in a serious case the symptoms can be seen to move on to the left side. Only rarely will they move back again. The headache is typically above the right eye, the tonsils are typically swollen on the right side, in mumps the glands are swollen on the right side. The perspiration may flow from one side. This is a Strange, Rare and Peculiar symptom. In the joints the pain wanders from side to side and from leg to arm, and back again. There is no direction which is why we call them wandering pains.

The Reproductive System

Many Pulsatilla health problems are related to the reproductive system. This is not surprising when we consider that the greatest changes in the body are in this system as we grow, and that each month the female goes through very radical changes in this system. Modalities of Pulsatilla that fit in with this are:

< puberty
< before menses
< childbirth
< menopause.

Many Pulsatilla women suffer from PMT as the hormone levels build up, increasing as congestion increases because of the added work required of the liver to clear them out of the system. Cramping pains, dull headaches and depression are common.

During pregnancy, the extra weight and pressure give rise to piles and varicose veins. These often disappear after childbirth but may accumulate after each pregnancy, never quite getting back to the old form. The internal organs similarly slacken.

At puberty, as the hormones appear, there may be acne, or problems with glands and catarrhs. Menses are often delayed for several years and even when they start, may be irregular or tend to disappear easily (amenorrhoea) after emotional crisis.

At menopause, the Pulsatilla patient may be plagued with severe flushes and migraines. At whatever level of disease the homoeopath still looks for the characteristic symptoms so the flushes will move upwards, be > fresh air and < emotion. The migraine headache will be pulsating over the right eye, < in warm rooms, < tobacco, < before menses and > in the fresh air.

ACTIVITY 6 How is the changeability expressed in the reproductive system? Where possible use the keynote and characteristic symptoms.

ACTIVITY 7 Describe a scenario where a Pulsatilla patient receives news of the spouse's death. Five years later how has he/she adapted?

Similar Remedies

Pulsatilla is such a broad polycrest it can resemble so many remedies.

Silicea has the meekness and catarrhal problems of Pulsatilla. Both are yielding and tearful. Silicea is left-sided and more stubborn. It is also less dependent on others and more analytical in thought than romantic.

Mercurius is easily swayed by atmospheres. It is also a remedy of lax tissues, glands and catarrhs. However, it is not bland. Discharges are foul and bloody. Mercurius is a remedy of decay.

Antimonium crudum has the same romantic view and sensitivity. They are < grief and disappointed love. It is also a remedy of catarrhs and glandular problems. It is < pork and rich foods too.

Natrum Muriaticum

Common name: Sodium chloride

Origin

The remedy was prepared by Hahnemann from a trituration of common table salt.

Characteristics of the Salt

Salt is almost inseparable from water and since our body fluids have the same consistency as the sea, 70–80% of the body is closely associated with Natrum muriaticum.

The salinity of the seas varies causing some of the movement in the sea. In the body, much of the movement of fluid is caused by osmosis in which Natrum muriaticum plays a major role. Sodium is also associated with the nerves to create transmission of impulses in the Sodium pump. If we look at this role in the body we can understand why the essence of the remedy is *exchange*. The symptom picture of the remedy shows that the ability to exchange has been affected. In fact Sodium chloride *controls exchange*. To do this it must be very *sensitive* and *receptive*. These are the qualities we will see in the remedy. We will also see that the method used to control the exchange is its *bipolar nature*. Thus, there is a dualism in the remedy – it fluctuates from one state to another, e.g. it is one of the remedies of intermittent fever and of manic depression.

Essence

This is a remedy found at the *point of change*. Present in the symptom picture is an inability to complete the change smoothly, so there is a distinct tendency to *polarize* in the symptoms. There is lack of spontaneity because the change becomes a barrier.

Keynotes and Characteristics		
	• **< grief**	Such a great change that needs a lot of adaptation.
	• **< disappointed love**	This symptom also brings out their emotional vulnerability.
	• **Sadness**	May be severe depression.
	• Depression < morning	Before they become occupied with the demands of life. < if not occupied.
	• **Monomania**	Keep talking of just one subject.
	• **Hopeless – about future**	Everything looks so black and they feel they do not deserve anything.
	• **Desire to be alone**	So do not have to adapt to others.
	• **Feel forsaken**	That no-one wants them.
	• **Feel unlovable**	They have such a poor image of themselves.
	• **Suspicious**	They do not trust because they could be hurt.
	• Consolation aggravates	They can become quite angry when you sympathize.
	• Dream of robbers	They are sensitive to violation of their boundaries.
	• **Sleepless from tormenting thoughts**	They chew over everything when they are no longer occupied.
	• **Awkward in movement**	There is lack of spontaneous flow.
	• **Abrupt**	Speech, movements, manners are abrupt.
	• Clumsy before menses	Co-ordination is lost.
	• **Chilly**	Wears a lot of clothes.
	• **< sun**	The heat goes to the head and usually pain accompanies. **Exciting cause**.
	• **Great emaciation – while eating well**	This is a remedy of great disturbance of metabolism as in cancer, tuberculosis, malaria.
	• **Anorexia**	Usually because they are unloved, even self-loathing.
	• > going without meals	One of the differentiating symptoms from Lycopodium which is < fasting.
	• < bread	The abdomen bloats.
	• **Craves salt or averse salt**	This may occur at different places in the disease process.
	• Constipation	There is much straining for the first dry lump and then the stool is looser. This is a good example of the remedy's polarity.
	• Scanty delayed menses	And of course in another Natrum muriaticum patient we will find the opposite.
	• **Amenorrhoea**	From grief or disappointed love.
	• **Averse coition**	They would have to let down their boundaries.

• **Dryness of vagina**	It is the opposite of the next symptom.
• **Watery leucorrhoea**	Once again, we have the opposite – see next symptom.
• White of egg leucorrhoea	
• Cannot pass urine in the presence of others	They cannot cross the barrier to start. They are reserved types that hold themselves in many ways.
• **Back pain as if broken**	> lying on something.
• **Greasy face**	In others the face may be dry.
• Herpetic eruptions	Dry, then break down and weep.
• Cold sores on lips	At the muco-cutaneous junction.
• Urticaria	After exertion or overheating.
• Eruptions on hairline	On the edge!
• Dryness of mucous membrane	At other times there may be copious catarrh.
• **Violent palpitations shake the whole body**	< lying on left side. There is much similarity to Phosphorus.
• Pulsating headache, as if 1000 hammers	Starts 10 a.m. and increases in pain with sun, then decreases with sun.
• Blood flows upwards to head	This may be a remedy of high blood pressure.
• Headaches after work, illness at weekends or holidays	When they relax.
• Painful shortening of muscles	eg. hamstrings, anus during constipation.

Modalities

< **grief**   > open air
< **disappointed love**   > **fasting**
< **sun**
< **before menses**
< mental exertion
< quinine
< seaside
< **10–11 a.m.**
< **sunrise to sunset**

ACTIVITY 8 List all those symptoms that occur at the point of change. Divide them into 'space' and 'time'.

ACTIVITY 9 List those symptoms to do with water imbalance or fluid exchange. Label the type of symptom, e.g. Strange, Rare and Peculiar.

ACTIVITY 10 List those symptoms that show polarity. You may find some more to fit in here as we go through the lesson. Label the type of symptom, e.g. Strange, Rare and Peculiar.

The Point of Change

If we look at the areas of the body affected by Natrum muriaticum we will find that they are involved in change, in exchange of fluids, or that the organs involved function by means of fluid:

- skin
- eyes
- mucous membrane
- lungs
- spleen
- large bowel
- female organs
- nerves.

122

When we look at the Materia Medica we will see that there is a similarity in the way the remedy affects these organs or tissues. There may be copious fluid discharge, followed by dryness, or the organ may underfunction 'drying up' before suddenly gushing forth after a struggle.

The herpetic eruption is a good example of the Natrum muriaticum action. Tiny vesicles appear, then break to exude a watery discharge. The part may then dry and crust, or it becomes dry and raw then moist again.

The times when the Natrum muriaticum illness 'strikes' are periods of exaggerated change, especially of fluids or emotions. Change of hormones affect both body and emotions. Look at the following list and compare it to your findings in Activity 8, 9 and 10 above:

- loss of fluids
- before or during menses, or ovulation time
- eating – think of all the secretion necessary to eat
- < heat – especially of the sun, 10 a.m. and increases as the sun rises then > after the sun passes its zenith
- < sunrise to sunset, most living and intercourse is done in this period
- < exertion – mental especially
- < falling asleep – they start and have electric shocks, hear noises, etc. (In fact they are letting go at this time!)
- < in the morning and after sleep – things are getting going again
- insomnia and cannot sleep because they have great difficulty letting go
- dreams go on after waking
- < grief
- < disappointment, shock, trauma, fright.

ACTIVITY 11 Describe the common cold of the Natrum muriaticum patient. Use as many keynotes and characteristics as are appropriate.

ACTIVITY 12 Describe the eczema of the Natrum muriaticum patient. Use as many keynotes and characteristics as are appropriate.

The Personality

On the mental level this is one of the most easily recognized remedies.

Abruptness describes many of their symptoms. They are *frank* and come to the point when you are talking to them. There are few frills to their conversation. In writing, their sentences are short and clipped. Their gait is similar in that it is perhaps the most *determined* in the Materia Medica. It may be described as a stomp. If we look at their gait we get a few hints as to their personality. The head leans forwards in a hen-strut, and they have a determined look on their face. They look only to their purpose. Their inner insecurity is contained by their purpose – this remedy is *better for occupation*. If they stop, or are stopped, that action may carry on and be directed against the intruder or . . . the action disappears, they lose momentum and are consumed by their insignificance.

They are very *sensitive* people and very vulnerable to criticism – *easily offended*.

If in walking they stop to think of their action, they lose rhythm, cannot recreate it consciously, so they become *very awkward*. Co-ordination in general is affected so they become clumsy if they are anxious, or if they are worn down before the menses. Sodium affects the smooth transmission of nerve impulses.

This *lack of flow* is often a physical result of *mental trauma* which has caused *isolation*. Usually the Natrum muriaticum patient is conscious of this isolation, and has a *feeling of being unworthy*, of being *forsaken*. This gives rise to great difficulty in relationships because no matter how much they are loved, and are told this, they cannot reciprocate because they cannot believe that anyone could love such an unworthy person. For similar reasons, they frequently cannot respect others' motives and show much *suspicion*. They doubt the others' good faith or, knowing how they themselves can control and manipulate a situation, they doubt others' motives. Often in early life they have *lost their spontaneity* and the natural flow of human communication, so have created behavioural patterns they think are appropriate, but these are rationally created and *consciously controlled*. In relationships they are therefore keen to talk out all situations. (Look at Freud's anal type of person who is very retentive and suppresses natural emotions.) They will go to encounter groups and psychotherapy, where they learn to rationalize their feelings and where they are often taught to overcome their vulnerability by talking about it.

These are the patients who *rationalize all their symptoms* (Lycopodium also). In case-taking, they really confuse the beginner, because they never talk about what is really the problem – it is all dressed up in other language. They *cannot expose themselves*. Often the most important symptom is retained until the very last minute, as they are going out the door and will no longer have to face you. Sometimes they are *shy* and cannot cope with your response. Often they send everything in a letter afterwards. Frequently they have told you things they have never ever mentioned to another living soul. You are told simply by virtue of your role. In order to cope with the feeling world Natrum muriaticum is often a follower of the rule book.

They are often celibate, because they cannot face the pain of relating closely, or the ultimate rejection.

They cannot face personal judgement so will often hide behind ideals or causes. They achieve worth through merging their identity to that of an organization.

Being somewhat *aloof* and outside the normal stream, others often come to them for advice because they are rational and compassionate, and can empathize with others. They can have such deep insight and *sensitivity* ... this comes from their vulnerability. When dealing with problems they can empathize so well they can lose themselves, or they can exert such control on their emotions that they can rationalize the most traumatic problems, or can see them from all angles. This last has many advantages but can extol great suffering if their feelings are left behind the barrier.

Natrum muriaticum patients are basically *honest* and frank because they have carefully constructed what is the right form of behaviour that makes them feel safe. They have an ideal of correctness that gives rise to the stereotype of a prime spinster. They are *easily offended* if you step outside the bounds of propriety.

They are particularly *fastidious about time* because this marks the 'off' in a relationship and gives it borders.

The idea of correctness is often a means by which they exert control over others. Natrum muriaticum in its very vulnerable state exerts a lot of control in order to protect itself. They manipulate and rationalize so as not to reveal their true self.

ACTIVITY 13   This is a common stereotype, so look around you and make some notes of similar behavioural patterns. Ask yourself what does the person do at the point of contact with another? How is the body held? Listen to the tone of voice and the content of the sentences.

The Effect of Emotional Trauma

The feelings of Natrum muriaticum patients are often hidden – they cannot *trust* others with their vulnerability. This is when they build a barrier around themselves. When you meet them they are often very open and cheerful people. This is a mask. They may mobilize enormous energies in order to maintain this persona and, of course, this gives rise to even greater stress.

When they are offended, usually loss of self through *grief*, *rejection* or *criticism*, they *withdraw* and *erect* a *barrier*. They refuse to show feeling or to acknowledge feelings. 'I felt kicked in the teeth but I wasn't going to let him have the pleasure of knowing he had hurt me.' So they pretend nothing has happened, or they rationalize it swallowing their pain – hence the lump in the throat (see Ignatia). The tears and dejection will come once they are alone – the reaction is controlled to hide the vulnerable self. If the tears sneak out whilst others are present, you will be expected to ignore them. If you observe and expose the Natrum muriaticum's feelings, she/he will be angry. If you attempt to console, you are stepping over the threshold of self and she will turn on you defending her vulnerability.

Once the wound is open she will be vigilant to defend it and, unable to forget, she cannot forgive. The hurt is imprinted on her mind and will not die. She thinks of nothing but . . . *monomania*. And when she relaxes to go to sleep it floods back, gnawing at her and preventing sleep. She has suppressed the feelings that should flow outwards as a curative action, so the hurt is still there. Holding onto the hurt is *resentment* where hatred pushes out, trying to keep the hurt from hitting home. In reacting to the source of her pain she must cut the lines of communication. She *cannot speak to the person* or have anything to do with him/her because she would have to feel the hurt. So she remains unhealed.

The great mental effort of suppressing the emotions in this way may lead to total breakdown when the duality of the remedy asserts itself and we get *laughter alternating with weeping* or manic depression where the depths are alternated with exhilaration. It is at this stage that we may see the keynote *fears might be insane*, which stems from feeling that they are out of touch with the world or that the world is *unreal*.

Shock is often diverted into the body where years of *silent grief* eventually reap the harvest of cancer, or resentment becomes multiple sclerosis or rheumatoid arthritis. It may be that the effort of defending their vulnerability may yield to Crohn's disease. In any serious illness the homoeopath always looks for the exciting cause which will give a clearer indication of the required remedy than a list of physical symptoms.

In summing up, Natrum muriaticum is a remedy of *lack of love*, but not because the person has none to give. They do not feel safe enough to express their love.

ACTIVITY 14   Contemplate situations you have experienced, or seen others experience, regarding grief or disappointed love. What reactions did you notice? How did this relate to the symptom picture of Natrum muriaticum?

Similar Remedies

Ignatia is the most similar remedy to Natrum muriaticum in emotions, especially grief and disappointed love. Both may gush forth, or become reserved. Either remedy may lose themselves in noble causes. They do not let go of their feelings and cannot share them.

Lycopodium is often confused with Natrum muriaticum because both tend to rationalize so much. Lycopodium is basically a coward who can be deceitful to get out of situations, whereas Natrum muriaticum is bold and confronts reality. Whilst one thinks of self, the other is altruistic.

Arsenicum may be confused with Natrum muriaticum because of their correctness and desire to be in control. Both are armour-plated remedies who use a great deal of energy to defend themselves, so when illness comes, it is severe and degenerative. Both are fastidious and use organization to defend themselves. As in Lycopodium, Arsenicum is very self-centred, whilst Natrum muriaticum is full of concern for others.

Sepia

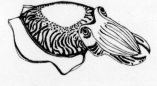

Sepia officinalis

Latin name: Sepia officinalis
Common name: Cuttlefish

Origin

Hahnemann is said to have noted the effects of the poisoning from an artist who used Sepia ink. Goullon, van Gersdorff, Gross, Hartlaub and Wahle did the proving from a trituration of the dried contents of the cuttlefish's ink sac.

Characteristics of the Creature

The cuttlefish is a primitive animal belonging to the Cephalopods, along with the squids. It swims by propelling itself through the water. If disturbed it shoots backwards at great speed. It is a clever predator that creeps up on its prey, changing colour to suit its environment. Then it rapidly shoots out a tentacle to grasp the prey.

The ink from which the remedy is made consists mainly of melanin. The cuttlefish squirts it out as a defensive mechanism hiding in the cloud.

Essence

The essence of this remedy is *sag*. They are such busy people consuming so much energy they are worn down. They lose their shape. They lose themselves in the cloud of business and their surroundings take the place of their identity! We will understand this more in what follows.

Keynotes and Characteristics		
	• **Sallow**	The skin loses its colour.
	• **Yellow saddle across the nose**	These are very worn down types.
	• Combination skin	Greasy down the centre.
	• **Liver spots**	It is often a remedy of the older woman, or of the menopausal woman, when this pigmentation appears.
	• **Busy**	She is a workaholic.
	• **> occupation**	It keeps her from her own needs and feelings.
	• **Fastidious**	About her house and environment.
	• **An organizer**	Always sorting out others.
	• **Irritable**	It is easier to do things herself than let others do them.
	• < after anger	This is especially directed to her partner.
	• **Irritability with indifference**	At this point they are reacting without really connecting.
	• **She wants to scream**	All is getting on top of her.
	• **Anxiety over trifles**	Everything has to be perfect. It becomes obsessive.
	• **Causeless weeping**	They are not connecting with their emotions.
	• **Total indifference**	This is sag at the mental level.
	• **Indifferent to her children**	This symptom frequently occurs before menses. When it occurs after childbirth it is associated with postnatal depression.
	• Dreads meeting people	Because has to find energy to be sociable.
	• **Indolent**	Wants to do nothing.
	• **< before menses**	A useful general symptom.
	• **Bearing down pains**	As if the internal organs would fall out.
	• Prolapse uterus	Ultimately the womb falls out.
	• **< menopause**	They cannot cope with the hormonal changes.
	• Flushes of heat upwards	All symptoms move upwards, < least motion.
	• **Palpitations**	Particularly at menopause, these pulse through the body.
	• **Tendency to abort 5–7 months**	Because of poor tone in uterus.
	• < after pregnancy	Because the body is tired.
	• Postnatal depression	It takes the form of indifference to the child and irritability with the husband.
	• **Averse coition**	Because so much < afterwards.
	• **Back pain < standing**	This is in the sacral area. < before menses.
	• Abdomen bloated	Because digestion is so slow.
	• **Desire vinegar**	The acid tones up the slack tissues of the digestive system.
	• Empty sensation epigastric	There are many sensations of emptiness in hollow organs.
	• **Sensation of a lump in abdomen**	Similar to Arsenicum. This is the opposite of emptiness.

• **Nausea at sight and smell of food**	With headaches in pregnancy.
• **Migraines**	Again < before menses, < at menopause, > exercise. Above the left eye.
• Zig-zag lines in visual field	Usually comes with headaches.
• **Constipation with sensation of lump left in anus**	There are a lot of lump sensations in Sepia.
• Piles	Sag of veins.
• Varicose veins	In state of sag.
• **Icy cold all day, hot at night**	Poor state of venous system.
• As feet become hot, hands become cold	**Strange, Rare and Peculiar.**
• **Love to dance**	They feel so good after it.
• Ringworm	
• Liver spots on front torso	Usually these occur on hands.

Modalities

• < cold, damp	> **violent exertion**
• < **standing**	> sitting with legs crossed
• < **coition**	> open air
• < after sleep, after eating	> warmth
• < hormone change	
• < before thunderstorms	

ACTIVITY 15 List all the symptoms of 'sag'. Separate the mental and physical symptoms.

ACTIVITY 16 Review the effects of sex hormones in the male and female. How does this relate to the Sepia symptom picture?

ACTIVITY 17 Study the role of melanin in the body. How is this reflected in the Sepia symptom picture?

Too Busy

A typical symptom picture of Sepia is of a mature woman with a large abdomen 'up front' and a 'combination skin', *greasy* over the nose and mouth area but dry elsewhere. Later on, the skin may be pasty and *dough-like*, with liver spots and/or a distinctive *yellow 'saddle'* across the nose. It is called the 'washer woman' remedy. Hahnemann saw her when she was so run down. He did not see her again until by chance he passed by and there she was by the river, washing clothes, too busy to come back to tell him she was better.

She is the busy housewife, who is *always on the go*, or today, she is the career woman, with a home to keep and a demanding job. She is a great *organizer* – she has to be to keep up the two jobs. She is very *fastidious* and *house proud*, so much energy goes into creating order. Her home or job is part of her self-esteem. It is the elaborate screen she has constructed around herself to hide in! These deflection shields will be many and any time she feels vulnerable, she flurries into activity creating around herself another screen, > *occupation*. These ladies are often found making the tea at the local women's institute. If her schemes are disrupted, she shows *irritability*. This increases before her period, when she is a bit more tired and can have severe PMT. Often it is directed against her children, or husband, who do not have the same needs to erect the screen and maintain it, as she does. Her behaviour is very similar to that of the animal that squirts ink into the water so it can disappear or hide from others, or it squirts its ink to enable it to prey on others! The Sepia patient often takes no tally of others in her magnificent schemes and this is a major difference from the Natrum muriaticum patient who is really very sensitive to others and cares, even if those feelings are disguised.

ACTIVITY 18

You must have seen women like this. Note some observations. Relate your findings to the Sepia symptom picture.

From Irritability to Indifference

The Sepia patient is very vulnerable and has a poor opinion of herself. Her *confidence is easily knocked*, so she is on edge and *worries constantly* and, of course, this wears her down. She is often described as *anxious over trifles*.

She worries about her health, her job and her home. She can thus resemble closely the Arsenicum patient. Her first answer to dissolution is to tighten the organization of the structure surrounding her but, of course, this creates more tension and gives her more to defend. She becomes irritable. Sepia contains a great deal of Natrum muriaticum and one similarity may be seen here when polarity appears under the symptom *irritability with indifference*.

She reaches the stage where she *wants to scream*, where she is so unsure of herself she wants something to hold on to, where she is afraid she will go off the deep end – again note the similarity to Natrum muriaticum who sees the goalposts shift as things appear unreal. Sepia patients do and say things that seem odd and out of place to others at this stage. She may become so irrational that the family do not know what she is going to do next. This describes many women with PMT or at menopause.

When the sag is complete she withdraws into *total indifference* and does nothing. It is difficult to get a response out of her. Her environment and person are uncared for. This is the same pattern that the poor Arsenicum patient will eventually take too, so the similarity is increased.

The Physical Response

The disease process in the Sepia patient is not a smooth progression. It is distinctly worse with each new crisis they have to deal with. The influx of hormones at various stages in the female cycle are often an added burden that acts as an exciting cause. Before the period she is *irritable* and *indifferent*.

There is much congestion which appears as a bloated abdomen and fluid retention. Pains are often dull and extend down into the thighs or may be severe and be described as *bearing down* and *as if all would fall out through the vagina*. Pain in the lumbar region of the back often accompanies the period and/or migraines occur in some patients. The headache is very distinct. It is left-sided and usually above the left eye, throbbing. Vision is frequently disturbed by zig-zag lines. With such PMT she is << *standing* as this further strains the abdominal muscles which are already in sag. She is worse when ironing, because not only is she standing but also she is in *damp, humid atmosphere*. Turkish baths are not for the Sepia patient! In fact she is *better for violent exercise* that increases the circulation. She may be slow to get going, in fact she sits around frequently doing very little, but once moving around she benefits greatly. Often Sepia patients are described as lovers of *dance* which is usually a violent but purposeful exercise! One more important point to note here is their *aversion* to *coition* and the aggravation afterwards. This is often an added burden to her marital duties! It involves the self she is hiding whilst the act leads to local congestion of a part which is already very congested.

Childbirth and pregnancy are times when the Sepia patient needs help. Often they have *never been well since pregnancy*. They may get worse after each pregnancy ending up very worn down. During pregnancy, she suffers terrible nausea and like Arsenicum cannot bear the sight or smell of food. After pregnancy the remedy is often indicated for postnatal depression. The main symptoms are *indifference to child* and *irritability with husband* and *loss of libido*. Prolapse is common in the Sepia picture. At first piles and varicose veins may be the only symptoms. Later on severe bleeding and *fibroids* often lead to hysterectomy. Menopause symptoms can be severe. It is one of the remedies of severe *flushes upwards*, of low thyroxin counts and of liver spots. At the menopause we see another strange symptom, viz, *she desires cold weather* and cold temperatures. This acts as a tonic on the skin. For the same tonic reason we see her desiring *vinegar* and sour things that perk up the flagging gut.

ACTIVITY 19 What effect does 'sag' have on the digestive system of the Sepia patient? Include as many keynotes and characteristics as appropriate.

ACTIVITY 20 Before 'sag' sets in, there is an excitable stage. Find symptoms for the common cold in a Sepia patient. You will find more similarities to Natrum muriaticum.

Similar Remedies

Arsenicum. Similarities to Arsenicum have been noted throughout the lesson. Both are great organizers who expend so much energy they ultimately collapse.

Natrum muriaticum. Sepia is often called the physical Natrum muriaticum. It has the same polar action but here we see the remedy so advanced into the physical symptoms that the collapse dominates. Like Natrum muriaticum the Sepia patient erects a barrier to protect the self and like Natrum muriaticum the Sepia patient is often selfless but not because of altruism.

Pulsatilla and Sepia have the same venous congestion and relaxation of organs. Both have a strong action on the reproductive cycle – Pulsatilla because of its action on glands and Sepia because of its action on hollow organs.

Nux vomica shares the irritability of Sepia. Both expend great energy in organizing. Both are fastidious remedies.

ACTIVITY 21 Create a table of comparison for Pulsatilla, Natrum muriaticum and Sepia using headings as follows:

Exciting causes
Modalities
Weather reactions
Mentals
Motivation
Headache
Food desires and aversions
Constipation
Colds
Reproductive system.

 SELF-TEST QUESTIONS

All the answers will be found in the text, and can be checked in the answer section.

1. Give three examples of Pulsatilla's changeableness.
2. What are the exciting causes of the Sepia symptom picture?
3. Which remedy has awkwardness of movements, < before menses?
4. Which remedy is fastidious?
5. Which remedy has the delusion of someone in bed beside them?

6. In which direction do the pains of Sepia move in the anus?
7. Which remedy sleeps on the abdomen?
8. What does Natrum muriaticum dream of?
9. In which remedy do palpitations:
   a. shake the whole body?
   b. pulse through the whole body?
10. Which remedy is indifferent to her children?
11. Which of the three remedies is most affectionate? Least affectionate?
12. Which remedy feels better when fasting?
13. Why does the Sepia patient tend to abort in the 5th–7th month?
14. Why is the Pulsatilla patient averse to the opposite sex?
15. Describe the menstrual symptoms of the Sepia patient.
16. Which remedy is so dry and stuffed up and yet thirstless?
17. Give four exciting causes of Natrum muriaticum.
18. Which two remedies are averse coition because of dryness in the vagina?
19. What are the fears of the Pulsatilla patient?
20. How would you differentiate the backache of Sepia and Natrum muriaticum?
21. Why does Natrum muriaticum desire to be alone?
22. Describe the constipation of Natrum muriaticum.
23. What are the food cravings and aversions of the Pulsatilla patient?
24. Describe the headache of the Sepia patient.
25. Why is the Pulsatilla patient so indecisive?
26. Which remedy feels unloveable?
27. What are the food cravings of the Sepia patient?
28. When is Natrum muriaticum most likely to feel depressed? Why?
29. Describe the headache of the Natrum muriaticum patient.
30. What happens when the Pulsatilla patient becomes heated?

Further Studies

Pulsatilla

1. Describe the role of 'change' in Pulsatilla.
2. Why would you consider Pulsatilla to be a childlike remedy?
3. Every worm turns. What would cause Pulsatilla to turn?
4. Discuss the role of Pulsatilla in childhood illnesses. Compare it to at least two other remedies.
5. Describe the Pulsatilla male.
6. How does Pulsatilla affect smooth muscle tissue?
7. Describe a first aid situation where Pulsatilla may be of use to you.
8. Compare Bryonia and Pulsatilla as sycotic catarrhal remedies.
9. If a child had fallen into the river, how would you distinguish between Pulsatilla, Rhus toxicodendron and Dulcamara?
10. Compare the causation of Pulsatilla that brings it to resemble Natrum muriaticum and Ignatia.

Natrum Muriaticum

1. How does Natrum muriaticum affect the water balance of the body?
2. Describe a chronic degenerative disease that might appear after the exciting cause, grief, in the Natrum muriaticum patient.
3. Describe the headache of Natrum muriaticum.
4. Which symptoms of Natrum muriaticum resemble Lycopodium and Arsenicum? How would you differentiate?
5. When would you use Natrum muriaticum in a skin problem?
6. When are Natrum muriaticum and Pulsatilla confused as remedies?
7. Can Natrum muriaticum be used on a self-help, first aid level?
8. Discuss the digestive symptoms of Natrum muriaticum. Do these resemble any other remedy/remedies?

9. When would Gelsemium be of use in the Natrum muriaticum patient? Describe the symptom picture.
10. Describe how the Natrum muriaticum patient copes with relationships.

Sepia

1. In what symptoms does Sepia resemble
    a. Arsenicum?
    b. Natrum muriaticum?
2. What is the relationship between Lachesis, Nux vomica, Bryonia and Sepia? Illustrate your answer with snippets of symptom picture.
3. How would you find Sepia of specific use in female problems?
4. Describe the migraine of Sepia. Repertorize these symptoms in your Repertory and then give similar remedies and differentiate between them.
5. Why is Sepia often of use in the pre-cancerous patient?
6. Compare Sepia with Lilium tigrinum and Pulsatilla.
7. When might you use Sepia in treating a child?
8. Why is Sepia of use in suppressed gonorrhoea?
9. Describe the Sepia male.

Three Nervous Remedies

Causticum, Phosphorus, Silicea

Aim: To illustrate how the essence of three sensitive remedies has such a profound, yet different, impact on the nervous system.

Objectives: To state the essence of the remedy in all its symptoms.
To describe in which way each remedy has a different effect on the nervous system.
To identify the areas and modes of action of each remedy.

Headings: INTRODUCTION
CAUSTICUM: Origin; Essence; Keynotes and Characteristics; Modalities; The Sensitive Worrier; Paralysis; Drying Up; Similar Remedies
PHOSPHORUS: Origin; Characteristics of the Element; Essence; Keynotes and Characteristics; Modalities; Hyperactivity; Hypersensitive; Too Much Wears Them Down; Similar Remedies
SILICEA: Origin; Characteristics of the Mineral; Essence; Keynotes and Characteristics; Modalities; Sensitivity; The Amorphous Stage; A Slow-acting Remedy; Similar Remedies
SELF-TEST QUESTIONS
FURTHER STUDIES

Introduction

Once again we have three major polycrests with remarkable similarity in essence and mode of action. In learning to differentiate them we will need to look carefully at the essence and how this is acted on by the exciting cause and which symptoms it then produces.

In looking at the nervous system remember it is divided into voluntary and involuntary and connects strongly with the emotions and the mind. Mind is a very misused term. In the context of the nervous system, it encompasses perception, cognition, understanding, imagination and will. All three remedies have a strong factor of imagination and each is a remedy of *fear*. In studying them you will see how understanding and sometimes perception is changed. You will see how the will of each is undermined by their lack of confidence. You will find it interesting to note how each remedy has a different personality and to see how this evolves from the different ways the component parts combine, or function, together. It reminds me that some see personality as the sum total of adaptations that enable a person to cope with his/her environment.

Causticum

Origin

Causticum is prepared from a distillation of calcium hydroxide and potassium bisulphate. The first symptom picture was produced by Hahnemann, but we no longer know the exact contents of the substance he used, because it contained impurities.

Essence

Vithoulkas describes this remedy as *gradual paralysis* on all levels. They are sensitive, over-excitable types who so overreact to impressions that their nervous system is exhausted. As the life force withdraws there is a drying up, so burning pains, cracks, and even ulcers are common.

Keynotes and Characteristics

• **< cold, dry weather**	So much so, that they are > damp weather.
• **< long-standing grief or anxiety**	The nerves are gradually worn down.
• **< loss of sleep**	Exhausts the nervous system.
• **< fright**	Strongly affects the nervous system.
• Hopelessness	Pessimists who always look on the dark side.
• **Foreboding – with an urge to stool**	As in Argentum nitricum and Gelsemium.
• **Worry over family and friends**	'Old worry guts'.
• Intense sympathy for others	But it is usually seen as smothering the other.
• **Suspicious**	This comes out of their fear of what might happen.
• **Confusion**	Mind and constitution break down because of the strain.
• **Fear < twilight**	The least thing makes the child cry.
• **Fear of the dark**	Because the imagination runs riot.
• **Easily startled**	Again, the imagination conceives awful things.
• **Timid**	Great lack of confidence.
• **Anxious while straining at stool**	**Strange, Rare and Peculiar** symptom.
• **Quarrelsome**	Their caution is so intense it must be imposed on others.
• **Censorious**	They can be so negative they are unpleasant to be with.
• **Peevish**	They are a bit of a wet blanket to others.
• **< thinking about complaints**	Because the imagination takes off to think the worst.
• **Spoonerisms**	Mistakes in speaking.
• Stammering	Paralysis of the tongue and vocal cords.
• Lack of co-ordination	They know they cannot think, or carry out their business.
• Tired from the vexations of business	Worrying turns everything into a negative experience.
• Sensation of empty space between the brain and cranium	There is a lot of loss in this remedy.
• Epilepsy	From fright, at puberty. They pass urine when unconscious.
	< full moon.
• **Restless**	
• Legs on the go all night	The nerves are agitated.
• Progressive weakness of muscles	The nerves are worn down.
• Indescribable fatigue and heaviness of body	They are now worn down on the general level.
• Heaviness of eyelids	
• Involuntary urination when sneezing or blowing nose	Because muscle so weak.
• **Trembling and debility of limbs**	They cannot hold things stable. All is falling apart.
• **Numbness of single parts**	Prior to paralysis.
• **Paralysis of single parts**	Always < cold, dry winds.
• Paralysis of extensor muscles	They have an inability to reach out.
• Shortening of flexor muscles	Pulling limbs inwards.
• **Tendons shorten**	Limbs are drawn up and out of shape.
• Ankylosis	From tightening up of joint – tendons and muscles.

• **Loss of voice**	< cold, dry due to paralysis of vocal cords.
• **Tearing, burning pains paralyse and numb**	All this shows action on the nerves.
• **Chilly**	< excess heat.
• **Cough > cold drink**	**Strange, Rare and Peculiar.**
• **Warts**	Especially on tip of fingers and face.
• Frequent abscesses of gums	Low vitality.
• Ulcers in mouth	Low vitality.
• **Burning as if lime in stomach**	This can be an ulcer remedy.
• **Desires smoked meat**	In fact they cannot take fresh meat.
• **Cracks and fissures**	e.g. the linings of the nose, the corner of the eyes, bends of the fingers.
• **Fissure of the anus**	
• **Thick, crusty eruptions on head**	May have yellow-green discharge.
• **Copious, thick, viscid catarrh**	From all mucous membranes.
• **Own words re-echo in ears**	**Strange, Rare and Peculiar.**
• **Stool passes > when standing**	**Strange, Rare and Peculiar.**
• **Menses flow only in the day**	Leucorrhoea may flow at night.

Modalities

< fats
< exertion
< change of weather
< **twilight**
< thinking about complaints
< new moon
< **right side**
< **cold dry winds**

> warm, wet weather
> gentle motion

ACTIVITY 1

Causticum is << drying up. List the symptoms that refer to the dryness of the remedy. Try to give examples on the physical and mental plane.

ACTIVITY 2

Paralysis occurs after exposure to cold, dry conditions. Describe the common cold of the Causticum patient, noting especially the tendency to overexcite then paralyse nerves. Which parts will be affected?

ACTIVITY 3

From your observations, note the different ways that people might respond to *fright*. How do you respond to fright?

The Sensitive Worrier

The Causticum patient is vulnerable and nervous, on the one hand *timid* and *peevish*, on the other, *censorious* and *argumentative*. The patient is much worse if allowed to internalize problems, i.e. < *thinking about things* (Ignatia, Aconite) because the imagination takes it all out of proportion. This accounts for the overwhelming impact of a major keynote < *fright*. Many problems of Causticum are brought on from fright – hysteria, convulsions, epilepsy, retention of urine, paralysis. The examples all show the profound effect upon the nervous system. *Great sorrow* (*disappointed love*, etc.) and *prolonged anxiety* also wear this patient down so much, because nerves are affected. Thus *night-watching* wears down nervous energy.

There may be a heaviness, which becomes a tendency to fall asleep. The patient may feel as if they have the world on their shoulders, as they grow progressively weaker. Under continued strain there may be a *trembling*, then *clumsiness*, as *co-ordination is affected*. In extreme tiredness their *speech may be full of mistakes*. Take away the cause and they will probably recover. When they reach the constitutional stage they may be called '*old worry guts*', always looking on the black side, the prophet of doom, especially as regards family and friends. In reality the Causticum patient *identifies too closely* with the situation of others. They are too *sympathetic* or *empathetic* and put themselves into the situation, so they are really saying that they cannot cope. This is very similar to the Silicea patient, who fears failure or his/her own vulnerability. However, Silicea takes control by being *stubborn*. The Causticum patient becomes *suspicious* and *distrustful*. As the nervous energy is drained, the mind becomes *confused* and then nerves unco-ordinated. As in Silicea, it is really themselves they do not trust. They suffer severely from a *lack of confidence*.

In the child, the weak ego boundaries and the enhanced imagination become *fear*, of the dark especially. The least thing makes them cry or they *startle easily* (like the Silicea patient). Causticum is also very similar to Phosphorus and as with Phosphorus the fear is < *twilight*. The great difference is that the Phosphorus patient is an optimist and always bounces back, but the Causticum patient has a marked degree of *hopelessness* and *foreboding*. The Phosphorus patient is also basically an egotist, whilst Causticum, like Silicea and Pulsatilla, easily loses him/herself. The quarrels, the argumentativeness and the censoriousness are projections of their fear and concern, rather than their ego (as in Nux vomica).

ACTIVITY 4 Causticum is a deep, chronic remedy. Aconite is an acute remedy. Compare how each affects the nervous system differently when frightened.

Paralysis

When the nerves break down there are a great deal of symptoms.

On the acute level, cold dry conditions produce *sudden paralysis*, usually of the exposed part. On a deeper, chronic level, the paralysis develops more gradually and is accompanied by rheumatism.

If the nervous system is assaulted intensely, paralysis results. Causticum is one of the most common remedies of paralysis. As in Aconite, the *paralysis is in single parts*, e.g. an arm or just one muscle in the arm. In the acute and chronic picture, the paralysis is brought on, or intensified, by *exposure to cold, dry winds*. It is interesting to note that it is the *extensor muscles that are subject to paralysis* and the *flexor muscles which are shortened*, so the patient *cannot reach out*. The Causticum patient is drawn into their own inner world. Thus, as we expect, emotional trauma is also a cause and aggravation of the Causticum paralysis.

Many parts may be affected by the paralysis. In particular, the sphincter of the bladder is affected giving rise to the keynotes:

- Has to wait before the flow of urine starts
- Urine flows better sitting down
- Involuntary flow of urine when coughing, sneezing, blowing the nose or walking
- Cannot tell in the dark that urine passes (wets the bed).

In the rectum, too, they may not know they are passing a stool, or may *pass the stool > standing*.

In the throat, paralysis of the vocal cords may cause *stammering* or *hoarseness*, especially in the morning (Phosphorus has this symptom in the evening).

When they are worn down, mentally, e.g. by worries of business, the brain is fatigued, so *spoonerisms* may be common, or stammering, or simply *inability to think*.

In older persons, where the disease is more chronic or has crept on more gradually, there is a *gradual fatigue* and a *gradual progressive paralysis*. There may be *heaviness* of the body and eyes, reminding us of Gelsemium, which also attacks the nerves. The older person may show the *grumbling, pessimistic nature*. They may be negative and critical, adding a wet blanket that dampens others' enthusiasm and spirits. As their mind lessens in stature, so does the body. The muscles and tendons shrink. The height shrinks as the spine is ankylosed. They are numb, chilly individuals, who appear to lack sensitivity, when the opposite is the case and they are *easily hurt*, or offended.

In the acute stage before paralysis comes excitement. The exciting cause < fright may bring on epilepsy, especially around puberty. The *fits often occur in sleep* and the unconscious patient often urinates. If not in sleep, they may be seen to *fall to the left*. Hysteria may be a result of fright, leading to *extreme sensitivity to noise, touch, excitement* or the unusual. *Starting* may then be exaggerated and the patient may *jerk and twitch*.

ACTIVITY 5   Investigate chorea and St. Vitus' dance. How do the symptoms resemble those of the Causticum symptom picture?

Drying Up

The burning sensations of Causticum accompany dryness. The keynote in the stomach symptoms is *as if slaked lime burning*. Causticum, of course, derives its name, like caustic soda, from its ability to take water molecules from another compound and thus burn. There is a *burning thirst for cold drinks*, the haemorrhoids burn, it is a remedy of cystitis, with burning pains and, of course, it is an excellent remedy for burns, where these are so deep and the *skin feels tight and shrinks*. There is then a risk of scarring.

In the older person we see more clearly the drying effect of Causticum. The skin dries producing *cracks at the corner of the mouth, nose or eyes*, or in the bends of the fingers, or anus.

In rheumatism and arthritis it is also as if the limbs dry up and shrink. In fact the *muscles and tendons shorten* and it is this that produces the *deformity of limbs* that points to Causticum in arthritis. Before this, there is much stiffness as if there were no lubrication.

When Causticum is a remedy of chest complaints, there may be a *dry tickle in the larynx* that becomes a *hoarseness* in the morning. The catarrh is tough because it is dry. The *cough is hollow and dry*, aggravated by cold air, but ameliorated by sips of cold water. As the disease deepens the patient cannot cough deeply enough to bring up the phlegm. Eventually, the chest is tight and dry, with a severe burning pain.

The Causticum patient is generally chilled and < excessive heat, because it further dries them up.

ACTIVITY 6   Describe the symptoms of the Causticum patient with sciatica. Use as many of the keynotes and characteristic symptoms as appropriate.

ACTIVITY 7   Causticum is often labelled the 'witch remedy', because of its shrivelled, crooked appearance, many warts and gloom and doom countenance. Outline the symptom picture that would enhance this stereotype. Refer back to the keynotes and characteristic symptoms.

Similar Remedies

Kali carbonicum is a fearful type who sticks rigidly to convention, yet still ends up with crooked arthritis because of the pressures to conform. It also has the burning in the chest problems and a lupus on the left side of the nose.

Arsenicum has many burning pains and tends to be very critical and fearful of the future. In later stages, it may degenerate rapidly, but it is less a remedy of paralysis.

Aconite has paralysis from cold and dryness and it has the fear of Causticum. It may even produce the burning pains in the chest. When well, Aconite is robust and full of life and not at all pessimistic.

Phosphorus closely resembles Causticum when we look at the fear and local symptoms, such as the hoarseness. Phosphorus bounces back as the eternal optimist and is less prone to paralysis.

Phosphorus

Red amorphous phosphorus

Origin

H Noah Martin did a proving from a trituration of red amorphous phosphorus. Much information had already been gathered before this from the poisonings and Hahnemann made use of these when writing in his Materia Medica Pura. Today the remedy is produced from yellow phosphorus in a saturated solution of alcohol.

Characteristics of the Element

This is a volatile mineral which bursts into flame on exposure to air, so has to be stored in a salt solution. The Phosphorus patient also has a desire for salt and has phlegm with a distinct salty taste. The 'phosphorescent' glow on a moonlit sea is due to the presence of phosphorus in the bodies of many microscopic organisms. The name means 'the light bringer'. This is most appropriate, since the main place we find phosphorus within the body is in combination with iron, in haemoglobin, which has the function of taking up oxygen to provide energy. Of all the ways in which energy is used in the body, oxygen has the fastest turnover. The healthy phosphorus patient bounds with energy, is quick witted, is quick in movement and is quick to move on. Interest shifts rapidly, as in a child, and often tasks are left undone. No other remedy can be better described as the 'eternal child'. Indeed the other major role of phosphorus within the body is in homoeostatic balance with calcium: in the bones, whilst calcium fossilizes, phosphorus adds resilience!

Essence

There is so much energy in Phosphorus, but it is spread in so many directions that it is quickly *diffused*. Then there is little energy, so exhaustion follows. Usually there is a quick recovery rate, so the patient bounces back, but chronic debility produces *indifference*.

Keynotes and Characteristics

• **Enthusiasm easily dissipated**	They put so much energy into things.
• **Hypersensitivity**	The body reacts quickly.
• Quickness of mind	They are lively, witty types, when well.
• Apathetic	No energy when ill.
• **Indifference**	To loved ones even, as in Sepia.
• **Anxious**	Live on nerves.
• Fidgety all the time	Can't sit still.
• **Fear of dark**	< on their own.
• **Fear of ghosts and supernatural**	Although they avidly watch horror films.
• **Fear of thunderstorms**	Although they can watch them in fascination.
• **See monstrous faces on wall**	So much imagination.
• **Clairvoyant**	They are sensitive beyond the norm.
• **Sense exalted**	Sight and hearing very keen.
• **Difficulty hearing the human voice**	**Strange, Rare and Peculiar** symptom.
• **Lack of modulation in voice**	They have problems orienting themselves.
• Re-echoing in ears	Usually when catarrh is present.
• **Desire company**	They are not happy by themselves.
• **Need of lot of reassurance**	Because they cannot set and maintain their own standard.
• **Like to be magnetized or stroked**	They love massage.
• **Sensitive to atmospheres**	Especially to electrical charge, but also to moods and emotions.
• **Gullible**	Easily influenced and taken in.
• **Affectionate**	Love is an energy that flows from them.
• **Sympathetic**	Also want sympathy.

• **Excitable**	Children can be overexcited. It often prevents sleep.
• **Highly sexed**	And they like plenty of variety!
• Expose themselves	They prefer the freedom of no clothes. They also enjoy their bodies.
• < **twilight**	Which is when the Earth's magnetic tides change. The light also enables them to see ghosts then.
• **Vivid dreams**	Often amorous.
• **Exaltation of fancies**	Escape into day-dreaming.
• **Want to escape**	They do not like to be pinned down.
• Love spicy food and salt	The energy of spices is fast-flowing through them.
• < spicy food	It produces hot diarrhoea.
• **Desire cold drinks**	They will only drink milk if it is out of the fridge.
• Vomit water as soon as it is warm in the stomach	When the stomach is disordered.
• **Averse fish**	
• **Empty sinking feeling in stomach**	Their energy can suddenly go.
• **Flushes upwards, beginning in hands**	Often seen at menopause.
• **Burning pains**	Between the scapulae, up and down the spine, on the palms, in the lungs.
• **Bleed easily**	Piles, expectoration. Nose bleeds.
• Small wounds bleed a lot	Blood easily diffuses.
• Blood bright red and often stringy	
• **Bruise easily**	It may be indicated in serious blood and spleen disorders.
• Violent ebullitions and congestions	Especially on putting hands in hot water.
• **Stool gets out of bed 5 a.m.**	As in Sulphur.
• **As if the anus remains open**	Sphincters remain open and closed.
• **Left-sided**	
• Upper right, lower left	Hence it affects the right lung and the left knee.
• **History of pneumonia**	The Phosphorus patient often has a weak chest.
• **Rapid growth spurt, then weakness**	Because they have outgrown their strength.
• **Polypi**	Especially in the nose.
• **Loss of voice < evening**	Opposite time to Causticum.
• Tickly cough < talking	A lot of chest and catarrhal symptoms are talking.

Modalities

< before thunderstorm   > **after sleep**
< **twilight**   > **being magnetized**
< **lying on left side**
< **fright**
< when alone

ACTIVITY 8 — List those symptoms that illustrate diffusion. Separate them into mental and physical symptoms.

ACTIVITY 9 — The Phosphorus patient is very sensitive to energy in many different forms. Which symptoms show this?

Hyperactivity

One exciting cause of the Phosphorus patient is when the child, or the adolescent at puberty, puts on a *growth spurt* that may add 6 inches to his or her frame. He/she outgrows strength so the weak organs show dysfunction. The weak organs of this patient are the lungs, which gives us the other serious exciting cause, pneumonia. You may also see this patient change drastically after a prolonged bout of study, so the young Phosphorus student will find examinations deal a severe blow to health.

In health, the Phosphorus patient is characteristically *tall*, with dark or red hair, long eyelashes and an open honest face! He/she is *well co-ordinated*, often athletic. When you meet them you often feel they bound up to you like a puppy. They will sit on the edge of the chair eager to communicate and will open up easily to tell you of their thoughts and feelings, even though they are often *shy* – give them a little support and they will swamp you with data floridly described. The Phosphorus patient is *very sensitive*.

The senses are overreactive. A headache may develop if there is too much light. Deafness is common in the Phosphorus patient and interestingly I have seen much industrial deafness amongst phosphorus steelworkers and – illustrating the Law of Similars – despite the fact that both ears are affected by noise it is the left ear that goes first, or is worse affected. Phosphorus is a *left-sided* remedy. One very unusual symptom is *deafness to the human voice*. All other sounds can be heard and any hearing test will record adequate hearing, but the brain can get confused, so it cannot distinguish speech. This extraordinary symptom does not appear until the nervous system is under some stress. Another hearing symptom peculiar to the Phosphorus patient is the lack of ability to sing or hear the difference between musical notes. They cannot hear the difference because they can hear so much more and have never settled down to concentrate on distinguishing or sorting out the sounds. The Phosphorus patient can be so scattered he *cannot focus attention long*. She/he cannot concentrate. Their strong desire to be with others, and the great lengths they go to to be accepted, is a need to earth their experiences and orientate themselves. This is more necessary when we meet the *clairvoyant* Phosphorus patient. The range of reception here is even wider and more in need of others to help modulate the experience.

ACTIVITY 10 Study the symptoms of the digestive system. Which symptoms show this system hyperacting?

Hypersensitive

The openness of the senses gives rise to a major characteristic, ≪ *fear*. The Phosphorus patient is *easily frightened*. He/she is ≪ *alone* and ≪ *in the dark*. In the dark the eyes see every little flicker of light and every shadow. The very active brain groups these into shapes, into faces, and monsters, then the *vivid imagination* takes over and fear overcomes the patients. The acute hearing, likewise, picks up all sorts of sounds in the dark and the imagination elaborates. The situation is often complicated by the fact the Phosphorus patient is often psychic. Their fascination with the supernatural does not help! They love horror films but will stay awake in terror for nights afterwards.

Another overactive sense is the ability to pick up changes in *magnetism*. This poorly investigated sense in humans is very obvious in the Phosphorus patient. He/she is *aggravated at twilight* when the magnetic tides change and he/she is *worse before thunderstorms* as electromagnetism builds up in the atmosphere. Other remedies suffer headaches, etc, before thunderstorms, but the Phosphorus patient is generally worse. And, of course, they are terrified of lightning, whilst still staying up half the night fascinated by the storm! Lightning is also 'present' in pains, like lightning or electric shocks, that shoot *up* limbs – Phosphorus pains move *up*. The lightning-like nature shows the activity of nerves. When really exhausted and unable to sleep because of excitement, lightning shoots through the head, frightening them. Phosphorus patients – many cats and horses – *love to be stroked* and magnetized.

The sensitivity is seen in the personality. These people can be very shy *introverts*, or *extroverts* who are the life and soul of the party. It is not explained in full by the philosophical tenet that every medicine has two actions and this appears to be a contradiction, so needs more careful investigation.

The Phosphorus patient is very sensitive, very perceptive, very sensuous. They are frequently artists, actresses/actors, or artistic people in design. They are very aware of the outside world and of others. This can make them self-conscious and frequently does or, since they are usually intelligent, they learn the ropes and put on a show, or mask, that hides their shyness. How many extrovert people do you know are really lacking in confidence? One notable raconteur showed a Phosphorus trait when it was said of him that it did not matter if 1000 people in an audience gave him a fantastic welcome, if one person disapproved. He was then devastated and depressed. Another example is the teacher who cannot keep order because he/she cannot risk his/her popularity by disapproving. Phosphorus is one of the most *egotistic* remedies in the Materia Medica, but it is not motivated by power so much as a need to be liked and to have a safe position which gives them an orientation. But like Pulsatilla, they have so little stability of themselves that they must be continually reminded.

ACTIVITY 11 This is a common type amongst artists and the performing arts. Note a few observations. Does this extrovert really need so much support from others?

Too Much Wears Them Down

Thus Phosphorus will work very hard, will take on anything, will promise anything to buy popularity but they take on so much, they do little of it. Phosphorus patients cannot modulate their activities. When they let you down, they will be distraught and will do anything to make it up to you. As this cycle continues, they become *exhausted* and *depressed*. The nervous system is exhausted so you may not recognize this worn-out gloomy person as the bright enthusiastic Phosphorus patient. They may try to bounce back as before. They make a performance of their tragedy. They may be so disillusioned they retreat from the world. *Indifference* is not a symptom we often associate with the Phosphorus patient, but it is common at this stage.

Grief and shock weaken the lungs, so they are prone to bronchitis or worse. In acute grief they may develop pneumonia. Young girls may develop pneumonia at puberty. Puberty is a shock to the body, especially when they grow six inches in one year to outgrow their strength. It may be they only have a tendency to take colds. However, the Phosphorus patient can be so weakened that more serious illness appears as the body collapses. There are many kinds of blood disorders including *pernicious anaemia* and thrombocytopenia. It is a remedy of cancer, especially of the oesophagus, ME and AIDS. Once so exhausted, there is a very long way back to recovery. They will often respond well, then the patient splurges out enthusiastically expending all that energy engendered for healing. The relapse comes rapidly and is so profound it is even more difficult to revive them.

ACTIVITY 12 What is the symptom picture of the Phosphorus patient with pneumonia? Give symptoms from the Mental/Emotional and General level as well as particulars.

ACTIVITY 13 Why would you use Phosphorus for a patient who could not sleep at night?

Similar Remedies

Arsenicum is a remedy of great activity. It resembles Phosphorus in the profundity of the collapse. Both affect the lungs, liver and blood though Arsenicum does the last through its effect on the heart. The Phosphorus patient is more sociable than the Arsenicum patient, whilst the Arsenicum is an organizer who finishes things. Both need a lot of approval.

Lycopodium resembles Phosphorus in its field of action in the respiratory and digestive systems. Whilst Lycopodium also affects the kidneys and the urinary system, Phosphorus affects the reproductive system. Both remedies are performers who need a lot of support. Both are irresponsible – Phosphorus with the best of intention and ingenuity; Lycopodium as a coward is deceptive. Whilst they are often difficult to tell apart in physical symptoms, it is more easy on the mental and emotional level.

Silicea

Origin

The remedy was first proved by Hahnemann from river clay.

Characteristics of the Mineral

The remedy is obtained from pure clay. Silicon is one of the most common constituents of the Earth's crust, forming a compound with aluminium (clay) called *sial* and with magnesium, called *sima*. It is the basic mineral in soil! In crystalline form it is present in many rocks from which it breaks down to form sand, or grit – quartz. Many semi-precious stones are made from silicon. It is a transmitter of light and energy. It may come as no surprise that many stone circles were constructed, by ancient peoples, of rocks with a high proportion of quartz and most computers are dependent on their silicon chips!

In organic compounds, it is found in the stem of plants, enabling them to stand erect and it is found in the hard seed casing encapsulating and protecting the life force. Silicea gives form and structure to life. Conversely, there was a period of evolution, before Calcium became the major component of organic life, when Silicea was the main ingredient. That time is characterized by *no* limit to growth. Plants did not have any set size. We shall find the opposite in the remedy – like Lycopodium it is a remedy of stunted growth and where the head early on becomes angular and fixed. Or sometimes in the child we find the large 'undeveloped' head as in Calcarea carbonica.

Essence

The essence of Silicea is *lack of grit*. There is no energy. There is no will. The symptom picture alternates between a rigid, fixed state and an amorphous, dissolute state. Sometimes, both of these states are present at different levels, i.e. it is possible the patient is very stubborn and rigid, whilst there is a catarrhal state in the tissue.

Keynotes and Characteristics	• **Easily exhausted**	There is no stamina.
	• **< mental exertion**	The brain is supposed to contain more silicea than any other part of the body.
	• **Aversion to work**	There is no energy.
	• **Mental confusion**	When exhausted.
	• **< on waking**	Because a lot of energy is needed for consciousness.
	• **Sluggish thought**	Cognitive processes involve organization.
	• **Lack of concentration**	There is no energy.
	• **Absent-minded**	They cannot hold things together.
	• **Irritable if spoken to**	Because a response is called for.
	• **Obstinate**	This is self-protective.
	• **Fear of failure**	So do not try anything.
	• **Mild, yielding types**	Similar to Pulsatilla.
	• **Timid**	Like Bashful of the Seven Dwarfs.
	• **Reserved**	They do not demand from others.
	• **Cries when spoken to**	The child prefers to be an observer.
	• **Dreams of corpses and dead people**	They can be a little morbid!
	• **Startle easily**	At anything strange.
	• **Oversensitive to noise**	To a marked degree.
	• **Fascination for pins**	**Strange, Rare and Peculiar.**
	• **Fear of sharp implements**	They will speak of injections, for example, with dread.
	• **Left-sided**	The opposite of Pulsatilla.

• **Slow to heal**	Operation scars are still open a year later.
• All injuries suppurate	And are slow to heal.
• **Leaves scars**	Acne is a good example that leaves a lot of scars.
• **Nails distorted**	Also a lot of pus beneath.
• **Tendency to take colds**	Resistance is poor.
• **Profuse, thick, yellow or green discharge**	Silicea has a strong impact on glands and mucous membrane.
• **Suppuration of glands**	Its major action is on the lymphatic system.
• **Induration of glands**	
• Abscesses at root of teeth	Especially on the left side.
• Pustular styes	Compare with Pulsatilla and Staphysagria.
• **Profuse night sweats**	This is a major remedy of TB.
• **Sweats on the head**	Like Calcarea carbonica. Both < night.
• Sweaty head with weak ankles	And poor at maths.
• **Foul foot sweat**	Smells of old cheese.
• **Curvature of the spine**	It is also a remedy of rickets.
• **Large-headed children with open fontanelles**	As in Calcarea carbonica.
• Ulcers on lips	
• **Caries of bone, especially mastoid**	After pustular ear infections.
• Desires only cold food	Like Pulsatilla and opposite to Lycopodium
• Distended abdomen	Full of wind as in Lycopodium.
• Fissure of anus	As in Causticum.
• **Bashful stool**	Comes out, then goes back in again.
• **Flow of blood from uterus when baby sucks**	
• **Child refuses mother's milk**	It is too poor in quality.

Modalities

< cold, damp weather	> warmth
< **new moon**	> wrapping the head
< loud noises	> from being rubbed or massaged
< **mental exertion**	

ACTIVITY 14 List those symptoms that show the amorphous stage and a breakdown in integrity.

ACTIVITY 15 Silicea is described as a scrofulous type. What does this mean? Study the nature of Tuberculosis and how the organism that survives is changed by the disease.

Sensitivity

The Silicea patient is known to be *very sensitive* – like the silicon chip. He/she is *shy* and *introspective* and easily dissolves into an amorphous state of *no confidence*. At the party, the child will hold back from joining in. He/she will observe, think about it and join in in his/her own time, once he/she has given form to what is expected in the situation. There is much of the sensitivity, *fear* and shyness of the Phosphorus and Causticum patients. One main difference is that Silicea uses the rational mind to organize the sense data. Until he/she has done that there is no reaction. In fact until he/she has organized the data, the Silicea patient can become very *stubborn and fixed*. She *will not* join in. At other times they are open, interesting and curious. The child can have very mature thoughts, can contemplate abstract subjects like death, the stars, etc. and you will not fob them off with childish answers. Traditionally they are poor at maths and logical thought, but you will find that this only occurs when the mind is in the amorphous stage, which is an advanced stage of the disease process.

143

The modern child brought up without the overbearing, formal discipline of past times, is more sure of himself, so shows curiosity and a lively inner world. Whether large-headed or small-headed, they are *refined by nature*. The small-headed has *translucent skin*; the large-headed has the rosy cheeks and cheeky disposition that often reminds of Calcarea carbonica.

They are gentle and mild-mannered though persistent in their opinions. They are vulnerable. The sense organs, as in the Phosphorus patient, are open and sensitive. *Noise especially startles* the Silicea patient. They will play quietly but you will notice their play is *intelligent* and experimental, as well as *imaginative*. Watch them play and listen to their questions and the interesting, imaginative dialogue. Watch how they use their toys.

ACTIVITY 16   If you have the opportunity to watch children, look for the sensitive Silicea type. Note your observations.

The Amorphous Stage

The amorphous stage shows most of the keynotes of the remedy. You will find this in the older person when age is catching up on him/her. The picture is summed up as a *lack of grit*, a lack of central organizing power. You will find this at the end of the process with gross pathology of a glandular or respiratory character.

The person is *easily exhausted* and, as it is the most highly evolved parts that are being reduced to an earlier mode, the person is especially exhausted by mental pursuits such as reading and writing. There is much *mental confusion* after such activities and *after waking*. The patient is generally worse on waking, at that *point of change from subconsciousness to consciousness*.

As the situation deepens we will see *sluggishness of thought* and *lack of concentration* which may then deepen into *inability* or sheer *lack of intellect*. Other characteristics of Silicea arise out of this mental affliction, i.e. aversion to work, absent-minded, irritated especially by conversation and consolation – activities that require a response.

When the Silicea situation becomes chronic, we find the lack of grit stamped on the personality of the patient, so we see the *mildness, timidity, reserve* and *tearfulness* that closely resemble Pulsatilla. The person is introspective and does not waste energy being exciting or adventurous – this stage most resembles Calcarea carbonica – the amorphous oyster that retreats into its shell, defined in its limits by obstinacy and showing activity as irritability – when a piece of grit does enter, it is harmlessly encrusted as a pearl. Only a homoeopath could possibly liken a pearl to a TB cyst!

Calcarea carbonica is an easy-going amorphous lump until pushed, when it turns (like every Pulsatilla worm) into a tiger. Silicea, like Pulsatilla most of the time, under pressure will be flattened into a tearful puddle, becoming totally dependent and hopeless. Like Pulsatilla they will rescue themselves by taking on the structure of an outside force, but they can stand alone.

Beyond *irritability*, two other reactions are central to Silicea. One is *obstinacy* – digging in the heels as a protection to take the pressure off themselves. Another is the peculiar *dread of failure* which causes such anxiety that frequently they will not even attempt a situation. If they can be got past the obstinate stage, and their fears allayed, they often overcome their dread or aversion.

ACTIVITY 17   Describe the behaviour of the Silicea child at a party. Use keynotes and characteristics to illustrate your answer.

A Slow-acting Remedy

Silicea is a slow-acting remedy – as Kent says, the symptoms develop slowly in the proving. This is as you would expect in a substance that represents more than any other the very rocks beneath our feet – the slowest form of consciousness. We do not see rocks move, or grow, but they do move and change, aided by water.

Kent quotes (*Lectures in Homoeopathic Materia Medica* p 925 para 1) that 'these slow-acting remedies are deep and long acting and, therefore, capable of going so thoroughly into the vital order that they can route out hereditary disturbances'. In modern days, it has been noted that the speed of the remedy has changed, and whereas Calcarea carbonica was only given once in the lifetime of an adult by Tyler, it is now often necessary to repeat it.

This deepness is seen in the TB pathology, the emaciation, cysts and broken mucous membrane coughing up blood.

Silicea is described as a *slow healer*. Kent (*Lectures in Homoeopathic Materia Medica* p 926, para 5) states this is due to poor nutrition, but it could be better described as an inability to reform the pattern, because somehow the octave has changed to a lower level than appropriate (see Philosophy Lesson 8). Another way of putting this is that the Silicea patient lacks energy! A common and simple example is *scar tissue*. The epithelial cells are replaced by more fibrosed tissue which is inappropriate and does not fit into the original pattern. The form at one level has broken down, but reappears at a lower level. There appears to be a tendency for run down body tissue to fibrose, or change, from epithelial to connective tissue. *Fibroids* are a prime case of this, and Silicea is very useful in fibroids, as is Calcarea carbonica. 'Fibrositis', knotty muscles, should be familiar to you, and indicate a run-down rheumatic constitution. Rheumatism is primarily of the tuberculoid miasm to the homoeopath, and as such, is worse for cold and damp as is Silicea. A rheumatic person is not just run-down. He/she is phlegmatic (lymphatic) and Tuberculinum, the nosode of Tuberculosis, has as its target organ, the spleen, which controls the lymph system. The lymph, the great sea of the body, is closely involved in the interchange of nutrients and waste products, though at a much slower rate than the blood. Silicea works through the lymph system and its controlling glands, whilst Phosphorus works through the blood.

The slower acting defence mechanism is suppuration. Thus in the Silicea patient *every wound suppurates*. *Abscesses* are common and even ulcers. The glands are a rich area of activity. These suppurate. Thick catarrhs are common, usually *yellow*, but *green* in respiratory disease. *Sweats are often profuse*, but notable for their *foul smell* of *old cheese*. When the process deepens further, as in the ear, the *bones are attacked* and *caries* result. Mastoiditis and abscesses under the teeth are common. *Rickets* and *curvature of the spine* are common in children within TB communities.

ACTIVITY 18 Describe the symptoms of earache in a Silicea child. Use keynotes and characteristics where appropriate.

ACTIVITY 19 Trace the symptoms as the disease process deepens from a cold through a throat inflammation into the lungs in the Silicea patient. What distinguishes Silicea in a case of Tuberculosis?

Similar Remedies

Pulsatilla presents a similar symptom picture of shyness and yielding. It is also a remedy of the lymphatic system, producing many catarrhs. Pulsatilla seldom goes into the lungs though. It is a right-sided illness, whereas Silicea is left-sided. The picture is complicated when both move to the other side as the case deepens.

Hepar sulphuris has festering wounds like Silicea. Both have a strong effect on the glands. Hepar sulphuris tends to be more active and irritable and more sensitive to slight draughts and touch.

Phytolacca is a major remedy of glands which suppurate. It also has tumours. Like Silicea, it has foul discharge and a strong effect on fibrous tissue. It has the same indifference as the disease deepens.

Mercurius strongly resembles Silicea in its effect on glands and bones, rotting away and producing foul discharges. Like Silicea, Mercurius is easily swayed and is sensitive to the atmospheres surrounding them. Mercurius tends to be more bloody and more rapid in its decay.

ACTIVITY 20

From reading the lesson and the recommended textbooks you should be able to make a table for Causticum, Phosphorus and Silicea showing the following:

Exciting causes
Modalities
Fears
Effect on nervous system
Effect on glands
Weather reaction
Personality.

 SELF-TEST QUESTIONS

You will find the answers to these in the text, and they can be checked in the answer section.

1. How does fright affect these three remedies?
2. When is the Silicea patient obstinate?
3. Where are the warts to be found on the Causticum patient?
4. Where does the Phosphorus patient usually escape to?
5. How would the Silicea patient demonstrate its fascination for pins?
6. Give four exciting causes of Causticum.
7. What is strange about the Silicea patient's sweat patterns?
8. Which remedy desires smoked meat?
9. Of what is the Phosphorus patient afraid?
10. Which remedy dreads failure?
11. Compare the sidedness of all three remedies.
12. Which remedy is irritable when spoken to?
13. What is significant about the paralysis of the Causticum patient?
14. What sometimes happens when the Phosphorus patient takes a cold drink?
15. What are the results of mental confusion in the Silicea patient?
16. What is peculiar about the nosebleed of the Phosphorus patient?
17. Why is Causticum called 'old worry guts'?
18. Which remedy has cracks at the corner of the eyes and nose?
19. What kind of food does the Silicea patient desire?
20. How would you describe the pains of the Phosphorus patient?
21. Of what is the Causticum patient afraid?
22. What stops the Phosphorus patient from sleeping?
23. What is peculiar about the stool of the Silicea patient?
24. What is interesting about the hands of the Phosphorus patient?
25. Which remedy is anxious whilst straining at stool?
26. Describe the acne of the Silicea patient.
27. State the modalities of Phosphorus.
28. What happens to the Silicea mum when baby is suckling?
29. Describe the voice symptoms of Phosphorus.
30. What happens to the legs of the Causticum patient at night?

Further Studies

Causticum
1. Discuss how fear affects the Causticum patient.
2. Compare and contrast Causticum and Phosphorus.
3. Describe the paralytic state of Causticum and, especially, how this may have arisen.
4. Which are the main remedies whose causation is cold dry winds? Name at least *four* and write a few lines on how each is commonly disturbed by this exciting cause. How do you differentiate between them?
5. Through what stages does the mental state of Causticum develop?
6. State how the rheumatism of Causticum differs from that of Rhus toxicodendron.
7. In what symptoms might Causticum resemble Arsenicum in digestive disorders?
8. Compare Causticum and Thuja.

Phosphorus
1. Phosphorus is seen often as the lightbearer – how is this reflected in the symptom picture of the remedy?
2. Phosphorus often comes up in treating a case of Lycopodium or of Arsenicum. How can this be?
3. Why is Phosphorus of use in bleeding?
4. Phosphorus bruises easily. Compare it to at least two other remedies that bruise easily.
5. Compare the delusions of Phosphorus with those of Belladonna and Stramonium.
6. What are the symptoms of Phosphorus in lung problems?
7. What is the similarity between Allium cepa and Phosphorus?
8. Compare Phosphorus and Pulsatilla in relationships.
9. How would you choose between Phosphorus and Aconite in fears? Are there any other remedies you would also consider in a similar case?
10. Compare Phosphorus and Sepia.

Silicea
1. Compare the lung symptoms of Silicea and Phosphorus.
2. Describe a wound that needs Silicea to cure it.
3. How might Silicea be of use for scars or adhesions? What is the difference between these?
4. Compare the Silicea and the Calcarea child in behaviour and appearance.
5. Outline how the essence 'lack of grit' appears in the Silicea symptom picture.
6. Silicea is often considered a chronic of Pulsatilla. Look at the symptom picture of both and state any similarities you see.
7. When does Silicea resemble Lycopodium?
8. Describe a person that might respond to Silicea.
9. Review how Silicea affects the nervous system of a patient.
10. List the modalities of Silicea.

Three Remedies from Animal Sources

Lachesis, Tarentula, Cantharis

Aim: To determine how the behavioural characteristics and idiosyncracies of the animal are reproduced in the patient needing the remedy.

Objectives: To outline the characteristics of the poison and of the animal behaviour.
To link the characteristics of the animal to the proving symptoms of the remedy.
To describe the patient in terms of the animal characteristics.

Headings: INTRODUCTION
LACHESIS: Origin; Essence; Nature of the Snake; Keynotes and Characteristics; Modalities; The Personality; Overactivity or Sluggishness of Mind; Congestion; Sepsis and Ulceration; Similar Remedies
TARENTULA: Origin; Essence; Nature of the Spider; Keynotes and Characteristics; Constant Movement; Intensity; Local Affections; Similar Remedies
CANTHARIS: Origin; Essence; Nature of the Fly; Keynotes and Characteristics; Modalities; Frenzy; Inflammation; Burns; Similar Remedies
REVIEW APIS: The Character of the Bee; Effect of the Bee Sting
SELF-TEST QUESTIONS
FURTHER STUDIES

Introduction

Primitive cultures have long held beliefs in such things as animal totems, in which an individual, or a tribe, put themselves under the protection of an animal deity. In so doing they emulated the behaviour of the animal. Whilst usually they avoided killing members of that species, some ritualistically ate parts of the animal in order to acquire its prized attributes. Martial arts, such as Kung Fu and Tai Chi have studied and adapted animal behaviour to enhance their art. Many Hatha yoga positions are based on animals.

Our language is full of allegories of animals: as sly as a weasel, as cunning as a fox, as stubborn as a mule, as agile as a monkey. These refer to mental skills, personality types and body attributes.

When you study homoeopathy you will find that this goes much deeper. You will be amazed at how closely the human can resemble the animal. There are reasons for this. Many of our remedies are specialized life forms. Some have peculiar adaptations, like the ink sac of the Sepia, or the poison of the snake. Many belong to a particular phase in evolution where they developed special mutations like the Lycopodium moss and the Equisetum fern. Others had specialities like the organized social life of the bee.

I think you will find this lesson quite fascinating. It should lead you to a new study of life that will enhance your understanding of Materia Medica.

Before we begin though, I want to point out that the homoeopath does not persecute or torture animals. Many of the animal products used by the homoeopath are venoms, so the animal does not have to be killed to obtain them. If the animal is killed, only one is needed because the remedies are diluted. They contaminate other materials, so even a very small amount goes a long way. When we come to study Tarentula Cubensis, we will see that it was only one spider and when the bottle was dropped, all sorts of impurities got into the bottle, so there is no way the remedy can be repeated, but because the homoeopathic remedy is diluted continually that is not a problem.

Lachesis

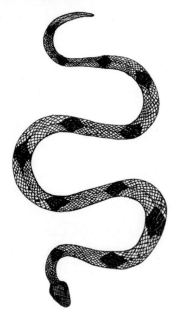

Lachesis muta

Latin name:	Trigonocephalus lachesis
Common name:	Surucuccu or bushmaster
Genus:	Ophidia
Habitat:	The humid forests of tropical South America and the Caribbean

Origin

Constantine Hering proved the remedy. He first developed symptoms whilst handling the crude venom.

Essence

The peculiar characteristic of the snake is the venom which is produced from a specialized digestive gland. Its purpose is destruction through coagulation of the blood. The theme that runs through this remedy is *digestion*. It destroys insidiously, eating away, creating much sluggishness and congestion.

Nature of the Snake

This is a very striking black snake with red or yellow diamonds along its back. It is found in the jungles of tropical America. Its character is also quite striking. I am told that it lurches at the genitals when it strikes and that it is one of the few snakes that coil to the left. I have never been able to validate these facts but retain the thought, because the myth is useful to help students to remember this remedy.

The nature of any snake is that it is very vulnerable around the neck – if you hold the snake's neck it is almost harmless, unless it is a rattlesnake, or a spitting cobra. The Lachesis patient we will find is also very vulnerable around the neck. The snake has a venomous tongue, and the Lachesis patient is very loquacious and has a good line in sarcasm. He or she is also inclined to stick out the tongue, or even to flick it in and out like a snake!

The most developed sense organ of the snake is touch. The Lachesis patient has a strange, rare and peculiar symptom regarding touch. He or she is worse for slight pressure and better for firm pressure. They are also very *touchy* people who become very suspicious and jealous.

I am using the word 'very' a lot in this remedy. It is a remedy that has strong characteristics, or that strongly expresses its characteristics.

The snake is an elongated tube that specializes in digestion. Once the snake eats, it is almost incapacitated. It has an enormous lump which grows smaller as the meal progresses down the alimentary canal and after eating, the snake is very sluggish. The Lachesis patient has strange, rare and peculiar symptoms of lumps especially in the chest and abdomen and he/she is much worse after eating.

The snake is a cold-blooded animal which takes on the temperature of the surrounding area. The Lachesis patient is chilly and does not care much for heat. There is such a sluggish flow that he/she cannot stand the heat, or motion, or digestion or anything that increases the rate of activity. He/she is particularly worse after sleep because on waking they have to move about.

Keynotes and Characteristics

• < **after sleep**	Because they become more and more dopey in sleep. This is one of the few remedies that sleep into the aggravation. Most are better sleep and rest.
• < **autumn**	When everything slows down. The sap falls in plants.
• < **sun**	Because it requires more activity of the blood.
• < **heat**	As above.

The above four symptoms are more than modalities. They are generalities because the whole person is affected.

- **Ascending symptoms** — Flushes, etc., upwards.
- **Left-sidedness**
- **Left side to right side** — The opposite of Lycopodium.
- **Sensitive to touch** — Touch is the most evolved sense of the snake.
- **< slightest touch, > firm touch** — The first excites whilst the second supports and controls.
- **Cannot bear anything around the neck** — This is the most sensitive part of the snake. They never wear a scarf.
- **Cannot bear tight clothing** — i.e. around the abdomen in digestive complaints.
- **Constrictions** — The movements of the snake are repeated constrictions and relaxations of circular muscle.
- Pains come in waves — Like a ripple of locomotion along the snake's body.
- **Spasms**
- Constipation — Because of paresis.
- **Sensation of balls** — Particularly in the chest.
- Ball in throat rises when they swallow — Sepia has this too.
- Ball rolling about in the abdomen, bladder, etc.
- **Venous congestion** — Circulation is very sluggish and congested.
- Blue, mottled skin — As the veins are engorged.
- Varicose veins — That look blue and bulbous.
- Thrombosis — The ultimate of venous congestion.
- Haemorrhoids with hammering pains — Because of congestion.
- **Black blood, soon coagulates** — You can see this in great clots with menses.
- Ulceration — Mottled purple because gangrenous.
- Sepsis — In wounds, suppuration of glands, ulcers.
- Foul discharges — Wherever discharge occurs.
- **Small wounds bleed profusely** — The blood will not coagulate. This is the opposite of coagulation.
- **Haemophilia** — The clotting factor is affected.
- **Palpitations** — The heart thuds when overexcited in any way.
- **Throbbings** — As veins are engorged.
- **Flushes upwards** — Particularly at the time of menopause.
- **Heart feels too big** — The heart is the target organ behind the circulatory system, so it is eventually disordered.
- As if the heart hanging by a thread — **Strange, Rare and Peculiar.**
- Wants to be fanned slowly, at a distance — So sensitive to touch of air.
- **Stops breathing as soon as falls asleep** — Stupor so overcomes them even the brain sleeps.
- Tongue trembles when protruding — There is a lot of muscular weakness in the remedy.
- **Tongue sticks out** — Like the snake.
- **Tongue flicks in and out** — As above.
- **Excitable** — This remedy has many similarities to Phosphorus.
- **Easily startled** — The nervous system is very sensitive.
- **Touchy** — They are so unsure of themselves they take offence easily.
- **Suspicious** — One patient described herself as a snake in the grass.
- **Fear of being poisoned** — Like the snake they expect to be hunted. They may say they are full of poison.
- **Cynical and mocking** — They erode reality.
- **Jealous** — They need so much themselves they cannot spare any good thoughts for others.
- **Malicious** — Especially with the tongue - sarcasm.
- Project poison into the atmosphere — So destructive of others.

- **Indifferent**
- Averse to talking

Life is so hurtful they lose interest in things.
People with pent-up emotions explode in a flood of words

- **Loquacious**
- Flick from one subject to another
- **Delusions**
- Think they are under control of a superior being.
- Hear voices telling them to do strange things – like kill someone.
- Dead relatives appear before them and they speak to them, yet know they are dead.
- Fear damnation
- Feel they have sinned away their hour of grace.
- **Guilt**
- **< before menses**
- **< when menses just about to start but won't start**
- **< menopause**

- Errors in perception
- **Religious insanity**

- Voluptuous thoughts
- **Vivid dreams**

- Dreams of revenge, of lust, ghosts, quarrels, snakes
- Dreams of the dead

It is a form of discharge.
Like the tongue!

You will see this remedy in psychopathic killers.

This takes away what little confidence they have.
In sluggish types where there is congestion.
Sluggish but > discharge.

There are so many symptoms here including flushes and congestion. It is seen here because this is the end of the discharge.
Time passes slowly.
In this remedy, the expectations of any authority evoke guilt and self criticism that further destroy confidence.
Yet do not always have the confidence to act.
Denied a full life outside because of lack of confidence, they retreat within.

They see dead bodies, dead relatives. They dream they are dead themselves. They dream of their own funeral. The decay is visible in the subconscious.

Modalities

< **after sleep**
< **slight touch**
< **sun**
< **autumn**
< **heat**
< **suppressed discharges**
< **before menses**

> **discharges**
> firm pressure
> commencement of menses

ACTIVITY 1   List the symptoms of sluggish circulation. Are these different from the symptoms of congestion?

ACTIVITY 2   List those symptoms that indicate decay and perversion of function or structure.

The Personality

They are basically *shy* people who *lack confidence*, who are yet sensuous with a lot of pent-up emotion. When the *feelings are suppressed*, or there is a trauma such as *grief* or *disappointed love*, the need is more release of thought and feeling. Anger and temper may be explosive, or there is an acceleration of the mental faculties, so they sit up late with *many thoughts*. There is *increased power of originality* and *imagination*. A discharge on the mental level is the best sign here that the patient is coping though it may not be nice for those around, because they may *prattle* on without allowing others a word in edgeways and they may *jump from one subject* to another which makes them very difficult to keep up with. Unfortunately, the vivid imagination more often leads to *suspicion* and mistrust because they are so unsure of themselves. They expect to be hurt and go out to meet it as it were. They are *quarrelsome*, *touchy* and nervous. We could, in fact, say that they are their own worst enemy and destroy themselves with their imagination and suspicion which comes out of their lack of confidence that anything good could possibly happen to them. Their mistrust of the world makes them *self-centred* and defensive. This often makes them *cynical* and mocking. If they fear they are not good enough in themselves, they will attack others before they can be attacked. This is another aspect of digestion and destruction – they turn their powers on to others and can become very nasty people indeed.

You must understand them as shy people who are defending themselves, like the snake. Thus they hold to loved-ones tenaciously and can be very *devious* and *inventive* in their schemes. One Lachesis patient I treated described herself as a snake in the grass because she was too shy to attack directly to get what she wanted, but she set out like the snake to track down what she wanted and made sure she got it. It is one of the remedies of *insane jealousy*. No other remedy has such jealousy or intensity.

ACTIVITY 3 You will have observed characters like this. Note some observations as to how they cope with crisis. What did you hear them say? What was the tone of the voice? Describe their posture. What emotions did you see?

Overactivity or Sluggishness of Mind

On the mental level, the remedy breaks down in two ways – the overactivity becomes *insanity* and the sluggishness becomes *immobility*.

If the pressure is mental, insecurity is created by their own thoughts that eat into them. They will spit back and weave others into a web of emotional blackmail. They are *easily moved to laughter* and tears and *will rage at trifles*. Their *frustration* and *dissatisfaction* will lead to an escapist dream life, where they can control and feel safe. The delusions will eventually escape into everyday life. First will come the *imaginings* and *suspicions*, the *insane jealousy*, the *fear of being poisoned*, then the *delusions*. They dream of being dead, even during waking hours, and can even see the preparations for their own funerals. They see the dead loved one sitting there and will have a conversation with them right in front of you.

The immobility shows as *indifference* and *aversion to talk*. They are simply not interested in their work or business. As they withdraw inwards, once again you may see the dreams that fulfil what everyday life cannot, but you also see the *depressions* which become *suicidal*. They do not wash, or care for themselves. They make sly demands on others, or have caustic conversations in which they sneer at others through their cynicism. You will find these people in the novels of A J Cronin (*Hatter's Castle*) or in George Douglas Brown's *The House with the Green Shutters* – it is very Calvinistic.

The paranoid state of Lachesis is quite frightening. They may feel themselves *under the control of a superior being*, or may *hear voices telling them to do things*, even to kill others. There are some famous criminals that might have benefited from Lachesis! They may have *religious insanity*, but even this is turned inwards to destroy, so they *fear damnation* and *feel* they have *sinned* away their *day of grace*. Back comes the depression.

ACTIVITY 4 Make two lists, one of overactivity of mind and the other of sluggishness. Can you find these symptoms in the *Mind* section of the Repertory?

Congestion

Before the breakdown stage there is a phase of overactivity of the blood, producing *throbbings* and *pulsations*, *palpitations* even, and *flushes upwards*. Some of these are only present when there is organ dysfunction – then there are many other symptoms.

The headache is an example of a minor ailment that shows *congestion*. There is a *fullness* with throbbing pains and sensitivity to light. This may appear *after an over-rich meal* when it may be accompanied by *black flickerings* before the eyes. Here the liver is congested. If the situation were chronic there would be troublesome *constipation*. The headache may also appear *before menses* when the blood is thickened because the liver is again slowed down. This is a major remedy of liver disorder in alcoholics, so there may be more symptoms than simply headaches. The headache often appears in the morning because they seem to become more sluggish and congested the more sleep they get.

Where there are glandular problems, there is fullness, dark *discoloration*, throbbing pains, *sensitivity to touch*. Some glands are less able to discharge. Others such as mammae and ovaries may be worse before the menstrual flow starts.

Systematic congestion is seen in venous stasis which could be a *swollen abdomen* that *feels bruised* and very sensitive to touch. Often the result of abdominal congestion and constipation is *piles* which throb *as if a thousand hammers* affected them. Varicose veins often build up in pregnancy and disappear after delivery, or they may appear later in life, giving a *blue mottled appearance* to the leg, there can be ecchymosis, and a troublesome throbbing. Once again, they are sensitive to slight touch and better for firm support.

The heart problems of the Lachesis patient are mainly due to congestion. Palpitations and flow of blood to the head are examples. Much later, they may suffer from congestive heart disease with pulmonary oedema, or oedema in the extremities.

ACTIVITY 5 Describe earache, or a congestive problem in the Lachesis patient. Use as many keynotes as appropriate.

Sepsis and Ulceration

On the physical level the action of the remedy, like the snake venom, is to produce sepsis on an acute level, then on a deeper level, to produce sluggishness that becomes ulceration. In both instances the mode of action is through the blood.

The main acute complaint is in the throat. There is inflammation and swelling, producing the typical Lachesis *burning pains*. The glands, especially the tonsils, suppurate, producing *foul breath*, then there is a liability to ulcerate. The person feels as if he/she is choking although solids can be swallowed easily there is *great difficulty in empty swallowing* – a very strange symptom. Once again, this is the nature of the snake which just opens its jaws and swallows anything! Each time the patient swallows, there is a *shooting pain up to the left ear*. And, as this is the neck area, we see that other snake symptom of *great sensitivity to touch*. Lachesis is one of the major remedies for true diphtheria, when a membrane is exuded like a second skin to close up the throat and cause death by blocking the airway. When it is the right remedy, you will see many of the symptoms in italics.

The other major area affected by the remedy is the genitals. In the female, in particular, there is much trouble with the uterus. Each month the uterus grows a skin, the endometrium, and each month if she does not become pregnant, this is sloughed off. In the Lachesis patient there is much pain before menses, because the endometrium comes off in large pieces, which are passed with difficulty. *Once the flow of blood starts she gains much relief.* This is called *membranous dysmenorrhoea*. It is a serious condition that can cause *sterility*. Another menstrual symptom is the *black, offensive blood* that can be passed. This is like the congealed blood produced by the snake venom. At menopause we see other keynote symptoms, *flushing upwards* and into the head which feels congested – this is one of the remedies of HBP, especially around menopause. There may also be palpitations then and *heavy bleeding* from the uterus, often associated with *fibroids* which grow in the uterus and are a sign of the slowing down of the life process which breaks down into a fibrosed state. The women who produce these are often slowing down in many ways. Look carefully at the full expression of the life force in each patient, i.e. take the total symptom picture.

154

ACTIVITY 6 Describe the Lachesis symptom picture in a case of diphtheria. Use as many keynotes as appropriate.

There is so much one can say about this polycrest. I will finish with two of its peculiar symptoms. It is common to find lump sensations in Lachesis. This might be a lump in the throat during tonsillitis, or a ball sensation in the rectum with piles, or it can be the *sensation of a ball rising from the stomach to the chest* in digestive or respiratory complaints. This sensation is very common in acute problems, or in inflammatory complaints. Another symptom that is also common in these situations is the *movement of symptoms from the left to the right*. Many of the symptoms of Lachesis move upwards.

ACTIVITY 7 Compare the Lachesis and Sepia symptom picture in a menopausal woman. Use appropriate keynotes and characteristic symptoms.

Similar Remedies

Sepia There is a strong relationship between Sepia and Lachesis. Both have venous stasis and the ascending movement of symptoms, including lump sensations. It is possible to find the Sepia type as an intimidating dragon who can be vicious, but she is usually more irritated and defensive than vengeful. Both have a strong effect on the reproduction system.

Lycopodium is closely related to Lachesis, as a liver remedy. The inertia of Lycopodium produces a stasis, particularly in the kidneys and digestive system. Lycopodium is more a remedy of the lungs and lymphatic system than heart and circulation as in Lachesis. Both lack confidence and are not honest and open. Lycopodium tends to show the vindictive side of their nature only at home. Lachesis may be careful about exposing their maliciousness.

Ledum may be difficult to distinguish from Lachesis in problems of circulation. Both are left-sided and symptoms move to the right. Both are blue and cold with burning, so here there is local congestion. Both are < heat, or anything that quickens circulation.

Carbo vegetalis is a sluggish, congested remedy of venous stasis. There is blueness and lack of vital heat. The varicose veins throb. One of its differences from Lachesis is its right-sidedness.

Tarentula

Latin name:	Lycosa tarentula
Common name:	Tarantula
Natural order:	Araneideae

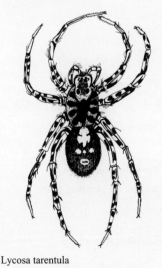

Lycosa tarentula

There are two Tarentula remedies – Tarentula Hispanica and Tarentula Cubensis. The story goes that Tarentula Cubensis was preserved in a bottle and on its way to a homoeopathic pharmacy in Europe the bottle was dropped and impurities got into the rotting mass, so it cannot be reproduced as a remedy, because no one knows what is really in the bottle. Tarentula Cubensis is thus used for more septic states – because it rotted! Because I want to compare the symptoms with the characteristics of the animal, I will concentrate on Tarentula Hispanica.

Origin

The proving was done by the Marquis Nunez from a tincture prepared from crushed, live spiders.

Essence

The remedy has a powerful effect on the nerves, creating *rhythmic, jerking movements*. It is a remedy of violent movement.

Nature of the Spider

It is a large hairy spider whose venom affects the nervous system. Have you ever watched a spider move – very fast, it scuttles, or like a clockwork toy it jerks and twitches. They silently await their prey, or scurry about in all directions if disturbed.

Keynotes and Characteristics	

• **Extreme restlessness**	They can't stop.
• **Fidgety**	
• **Hurried motion**	Spiders are always moving fast.
• **Constant motion, through < motion**	
• Muscles twitch and jerk	Think of the movements of the Flamenco dancer.
• Restless legs want to walk	
• **Chorea**	Jerky, spasmodic movements.
• **Rhythmic movements**	These may be subconscious.
• Roll on ground from side to side	During intense laughter or tears.
• Can run better than walk	**Strange, Rare and Peculiar symptom.**
• Sensitive to music	They may dance whenever music is heard.
• **Impulsive**	The energy within erupts.
• Cunning	Will put on a show only when you are looking.
• **Discontented**	They have strong emotional needs but are frustrated in feedback and support.
• **Moods suddenly alternate**	They will laugh then cry. See above. A slight cause may change their direction.
• < disappointed love	**Exciting cause.**
• < bad news	**Exciting cause.**
• < scolding	They have a pride which is insulted.
• **Hysteria**	When the doors to emotion open, there is a flood.
• **Aversion to black/yellow/red/green**	**Strange, Rare and Peculiar.**
• **Destructive**	Tears clothes, etc. Even hurt themselves.
• **Kleptomania**	Is it attention seeking?
• **Periodicity of symptoms**	Yearly, or at same hour.
• **Chilly**	Fire is created in the movement.
• Hyperaesthesia	< least excitement. The nerves are further over-stimulated.
• Tips of fingers very sensitive	Like the toes of the spider.
• **Spine sensitive to touch**	Causing spasm in chest. **Strange, Rare and Peculiar.**
• Burning, stinging pains	In particular symptoms.
• **Numbness with prickling**	The nerves are involved.
• Sexual excitement	As soon as genitalia touched.
• **Voluptuous itching**	That drives the patient mad.
• Headache > rubbing head on pillow	< least noise, < stooping.
• Photophobia with headaches	Right pupil enlarged.
• Flatus from vagina	**Strange, Rare and Peculiar** symptom.
• Menstrual flow profuse with erotic spasms	Once again the reproductive organs are strongly affected by spasm.
• **Crave raw food**	
• **Crave cold water**	
• **As if cold water poured on the head**	**Strange, Rare and Peculiar** symptom.
• **Sepsis**	With purple discoloration and burning pains.
• **Fibrous tumours**	
• **Copious sweat at night**	With pain in the spleen.
• Cough at night > smoking	**Strange, Rare and Peculiar** symptom.

156

Modalities

< motion   > open air
< touch   > music
< noise   > smoking
< **periodicity**   > rhythm – massage, dance, riding

ACTIVITY 8   List those symptoms of restlessness.

ACTIVITY 9   How does spasm show in respiratory symptoms? Use as many keynotes and characteristic symptoms as appropriate to illustrate your answer.

ACTIVITY 10   Research the effect of spider poison on the nervous system. How does this relate to the symptom picture of Tarentula?

Constant Movement

Restlessness is the first symptom of importance. It is very noticeable in acute problems, or in children. There is *constant movement*. On the mind level this translates as busyness – they need to be on the go. Physically, the limbs and muscles *twitch and jerk* often showing *cross laterality*, so it is the right arm and the left leg that twitch (See Phosphorus). There is a *macabre rhythm* to the movement, so it is often called dancing. The myth surrounding the Tarantula is that the victim once bitten dances till death. The patient is very *sensitive to rhythm*, as in music.

The rhythm can be seen also in the *periodicity* of the remedy, or even in the *alternating moods*. The moods can vary between anger and sadness, but the *anger can be violent* and consuming, threatening. She/he can be *angry if contradicted*. The sadness consumes her. She will not be spoken to, *tears her clothes* and *weeps if consoled*. *Hysteria* is the word used to describe sudden and unaccountable changes in mood. The passion and *impulsiveness* is the unsmooth dance on the emotional level. The emotions reach, like the spider, to consume those around. Emotional blackmail is seen in its full meaning in this *possessive* woman. The spider spins a web to trap things and destroy their motion. The hunter nature of the spider is seen in the way this patient *feigns illness*, especially *fainting*, then is OK when your back is turned. She is described as *cunning* and *destructive*. It is also one of the few remedies for *kleptomania*!

On the physical level the activity is seen in the *fidgetiness* and restlessness, in jerking and twitching, and in *itch*. The itch may be creeping and *crawling all over the body* or mainly in the soles. This is one of the remedies of violent *cystitis* which is described as a *voluptuous itch*. An *acrid discharge* is often present. As the nerves are affected the itch may become a *burning* in the parts, or on an even deeper level, there may be *neuralgias*, with *prickling* as of a *thousand needles*. *Chorea* is then the general state which arises when the disease deepens to the general level.

Intensity

The intensity will eventually lead to *insanity*, < *after grief, disappointed love* or *intense excitement*. Even here, there is a rhythm as the insanity comes in *paroxysms*! There are phases of *intense activity, then quietness*. In the active phase, she will sing and dance, and weep at any slight excitement. She may explode with violence if she even thinks she has been insulted, or she will petulantly *refuse to answer*. A mental picture of the flamenco dancer helps to conceive a vision of the Tarentula patient in this phase.

The passion may be very sexual, so much so that she may become very provocative and '*lose all shame*'. At the height of her hysteria she may laugh and scream. She may also have a strong *aversion* to the colours *green*, *red* and *black*, especially where they appear together. This may excite her and bring on the hysteria. Sometimes she may *see monstrous faces* and *ghosts*, or she may *see strangers in the room*. On the one hand, she can hit her head against a wall, or launch forth at others, or she can sink into such dire depression she *wants to hide*. More normally, she is described as *flighty* with a tendency to overreact. Anxiety is the main mental/emotional symptom and this affects the heart, so we get what is called *cardiac anxiety*. Arsenicum also has this. Aconite and Phosphorus are more likely to feel anxiety in the stomach.

ACTIVITY 11   Describe the intensity of the Tarentula child in fever.

Local Affections

Tarentula Hispanica is more a remedy of inflammation and irritation than sepsis. It has a more powerful effect on the nerves, causing neuralgias, with numbness and prickling pains. The cystitis is characterized by voluptuous itching and burning pains when the labia touch.

When the eyes are affected there is itching and spasmodic opening and closing. Abscesses are cold and purplish, but occur less than in Tarentula Cubensis.

ACTIVITY 12   List at least eight Strange, Rare and Peculiar symptoms of Tarentula.

Similar Remedies

Agaricus has the itching and inflammation of Arsenicum, but is a cold and blue remedy like Tarentula. It has a powerful effect on the nerves, producing irregular, angular motions – jerks and twitches. It also has the sensation of being pricked by needles. They throw things and prattle. Agaricus is > for gentle motion.

Ledum may resemble Tarentula in local affections. It has jerking, coldness and blueness. On a general level it is more a remedy of circulation than of the nerves.

Cantharis

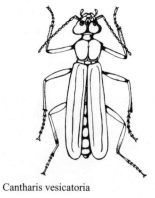

Cantharis vesicatoria

Latin name:	Cantharis vesicatoria
Common name:	Spanish fly, blister-beetle
Natural order:	Caleoptera
Habitat:	It is found amongst the trees and shrubs of south and central Europe

Origin

The remedy was proved by Hahnemann from a tincture prepared from the dried powdered insect. The active ingredient is cantharidin. Uric acid, formic acid and acetic acid are also present.

Essence

This is a remedy of *violent irritation* producing heat, burning pains and oedema.

Nature of the Fly

Flies flit about creating irritation. They eat and produce countless progeny. This particular fly also produces irritating vesicles when touched. It creates much excitement in the system. Urticaria and oedema are produced. In frenzy, the patient appears to bite, like a fly.

Keynotes and Characteristics

- **Burns blister**   Fluid-filled vesicles are formed.
- Skin is fiery and inflamed   This may occur in allergy.
- **Violent burning, especially in cavities**   **Strange, Rare and Peculiar** symptom.

158

• Burning at anus	At the muco-cutaneous junction.
• Burning all down intestines	This is inflammatory.
• Burning pains in urethra with urge to urinate	As in cystitis.
• Burning vesicular eruptions that turn black	There is necrosis in the remedy.
• Eruptions burn when touched	Think of an allergic reaction to the touch of a fly!
• **Stringy discharges from mucous membrane**	This is seen in colds.
• **Bloody, acrid discharges**	You expect this with the burning inflammatory reaction of skin and mucous membrane.
• **Biting pains as if raw**	At if the skin were removed.
• **Cutting sensation in inner parts**	This may be seen in the cystitis.
• **Prickling of inner parts**	The same raw inflammation is present in inner hollow organs.
• **Tearing and stinging from outside to inside**	As when pricked from without.
• **Sensitive to touch**	
• **Dryness in joints**	Usually a sensation of dryness.
• **Burning thirst but averse liquids**	**Strange, Rare and Peculiar** symptom.
• **Spasms < sight of water**	**Strange, Rare and Peculiar** symptom.
• **Thought of drinking produces spasms**	Even the sound of water is enough to cause spasms.
• **Retention of urine with spasm in bladder**	< drinking water
• **Constant urge to urinate, but only a few drops**	Main character of cystitis.
• **Stools like scrapings of intestines**	The inflamed lining of the intestines may be sloughed off.
• **Confusion**	Thoughts run riot.
• **Excitement**	< looking at dazzling lights.
• **Frenzied rage**	Cries, barks, bites.
• **Amorous frenzy**	Not > coition.
• **Strong sex desire**	It is a remedy of deep irritation/stimulation.
• **Priapism with painful contractions**	
• **Cutting pains along spermatic cords**	This is similar to cystitis – same symptom, same tissue as the urethra.
• **Sing lewd songs**	Similar to Hyoscyamus.
• **Restless**	Mental irritation.
• **Constantly attempt to do something but accomplish nothing**	Too irritable to settle.
• **Dissatisfied**	It is described as an uneasiness.
• **Contradictory**	A bit irritating!
• **Objects look yellow**	Eyes are inflamed.
• Debility	So severe is laid low. May lose voice.
• Sudden loss of consciousness	With red face.
• Slough off dead skin	It can be used to clear up burns.

Modalities

< **right side**
< before, during and after urination
< **sound and sight of water**
< **drinking**
< **touch**
< bright objects
< coffee

> rubbing
> warmth

159

ACTIVITY 13 Research the effects of cantharidin, acetic acid and formic acid. How do these relate to the Cantharis symptom picture?

ACTIVITY 14 Describe the symptom picture of Cantharis in a sore throat. Pay particular attention to the modalities.

Frenzy

The mental picture may not be present in burns cases unless the situation is severe but the *anguish* and suffering may be present in the cystitis as an *inclination to complain*. There is a great amount of energy in the remedy, so mental situations of stress become anguish rather than a passive whimper. The mind and body are *restless* moving irritably all the time. In such conditions as nephritis or pneumonia the restless mind may go into *delirium*, similar to Belladonna. More usually, the mind will rant on expressing great *dissatisfaction*, as in Nux vomica. In the cold North, frenzy is toned down. There is often a *strong sexual desire* or voluptuousness when the genital parts are inflamed. When this becomes more severe, the sexual desire may become *lewdness*, embarrassingly frank talk or actions connected with the genitals, which irritates others. We may choose to see this more as mania than frenzy, but it should be sufficient to remind you of the energy of this remedy.

ACTIVITY 15 Compare the symptoms of Cantharis in inflammation with those of Hyoscyamus, and Stramonium.

Inflammation

The process of the Cantharis disease is first *heat leading to dryness*, as in Belladonna, but in Cantharis the area afflicted then becomes sore, the specific sensation being *burning and prickling*. Belladonna could still be seen to cover the patient's symptoms at this stage, but not at the next stage, and there will be little confusion because Cantharis, like Belladonna, develops the full picture symptom very rapidly. Whereas Belladonna goes into fire and fever, convulsions and delirium, Cantharis nips and smarts then breaks down, so *exudate* is produced. On the skin this may be contained in *blisters*, on the mucous membrane it may produce mucus, in a burn this may be so much fluid that the child says 'I'm peeing from my legs'. The next stage is *contraction,* a *tightening of the skin* or mucous membrane, which may go on to tetanic spasms in sphincters. The final stage, *gangrene,* is seldom seen today.

The burning sensations should remind us that Cantharis, like Belladonna, is a remedy of *inflammation* and is, therefore, to be found in many ailments, both minor and deep. Where it is called for, we will find the keynotes and characteristic pattern of Cantharis. The tissues affected are well lubricated by lymph, or closely involved with the activities of lymph – mucous membranes especially but also intestines, lungs and respiratory tract, genitals, kidneys and urinary tract – the *tubes and cavities* of the body. Characteristic patterns will include:

• burning and throbbing	*Heat stage*
• cutting, prickling	*Dry irritable stage*
• sensation of dryness in the joints	
• tenacious mucus, rusty sputum	*Exudate*
• early, profuse menses	
• spasms – retching, vomit	*Spasm*
• sensitive to touch	
• retention of urine.	

Cystitis is a relatively minor but common ailment, that often requires Cantharis. The symptoms fit the picture of Cantharis well:

- constant urging for a few drops
- burning in the urethra on passing urine
- bloody urine, if more severe attack.

It may reach up to inflame the kidneys and may then lead to the more serious condition of nephritis affecting fluid metabolism, so no water is excreted. It is only at this point that we see the symptom < *even small quantities of fluid.*

Burns

The first aid use of the remedy in burns reflects the different stages of the disease process and shows the scope of the remedy from minor burns to those which are a very deep disturbance of the economy.

When the skin is *red and nipping* after lifting a hot plate, Cantharis 6, internally, or on the surface can bring instant relief and correct the situation before the blister stage develops. Once the *blister* stage arises, Cantharis 6 can still be taken internally and you should not be surprised to find the blister gone before you finish dissolving the pill in the mouth. This happens especially if the blister is still arising. The pain, of course, disappears within seconds. If the burn is deep and nerves are involved, Hypericum may be better, but when it gets to the stage where the *raw skin begins to tighten*, Cantharis is again beneficial (or Causticum) if the situation is more serious or involves deeper structures. Apart from the danger of infection, the greatest complication of burns is fluid loss and ensuing kidney failure. Cantharis 30, or even 200, can stop the exudate stage, so preventing fluid loss. In days past it may also have been used for the deep suppuration and *sloughing* of burns that turned to *gangrene*. Wounds seldom reach this stage today, because of better hygiene. However, Cantharis should not be used for deep burns which have been skin-grafted, as it may cause rejection of the skin graft.

The relationship of Cantharis to sunburn is an interesting case, illustrating the uniqueness of homoeopathy. A patient who needs Cantharis is easily affected by the sun, so exposed parts go red, raw and blister – just as in sunburn.

ACTIVITY 16 Compare the use of Cantharis, Urtica urens and Hypericum in burns.

Similar Remedies

Urtica urens is one of the closest remedies to Cantharis. Both produce intense irritability and fire. The skin of Urtica tends to be more dry whilst Cantharis has vesicles or moisture.

Tarentula has the restlessness and sexual frenzy of Cantharis, but it is cold where Cantharis has burning.

Review Apis

It is fascinating to talk to a beekeeper about the habits of the bee, then to relate these to the characteristics of the homoeopathic remedy.

The Character of the Bee

Bees are *busy* and *fidgety*, always on the go, easily angered in certain conditions such as heat. The queen bee is the busiest of all bees, she is the only one who can fulfil certain tasks, so she is important and she is the only queen. If she does not kill her rivals, she leaves the hive, so jealousy is a marked feature of the personality of the remedy. She is *suspicious*, she is *hysterical*, she *cannot bear to be alone* yet she will become *indifferent* and turn her back on others who might help.

Effect of the Bee Sting

The bee sting is how most of us first experience the bee intimately. The sting causes *burning, stinging pains* and a great deal of *local oedema*. These two keynotes characterize the remedy wherever there is inflammation. The third keynote that goes with them is the *red shininess* usually seen around the area of the bee sting. On the organ level this remedy affects all the parts where fluid is important. It is a major remedy in cerebro-spinal meningitis where there is an increase of cerebro-spinal fluid causing violent *opisthotonos* and the keynote the *head bores back into the pillow and the patient shrieks*. The patient also *shrieks before urination* because the mucous membrane is raw and the urine stings and burns. *Urine is retained in the new-born* because of fright, or this patient can pass more urine than she drinks. There is a strong effect on the kidneys which can be seen in certain types of HBP and in some older rheumatic types where fluid collects in the legs. The remedy may also be found in acute inflammation of the mucous membrane or serous membrane, or where there is *fluid effusion* as in pleurisy, diphtheria, hay fever and *anaphylactic shock*.

One organ particularly affected by Apis is the ovary, especially the right, which comes as no surprise, since most bees are female and divided into queens or workers, depending on whether or not they are fertile.

ACTIVITY 17 Review Sepia and Calcarea carbonica in the light of this Lesson. Look at the behaviour of the animal. How is it specialized, or what part or behaviour is unique? How does this affect the character of the ailments? How does the character of the patient reflect the animal's behaviour?

? SELF-TEST QUESTIONS

Answers can be found in the answer section.

1. Name four modalities of Lachesis.
2. Which remedy has prickling in the inner parts?
3. What happens when you touch the spine of the Tarentula patient?
4. How is Cantharis sometimes of use after miscarriage?
5. Name three general symptoms Lachesis shares with Sepia.
6. What is peculiar about the thirst of the Cantharis patient?
7. Describe the delusions of the Lachesis patient.
8. In which remedy do the eruptions burn when touched?
9. Describe the movements of the Tarentula patient.
10. When do objects look yellow to the Cantharis patient?
11. What is peculiar about the neck of the Lachesis patient?
12. Describe the cystitis of the Cantharis patient.
13. Which remedy is > smoking?
14. Why is Lachesis > after the menses start?
15. Which remedy barks in rage?
16. What is strange about the tongue of the Lachesis patient?
17. What do we mean by religious insanity?
18. Which remedy cunningly demonstrates distress only when you are watching?
19. What happens when the Cantharis patient is dazzled by bright light?
20. How is venous congestion expressed in the Lachesis patient?
21. What is the periodicity of Tarentula?
22. Describe the dreams of the Lachesis patient.
23. In which remedy is the right pupil enlarged with the headache?
24. How would you distinguish the ulcers of the Lachesis patient?
25. Name two exciting causes of the Tarentula symptom picture.
26. Which remedy is < slightest touch and > firm pressure?
27. When is the Tarentula patient chilly?
28. Give two peculiarities of the heat symptoms of Lachesis.

Further Studies

Lachesis

1. Name at least three other remedies you have studied that have a marked blue coloration. Where is this likely to be found in each?
2. Describe how the pathology of Lachesis resembles the characteristics of the snake, e.g. when striking, the snake lurches at the genital area.
3. Describe the suspicious Lachesis character and compare it with that of Natrum muriaticum and Hyoscyamus. How do they get into this state?
4. A snake is little more than a specialized digestive tract - how is this reflected in the pathology of the Lachesis patient?
5. Explain how Lachesis disturbs cognitive processes.
6. List the modalities of Lachesis and try to explain these.
7. Summarize how Lachesis affects the menstrual cycle.
8. Compare Lachesis, Lycopodium and Ledum in rheumatic patients.
9. Describe one episode of acute disease in a child to which Lachesis may be applied.
10. State four Strange, Rare and Peculiar symptoms of Lachesis.

Tarentula

1. Describe how the restlessness of Tarentula presents in a cystitis case.
2. What is chorea?
3. Describe the temper tantrum of a Tarentula child.
4. Compare the impulsiveness of Tarentula and Nux vomica.
5. Describe the digestive symptoms of Tarentula.

Cantharis

1. In a burns case, distinguish the use of Cantharis, Causticum and Kali bichromium.
2. Describe the onset and progression of a case of cystitis which could respond to Cantharis. Underline the distinguishing symptoms.
3. Compare Cantharis and Causticum in urinary system symptoms.
4. What are the similarities between Cantharis, Tarentula and Kreosotum?
5. Differentiate clearly between Belladonna, Rhus toxicodendron and Cantharis. Under what circumstances could these remedies be confused?
6. When could Cantharis be used instead of Apis in a dropsy condition associated with a kidney disorder?
7. Give three characteristic symptoms of Cantharis.
8. Describe the mental state of the Cantharis patient who has just been scalded.

An Acute, Constitutional and Pathological Remedy

Allium Cepa, Argentum Nitricum, Phytolacca

Aim:	To discover how a remedy might function within a particular phase of the vital force's action.
Objectives:	To outline the acute symptom picture of Allium cepa. To distinguish the essential nature of the constitutional symptom picture of Argentum nitricum and in particular how this affects the mucous membrane. To identify when the symptom picture of Phytolacca can cure pathological states in the lymphatic system.
Headings:	INTRODUCTION ALLIUM CEPA: Origin; Characteristics of the Plant; Essence; Keynotes and Characteristics; Modalities; The Common Cold; Congestion; Neuralgias; Similar Remedies ARGENTUM NITRICUM: Origin; Characteristics of the Mineral; Essence; Keynotes and Characteristics; Modalities; Perpetual Agitation; The Disordered Stomach; The Acute Symptom Picture; Similar Remedies PHYTOLACCA: Origin; Characteristics of the Plant, Essence; Keynotes and Characteristics; Modalities; Catarrhal Discharge; Overactivity; Similar Remedies SELF-TEST QUESTIONS FURTHER STUDIES

Introduction

The three remedies in this lesson each have a profound effect on mucous membrane, but they work in different ways. Previously we have looked at different exciting causes, different essence, different levels of the disease process. In this lesson I want to introduce you to an acute remedy, a constitutional remedy and a remedy that can act on pathological states.

There is only one vital force so, at any one time, there is only one symptom picture. The basic nature of an organism is represented by a constitutional remedy. We do not really change the character of a person with homoeopathic treatment. We free the energy to allow the potential to be realized. The basic nature contains weaknesses which predispose the individual to certain patterns of ill health. The constitutional remedy strengthens these weaknesses so the vital force can respond more effectively to disturbances.

When disturbed the vital force produces a symptom picture. This may show the weakness of the constitutional remedy so we may use this to cure. More often though the vital force accelerates when disturbed. This may produce a slightly different symptom picture as the energy level is now more volatile. This is the symptom picture of the acute remedy. There is a clear relationship between the acute and chronic remedies. The same areas of weakness are affected by a similar essence. Some remedies, like Argentum nitricum have an amazing range of action that includes the acute, constitutional and pathological levels. Some, like Allium cepa, seldom go very deep. They work at the level of sensation and dysfunction. When disturbed the vital force throws out acute ailments of an inflammatory or suppurative type to clear out toxins and restore balance.

Sometimes the energy of the vital force is low. It may have been so exposed to stress, illness, shock, pollution that the parts are weakened, that the vital force has to localize the disorder. When this happens the disease is different from the constitutional picture but could not be described as an acute as above. It is called the acute of the chronic because the chronic level is so overloaded that it spills out. This can happen when there are recurrent colds, sore throats, tonsillitis, etc. When the continual wear and tear affects an organ, structural change may occur – we call this pathology. Whilst it is often possible to use the constitutional remedy here, the energy may shift to enhance only part of the total symptom picture. Thus Phytolacca may be a constitutional remedy or it often appears in cases where the glands are disturbed. If mucous membrane is the surface of the great sea of the body, the lymphatic system, the glands are the gateways to it, the focus of action. When localized the rhythm of the disease may change to overfunction, overproduction of mucus, then structure may change so, in this remedy, cysts and cancers result.

To gain deeper understanding of this theme you may find it useful to study those lessons on disease in the companion text *An Introduction to Homoeopathic Philosophy*.

Allium Cepa

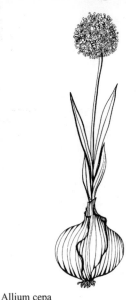

Allium cepa

Latin name: Allium cepa
Common name: Red onion
Botanical family: Liliaceae
Habitat: Red onions have a long history as garden vegetables.

Origin

A tincture was made of the whole fresh plant.

Characteristics of the Plant

The edible bulb of the onion contains sulphide of allyl which gives it an acridity. If you have ever cut a raw onion you will be aware of the excoriating effect on mucous membrane. The eyes sting and burn and water profusely, the nose burns causing coryza and sneezing. You do not even need to touch the onion. It is sufficient to be exposed to the surrounding air.

To the Chinese, onions are powerful herbs that help digestion and warm the body. When added to soups and stews, like tomatoes, they retain their heat whereas more farinaceous vegetables cool quicker. Onions and garlic (Allium sativum) are often taken as a folk cure at the start of a cold and you will find that, along with Aconite, Allium cepa is commonly used by routine prescription at the start of a cold. The onion works by increasing flow from the mucous membrane which thus increases discharge and expulsion of toxins as it heats up the cold phlegmatic constitution.

Essence

There is a violence to this remedy as if acid burns and tears at the parts affected. *Acridity* accompanies all symptoms. This stimulates mucous membrane to secrete copiously producing watery discharge in less serious cases, thicker catarrh where the disturbance is greater.

Keynotes and Characteristics

- **Watery discharge from nose, bland from eyes** — The opposite of Euphrasia.
- **Profuse bland lachrymation** — When in a cold wind.
- **Discharges burn and excoriate** — Wherever the skin is touched.
- < left nostril — There is a little raw excoriated patch beneath this.
- Symptoms start left and move to right — As in Phosphorus, the opposite of Arsenicum.
- Eyes red and itchy — This can be seen in many allergic reactions.
- **Violent sneezing** — In a cold, hay fever, or allergy.
- As of a lump at the root of the nose — This is found in hay fever.
- **Sensitive to the odour of flowers** — **Strange, Rare and Peculiar** symptom.

166

- **Tickle in the larynx** — < cold air, > in a warm room as in Phosphorus.
- Rough, raw throat — The mucous coating has been removed so it burns. Extends to the ear.

- **Grasps the throat as if torn** — The pain is tearing. The spasm is so violent.
- Rattling cough — There is so much mucus.
- Incessant hacking cough — Spasmodic, it is worse breathing deeply.
- Pains in long threads — Tear along the nerves as in Aconite.
- Rending, tearing pains — Where nerves are involved, e.g. where flatulent colic attacks the navel.

- Burning stinging pains — Where parts raw, e.g. when the heel is skinned.

Modalities

< evening	> **fresh air**
< **cold air**	> menstruation
< stuffy room	
< getting the feet wet	

ACTIVITY 1

Define the typical symptom picture of a hay fever case. How do these symptoms correspond to the symptom picture of Allium cepa? Use the keynotes and characteristics above to illustrate your answer.

The Common Cold

The cold of the Allium cepa patient is a profuse watery discharge from the nose and eyes. There is a particular pattern from which we derive some of the keynotes.

The *nose discharge is watery and acrid* (as in Arsenicum) but there is also a *profuse bland lachrymation* from the eyes (Euphrasia is the opposite – the nose discharge is bland and the eye discharge is acrid).

The nasal discharge burns and corrodes the upper lip and below the nose where it touches the skin (Kent says it burns like fire). Often it may come only from the *left nostril* – Arsenicum affects the right nostril. The Allium cepa nasal discharge *starts on the left and goes to the right* – like Phosphorus.

The eyes are usually *red* with the discharge. They may *itch and burn and sting* as when you peel an onion. *Note*: This is very different from saying the lachrymation excoriates.

The cold is further distinguished by *violent sneezing* particularly on entering a warm room, as in Pulsatilla. The cold often starts after damp cold as in Pulsatilla and we could even say they both share the unusual exciting cause, *worse getting the feet wet*. Rhus toxicodendron has a similar symptom picture *worse getting soaked*. All the symptoms of the cold are worse in a warm room except the *tickle in the larynx* which is worse for cold air. Phosphorus has a tickle in the larynx worse for cold air or talking. As in Phosphorus the tickle leads to a cough and this and all other symptoms are worse in the evening, as in Phosphorus and Pulsatilla. The cough is *incessant and hacking*. The throat may be *rough and raw* as when peeling onions. When coughing the patient *grasps the throat as if it would be torn* – compare with Bryonia and Aconite which both grasp the throat.

The excessive secretion of mucus produces a *rattling cough* in bronchitis or catarrhal hoarseness or laryngitis.

ACTIVITY 2

Make a table of comparison of the cold symptoms of the remedies mentioned above, i.e. Allium cepa, Arsenicum, Aconite, Pulsatilla, Phosphorus and Euphrasia. Pay particular attention to modalities and exciting causes.

Congestion

The effect on the mucous membrane at a deeper level is to cause congestion. This *engorgement of the tissues* gives a *sensation of fullness* or of *throbbing* and heat (*burning*) and, as in Phosphorus, may lead to diffusion of blood and/or *nosebleeds*. A congestive headache often accompanies the coryza. It starts through the sinus of the jaw and face and is *worse for winking*! Winking of course is movement. The coryza often spreads to the ears so Allium cepa can be a useful remedy in earache when there is inflammation of the lining of the eustachian tube, engorgement and mucous discharge. There is a sensation of fullness and throbbing up the eustachian tube to the left ear *after exposure to damp cold*. The pain is worse in a warm room. This congestion is seen in the urinary system as pressure on urinating. There is also burning as the urine is passed. In the digestive system the swollen, engorged intestines cannot absorb food so much flatus is produced. The spasm is seen in the colic which is worse when the patient is sitting or moving about, i.e. the area is sensitive, like the tickly throat, so stimulation or pressure sets off a reaction, colic in the abdomen, cough in the throat.

ACTIVITY 3 It is said that Allium cepa is especially adapted to phlegmatic patients. What do we mean by a 'phlegmatic' patient? Does this describe the Allium cepa symptom picture?

Neuralgias

Allium cepa closely resembles Aconite in its action on the nerves. *Tearing* pains stretch along the nerves to give the keynote *pains in long threads*. This is also similar to Hypericum, both can be used for the damaged nerves after amputations. More commonly the nerves of the Allium cepa patient are sensitive to cold. When exposed neuralgic pains arise. The left trigeminal nerve is a favourite site, as in Aconite. The difference, if you take the case in enough detail, is that Allium cepa is sensitive to damp cold whilst Aconite is sensitive to dry cold.

Allium cepa is useful when nerves are traumatized and pain remains long afterwards. Toothache, notably one of the most severe 'neuralgias', responds well to Allium cepa when there is an amelioration from cold, even though cold damp may be the causation!

ACTIVITY 4 Read the chapters on Allium cepa in J H Clarke, 1977, *A Dictionary of Practical Materia Medica*, Health Science Press, Devon and in E A Neatby and T G Stonham, 1987, *A Manual of Homoeo–Therapeutics*, Foxlee-Vaughan Publishers, London

---

Similar Remedies

Aconite has the same level of energy in an acute disorder to affect the mucous membrane of the upper respiratory tract with copious fluid discharge. It also affects the nerves in a similar way to produce tearing pains. Aconite is worse cold dry weather whilst Allium cepa is worse cold wet weather.

Arsenicum. Allium cepa is considered the vegetable analogue of Arsenicum. They share many symptoms and it is difficult to separate them in colds, hay fever and allergies(!). Profuse excoriating lachrymation is produced by both. Whilst they start on different sides of the body they can cross over, so either may appear on the other side. Both have burning pains but Allium cepa has more action on the nerves than Arsenicum.

Phosphorus patients have a strong liking for onions. Both have burning pains and a strong sensitivity to smells which may bring on sneezing and coryza. Phosphorus is often found in hay fever or at the start of a cold like Allium cepa.

Argentum Nitricum

Silver nitrate

Origin

The nitrates of all metals are soluble so it is possible to triturate and prepare a solution.

Characteristics of the Mineral

Silver is an impressionable metal. It conducts heat rapidly, it heats up quickly but it cools just as quickly. Its use for mirrors and photography shows its ability to reflect rather than hold on to light. It is associated with the moon which has long been seen as the world of illusion. The Argentum nitricum patient is one of the most imaginative. They are also elusive types who flap about like mad hatters.

Silver has an affinity for organic tissue reacting with the sulphur of protein to cause a black discoloration – think of the effect of egg on a silver spoon. It is used medically to burn off warts. When silver nitrate is taken internally it has a strong effect on the mucous membrane lining the digestive system causing over-secretion, vomiting and diarrhoea. The mucous membrane can then be protected by ingesting milk, soapy water or white of egg.

Essence

This is often described as the white rabbit remedy (from *Alice in Wonderland*). The white rabbit rushes through its scenes chanting 'I'm late, I'm late, I'm late'. The Argentum nitricum patient rushes too. *Haste* describes the speech, how they eat, how they walk. He goes so fast he trips over himself, stuttering, jerking and twitching, he gets into a fluster. *Perpetual agitation* describes this individual who does not stop.

Keynotes and Characteristics

• **Walks faster and faster**	Until he drops. He does this whilst gnawing a problem.
• **Haste in speech, walking, eating**	Their momentum is onward without a pause.
• **Impulse**	To throw themselves off high buildings, etc. so they hold on fast.
• **Constant flow of thoughts**	The mind flows onwards in haste and thus often superficially.
• **Tormenting thoughts**	The opposite of the above – some thoughts stick and worry away at them.
• **Anticipatory fear**	He has diarrhoea before the performance. The imagination runs on.
• **Fear tall buildings will fall over**	So they have vertigo looking up. Note, the buildings are on the move towards them.
• **Fear of heights**	They lose orientation and feel themselves going over.
• Fear of narrow places	They feel hemmed in and cannot move on. Panic results.
• Fear to cross bridges	The bridge and water level are different so confusing and disorienting them.
• Fear of passing a certain spot	They have a foreboding of evil.
• Fear of crowds	They cannot escape.
• Excitable	They easily anger.
• Vertigo – as if they turn in a circle.	< after opening the eyes.
• Lose their balance when the eyes are closed	They cannot orientate themselves.
• Buzzing in the ears with vertigo	It comes with much weakness.
• Time passes too slowly.	This will come in the chronic phase when they are confused.
• **Flatulence**	Everything they eat turns to gas.
• Violent belching	> warm food and drink.
• Simultaneous vomiting and diarrhoea	When the stomach is disturbed.
• Spluttery green diarrhoea	Looks like spinach!
• Sour-smelling diarrhoea	As in Chamomilla.
• Diarrhoea after milk	Compare with Chamomilla.
• < sugar yet crave sugar	Causes much flatulence.

- Desires strong cheese
- **Stick-like sensations in the throat**   So dry – chronic laryngitis of singers.
- Head pain > tight bandage   Unusual.
- **Thick, yellow, bland discharge**   Can be seen in the newborn infant exposed to
  from the eyes   gonorrhoea.
- **Palpitation**   The heart problems arise because the haste causes
  > pressure of hand   so much tension.
  < lying on the right side
  after excitement
  with nausea and fainting
- **Fullness of blood vessels**   Felt all over.
- **Crave fresh air**
- Lose sex drive because the organs dry   The life force is withdrawing from this patient.
  and shrivel.
- **Erection does not last**
- **Left-sided**

Modalities

< **anxiety**   > cold open air
< **apprehension**   > hard pressure
< closed rooms   > eructations
< **sugar**   > bending double
< heat   > cold, open air
< cold food and drink
< before and during menses

ACTIVITY 5   Describe the symptoms of colic in an Argentum nitricum child. Use the keynotes and characteristic symptoms where appropriate.

ACTIVITY 6   Describe an Argentum nitricum patient with angina pectoris. Use keynotes and characteristic symptoms where appropriate.

ACTIVITY 7   What symptoms of Argentum nitricum would you expect to find in one who was agoraphobic?

Perpetual Agitation

When troubled he goes walking and he *walks faster and faster* until he drops. He feels driven and has *impulses* to do things. If he puts himself in motion then he is in control himself. When the motion is stopped he is *impatient* – this comes with *anxiety*.

The mind never stops, there is a *constant flow of thoughts* and these may be of awful things that can happen to him, they *torment* keeping him awake. He has a wild and *vivid imagination* that runs away with him so he becomes anxious because he is always *thinking into the future* about what might happen. So he gets into a flap and *rushes around* doing so many things that nothing gets done. He uses a lot of nervous energy. This is one of the main remedies for *anticipatory fears*. Before he goes on stage or begins the driving test, he imagines vividly all the things that might happen and this frightens him. He breaks out in a sweat which may be profuse then if the anxiety goes further the bowels will move, urgently. There is a lot of *excitement* and a lot of fear. Excitement gives rise to *palpitations*, even *nausea and faintness*. The fears give an interesting insight into the way the remedy affects the mind. When the Argentum nitricum patient looks up at high buildings there is a fear the building will fall on them. This is similar to anticipation. The mind does not 'fix' objects, the objects keep travelling nearer to the patient. There is a *fear of heights* – when they look over the cliff edge their orientation goes and it is as if they will fall over. They feel *giddy*. *Claustrophobia* arises because the walls seem to close in. *Water and bridges frighten* them because their perception is distorted. There is a *fear of crowds* which seem to close in. Argentum nitricum can help *agoraphobics* who imagine all sorts of things happening to them out of doors.

Cognition and perception are distorted by anxiety. They anticipate then overcorrect to accommodate the distortion, then they find themselves *confused* and *disorientated*. This panics them. The personality that arises out of this is very unsure of itself – with good reason. They are *jittery, move jerkily*. There is no smooth flow so the patient has to think more to try to understand. The nervous system is worn down by all this activity. *Thoughts torment them.* Fed by imagination and their lack of confidence *they fear evil* will get them, or *an incurable illness*. They have no grip on the flow, so thoughts tumble out and they think the worst. When they are confused they become quite irrational and *do and say strange things*. They can become confused as the memory becomes defective. You have to hold ideas to allow memory to function and the Argentum nitricum patient cannot do that. The emotions flow easily too, so they are *easily excited* or angry.

The instability of the nervous system comes in the vertigo and in *palpitations*. In the vertigo it is *as if the patient is turning in a circle*. They are *worse closing the eyes*. The nervous disturbance can be seen in the *buzzing in the ear* which accompanies the vertigo. *Weakness*, with buzzing in the ear, shows the depth of the disturbance. The remedy is useful in *locomotor ataxia* when the patient loses balance when the eyes are closed because there is no reference point.

The nervous state continues until all organs in the body are disordered, but it always starts in the stomach.

ACTIVITY 8   You may have seen an Argentum nitricum patient before an examination or public performance of some kind. Make notes on what you observed. Use keynotes and characteristic symptoms, where appropriate.

ACTIVITY 9   Study the heart pathology of the Argentum nitricum patient. List the symptoms. How do these arise from perpetual motion?

The Disordered Stomach

This is one of the most flatulent remedies in the Materia Medica. *Everything eaten turns to gas.* When nervous there is much gas, which often makes the poor patient more nervous. Flatus goes up and down. There is often *loud* and *violent belching*. They easily produce *diarrhoea* which is *spluttery* with much *rumbling in the abdomen*. The abdomen is very *distended*. The gas is *worse after they consume sugar* which they have a craving for. It is one of the few remedies that *crave sugar and salt*. If the diarrhoea is serious it is *sour and green*. This is one of the few remedies that will have *simultaneous vomiting and diarrhoea* when the stomach is upset.

When we look at the stool – the end product of digestion – the green and sourness shows *lack of assimilation* due to the speed with which the food has moved through the digestive system. The acidity which produces the gas may produce a *mucousy stool* when the disturbance is increased. Thus the remedy is often used in colitis and Crohn's disease where there is excessive flow through the gut accompanied by much mucous secretion. The sufferer from these diseases frequently presents an anxious symptom picture of perpetual agitation. Note that when we talk of tormenting thoughts, we use words such as 'gnawing'. The worrying thoughts of the Argentum nitricum patient are felt in the stomach.

ACTIVITY 10   Study Crohn's disease and ulcerative colitis in a medical textbook. How do these reflect the keynotes and characteristics of Argentum nitricum?

The Acute Symptom Picture

The most common acute symptom picture of Argentum nitricum is a sore throat. This shows its strong effect on the mucous membrane. It is a major sycotic remedy which causes *excessive flow of mucus* so there may be a great deal of *catarrh*. In severe cases this invades the sinus giving a congestive headache but it moves into a dry phase where there is a feeling of *constriction* in the throat and the keynote symptom of a *stick-like sensation*. The excessive flow can be seen at an earlier stage of the disease process where it may simply be *rhinitis with itching* – the nervous irritability explains the process behind this symptom. In a more severe stage where it has gone deeper the catarrhal flow can become *copious leucorrhoea*. Inversely *violent dysmenorrhoea* may occur. The exciting cause of this brings us right back to the basic character of the remedy in that the dysmenorrhoea is caused by *excitement* and the pain comes because of *increased flow*.

Argentum nitricum differs from other sycotic remedies in that the mucous membrane also ulcerates and, as in other syphilitic remedies, there is tendency to haemorrhage. Both of these characteristics would appear to come from the nitric component of the remedy.

ACTIVITY 11   Compare the symptoms of rhinitis, a sore throat and leucorrhoea. Pay particular attention to the effect on the mucous membrane.

Similar Remedies

Phosphorus has the vivid imagination of Argentum nitricum producing fear. It is also an excitable remedy that wears down the nervous system to produce colds. It is not windy like Argentum nitricum though it can produce congestion of mucous membrane and copious catarrh. When the catarrh is severe in Phosphorus, there tends to be streaks of blood. Both remedies are used for haemorrhage.

Lycopodium has the agitation, haste and lack of confidence of Argentum nitricum. Both are remedies of anticipation that affect the gut to create wind and loose stool. Both are thinkers and make themselves ill thinking. Both crave sugar which makes them ill. Lycopodium tends to be more logical and rational and less imaginative.

Phytolacca

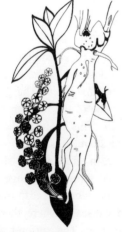

Phytolacca decandra

Latin name:	Phytolacca decandra
Common name:	Poke root, red ink plant
Botanical family:	Phytolaccaceae
Habitat:	The plant is a perennial bush common in North America and in Mediterranean climates, where it grows in damper areas, under hedgerows and along streams

Origin

The proving was done by the American School of Homoeopathy. There are two forms of tincture, one prepared from the root dug up in winter and the other produced from the berries.

Characteristics of the Plant

The plant has a purplish stem and purplish berries. Though poisonous, the berries are often eaten by birds which become emaciated. Active ingredients include oxalates, formic acid and large quantities of potassium. As a herb it enjoys a good reputation for helping rheumatism and cancerous growth. In particular it has an affinity for the mammary glands.

Gibson states that it promotes multiplication of mononuclear cells in tests and deduces it has a beneficial effect on leucocytes in the bloodstream.

Essence

The remedy acts to suppress the vitality causing a negative attitude to life. The lymphatic system responds with inflammation and copious secretion which becomes pustular and finally, as it breaks down further, glands and mucous membrane ulcerate producing a thin, excoriating discharge. On the general level the patient is exhausted then emaciates. The suppurative, congestive stage goes very deep and can last a long time in the glands before the final breakdown into ulceration.

Keynotes and Characteristics		
	• **Excessive secretion from mucous membrane**	
	• **Indurated glands**	< parotid and submaxillary. Also testes. It has a special affinity for the breasts. It can be acute or ongoing.
	• Sensation of lump in the throat as if a ball of red hot iron	They continually try to swallow this.
	• Pains shoot from throat into ear	
	• Pain at root of the tongue on swallowing	**Strange, Rare and Peculiar**.
	• Copious salivation	
	• Metallic taste in mouth	Plus salivation as in Mercurius.
	• **White spots on the tonsils**	There is a lot of suppuration in this remedy.
	• Ash-coloured membrane on the tonsil and throat	This can be a remedy of diphtheria.
	• **Ulceration**	On glands, especially breasts.
	• Breast has purple hue and hardens	Right side Bryonia, left side Phytolacca.
	• Sore fissured nipples < cold weather	
	• **Spasms in the breast as the child sucks**	May radiate to the back.
	• **Ichorous, foetid discharge from ulcers**	This can be disturbing for the patient especially on the breasts.
	• **Indifferent to work**	
	• **Indifferent to self**	She is sure she will die so gives up.
	• Prostration	e.g. in tonsillitis.
	• Nodules on breast	May be malignant.
	• **Emaciation**	All over.
	• Drawing pains in muscles	Especially in the back < heat.
	• Pains like electric shocks	Along the tract of the nerve like Phosphorus and Hypericum.
	• Rheumatism	Of fibrous and periosteal tissue < cold damp.
	• Sciatic pains moving down the outside of the thigh	
	• Bruised sensation all over body	You will recognize this in flu and glandular fever.

Modalities		
	< **cold, damp weather**	> work
	< swallowing	> lying on abdomen
	< hot drinks	
	< rising from bed	
	< when child suckles	

ACTIVITY 12 Using the keynote and characteristic symptoms describe the sore throat of the Phytolacca patient.

ACTIVITY 13 Which symptoms arise in the rheumatism of the Phytolacca patient?

ACTIVITY 14   List the digestive symptoms of Phytolacca, using keynotes and characteristic symptoms where appropriate.

Catarrhal Discharge

This remedy has a profound effect on mucous membrane especially in the respiratory system and digestive system. *Excessive mucus* is produced *when exposed to cold, damp weather* or when the vitality is lowered. This is a remedy of lower vitality than the Bryonia/Gelsemium type patient, so they can produce on-going catarrhal situations that may last years. In the acute phase it affects glands throughout the body, in the chronic phase it produces rheumatism.

The *glands inflame and swell* and then there is a lot of heat and pain. The parotid and submaxillary glands are particularly involved. The throat feels full *as if choking* or there is a *sensation of a lump* which causes the patient to continually swallow. *On swallowing, a pain shoots into the ears.* It may be there is a sensation as if there is a *ball of red-hot iron* lodged in the throat or the throat may feel raw. On swallowing there is a strange, rare and peculiar *pain in the root of the tongue.* There is also *much salivation* and a *metallic taste in the mouth.*

In tonsillitis, the suppuration can be seen as *white patches which gradually join up.* The breath can be foul. In an even more acute phase this symptom picture may describe diphtheria when the *grey membrane covers the whole of the back of the throat.*

Often the symptom picture will slip deeper into specialized glands like the testes and breasts. There may be *abscesses* or *hard nodules.* These are often *worse before menses* when the nipples may also be sensitive and sore. Or it may be that the nipples are sore when the temperature drops and it is cold outside. This is one of the remedies of breast cancer, or of *discharge from the nipples after weaning.* It is also one of the remedies one thinks of when there is a problem producing milk.

The cancer develops because of the tendency of the remedy to *form abscesses* and *fissures.* We are going beyond the suppurative stage here to produce necrosis with the *foetid thin discharge* that is found in the cancer. At this stage you will clearly see *drawing pains* in the glands.

ACTIVITY 15   Study the different forms of breast cancer in a medical textbook. Which correspond to the symptom picture of Phytolacca?

ACTIVITY 16   Describe how over-secretion affects the digestive system of the Phytolacca patient.

Overactivity

Although it inclines to overproduction and to overreact like Argentum nitricum, Phytolacca does not do this from nervous irritability. In this remedy the nerves produce spasm and contraction. The degree of sensitivity can be seen in the *breast spasm which extends to the back when the child sucks.*

Elsewhere the spasm may be seen as *drawing pains.* In rheumatism the muscle is drawn from its attachment. The sciatic pain may be drawing or shoot like an *electric shock* down the *outside of the thigh.*

On the general level there is *restlessness* that quickly passes into *indifference.* On the one hand they may be *irritable,* on the other they are *tearful and depressed.* These could be *mood swings* of PMS. It is confused with Sepia when the patient *cannot be bothered,* does not want to work and cares little of herself or her appearance. The patient may now feel *sore and bruised all over,* the brain even feels bruised, the eyes feel large with *pain on moving.* The *eyes may feel gritty* as in Sepia. This is a run down condition of the lymphatic system. It may produce *glandular fever* in acute situations, or ME when this is on-going and there is little energy to resolve the situation. In another patient rheumatism may take the disease into the extremities where it can become inflammatory.

ACTIVITY 17

Define glandular fever. How does the Phytolacca symptom picture resemble this disease? Relate the symptoms to the keynotes and characteristics where appropriate.

Similar Remedies

Silicea is a remedy of the glands which suppurate but may finally ulcerate. The discharges of both are offensive. Both produce abscesses, cysts, fibrosed tissue and cancers. Either remedy may appear to under-function – Silicea because of fear, Phytolacca because of hopelessness.

Mercurius also works on the glands to increase discharge. Both have excessive salivation and metallic taste. In both the suppurative state is foul smelling and may ulcerate. Like Silicea, Mercurius has no confidence because it has no energy to create any but Phytolacca has lost confidence through disappointment – this tarnishes their view on life.

Calcarea carbonica shares the indurated glandular problems leading to copious catarrhs, sour smelling discharges and fibrosis. Calcarea will not produce the ulceration or ichorous discharge. It may be well indicated in cysts and cancers of the breast.

ACTIVITY 18

Construct a Table of Comparison for Allium cepa, Argentum nitricum and Phytolacca showing:

Exciting causes
Maintaining causes
Modalities
Effect on mucous membrane
Effect on lymphatic system
Effect on respiratory system
Effect on digestive system
Mental/emotional symptoms.

 SELF-TEST QUESTIONS

You will find the answers in the text, and these can be checked in the answer section.

1. Describe the fluid discharge from the eyes and nose of the Allium cepa patient.
2. Why does Argentum nitricum walk faster and faster till they drop?
3. Describe the eye discharge of the Argentum nitricum patient.
4. Describe the ulcerated breast abscess of the Phosphorus patient.
5. Which two remedies are sensitive to the smell of flowers?
6. How does anticipation affect the Argentum nitricum patient?
7. Name two remedies with copious salivation.
8. Name at least four fears of the Argentum nitricum patient.
9. How does the discharge from the nose of the Allium cepa patient differ from that of Arsenicum?
10. Which remedy has the sensation of a red hot ball at the back of the throat?
11. Name three remedies that grasp the throat as if it were torn.
12. What happens to the breast when the child sucks the Phytolacca patient?

13. Describe the sciatica pains of the Phytolacca patient.
14. How does the direction of movement of the symptoms of Allium cepa resemble Phosphorus?
15. In which symptoms do you see the haste of the Argentum nitricum patient?
16. Describe the pains of the Phytolacca patient.
17. Describe the eyes of the Allium cepa patient.
18. Which remedy has pains like an electric shock?
19. Which remedy has a neuralgic pain < winking?
20. How do the gland symptoms of Phytolacca resemble Silicea?
21. Which remedy has the sensation of a lump at the root of the nose?
22. How does excitability affect the heart in the Argentum nitricum patient?
23. How does Phytolacca present in diphtheria?
24. Why does the cough of Allium cepa rattle so much?
25. Which glands are particularly affected by Phytolacca?
26. What is Strange, Rare and Peculiar about the pains of the Allium cepa patient?
27. Name two remedies with tormenting thoughts.
28. Describe the stool of the Argentum nitricum patient.
29. In which remedy does time pass too slowly?
30. Name four modalities of Allium cepa.

Further Studies

Allium Cepa

1. State the 'cold' symptoms of Allium cepa. How do these compare with those of Euphrasia? What other remedies have similar symptoms in a cold?
2. Compare the symptom picture that might arise in the Allium cepa patient's hay fever with that arising in the Arsenicum patient.
3. Compare the symptom picture of Pulsatilla, Chamomilla and Allium cepa in earache.
4. When would you use Allium cepa in colic?
5. When might you consider Allium cepa alongside Hypericum? Differentiate between the two. From the pharmaco-dynamics of Allium cepa try to discover the basis of this reaction.
6. Study the function and nature of mucous membrane and attempt to define the interaction of Allium cepa with this.
7. Give three Strange, Rare and Peculiars that might help you identify Allium cepa as the required remedy.
8. List five main characteristics of Allium cepa.

Argentum Nitricum

1. Name four Strange, Rare and Peculiar symptoms of Argentum nitricum.
2. How can Argentum nitricum be of use in diabetes?
3. Compare the symptom picture of Argentum nitricum with that of Lycopodium and Phosphorus.
4. Describe the growths Argentum nitricum produces as a sycotic remedy.
5. When would you use Argentum nitricum in a first aid situation?
6. Compare the tormenting thoughts of Argentum nitricum with those of Natrum muriaticum and Hyoscyamus.
7. List the modalities of Argentum nitricum and try to explain them in terms of the essence of the remedy.
8. Describe the symptoms of the Argentum nitricum patient with asthma. Pay particular attention to causation and to how the essence of Argentum nitricum expresses itself.
9. Describe the Argentum nitricum child as you find them after waking up from a nightmare.
10. Compare Argentum nitricum, Argentum metallicum and Nitric acidum.

Phytolacca

1. Study the role of oxalates in the body.
2. Compare the sore throat of Phytolacca, Mercurius, Lachesis and Silicea.
3. How does the disease diphtheria present? Compare the use of Phytolacca, Lachesis, Apis and one other in this disease.

4. How would you describe 'drawing pains'? Which other remedies have these?
5. Define sciatica. Compare the symptom picture of Phytolacca and Sepia in this disease.
6. What problems might arise during breast feeding that would respond to Phytolacca as a remedy?
7. Compare Phytolacca, Silicea and Mercurius.
8. How does the symptom picture of Phytolacca resemble that of Hepar sulphuris?
9. What problems might arise in old age that would respond to Phytolacca in particular?

LESSON TWELVE

The Antimoniums

Antimonium Crudum, Antimonium Tartaricum

Aim: To demonstrate how a remedy can produce a different symptom picture when one ingredient is changed.
To compare the symptom picture of remedies which contain Sulphur in their make-up.

Objectives: To define the difference in the symptom picture of Antimonium crudum and Antimonium tartaricum.
To outline the different level of action of Antimonium crudum and Antimonium tartaricum in stages of degeneration of disease.
To contrast and compare the symptom picture of Antimonium crudum, Sulphur and Pulsatilla.

Headings: INTRODUCTION
ANTIMONIUM CRUDUM: Characteristics of the Metal; Origin; Essence; Keynotes and Characteristics; Modalities; Wallowing in Emotions; Disordered Digestion; The Skin; Similar Remedies
ANTIMONIUM TARTARICUM: Origin; Essence; Keynotes and Characteristics; Modalities; Lack of Life; Relaxation; Similar Remedies
REVIEW SULPHUR: Self-indulgence; Areas Affected
REVIEW PULSATILLA
SELF-TEST QUESTIONS
FURTHER STUDIES

Introduction

There are over 2000 remedies in the homoeopathic pharmacopoeia. Some of these are very similar in their action and it may not be easy to see that which is unique in their symptom picture. Hahnemann tells us that each remedy has a separate identity, but already you will have begun to notice the overlap in the symptom picture of remedies. In this lesson we shall look deliberately at the overlap, asking what makes the remedy distinct.

Remedies are related to each other like a spectrum. There may be a basic core of redness, or anger, which links them, but each expresses anger in a slightly different way. One may have a tinge of blueness as it weeps. Another may shade into purple as the face is swollen and bloated. Yet another may be a bloody shade of red as the anger consumes and it wants to kill someone. To recognize the difference is to achieve greater resonance with the patient's symptom picture and therefore more efficient cure. What makes the difference? On what factors do we make our decision when the remedies are so similar?

In looking at a case, we ask first what is the point at which the vital force was affected, what affected the vital force, then what are the main symptoms around which the case hinges – what need we change to cure the patient? No remedy is exactly the same, so we must find the subtle nuances of expression, of sensation, modality and essence which correspond most closely to the symptom picture of the patient.

There is much similarity in the symptom picture of Antimonium crudum and Antimonium tartaricum. The same areas of the body are affected, the essence or type of energy flow is the same, but Antimonium crudum works on the general and dysfunction level whilst Antimonium tartaricum works more locally in organs pathologically but the energy is so low little activity is evident.

179

Antimonium Crudum

Sulphide of Antimony (Sb_2S_3)

Characteristics of the Metal

The name antimonos (Gk) refers to the fact the metal is seldom found alone in pure form. It is found naturally as stibnite (Sb_2S_3), a compound of sulphur and antimony which takes form as long black needles up to one metre in length. Antimony has a great affinity for sulphur. Indeed in its purest form it is yellow resembling sulphur, but in this stage it is highly reactive and unstable.

Its properties are strange. It is both a base and an acid. It neither conducts electricity nor is attracted by magnetism. When placed between the poles of a magnet it aligns itself at right angles to the lines of force.

Thus in anthroposophical medicine it is considered to have a special role as the energy in-between that allows form to come into being. (See Uyldest Mellic, 1980, *Metal Magic*, Turnstone Press Ltd, London.)

Origin

The remedy is prepared by trituration from the black sulphide of antimony. Hahnemann was the first to describe its effects homoeopathically in his Materia Medica Pura.

Essence

As in Silicea, the symptoms of Antimonium crudum vary between hard form, induration and cracks, and lack of form, softness or sentimentality. There is poor assimilation and substance so it appears there is a yearning for *connectedness*. The remedy is often given the uncomplimentary title 'The Greedy Pig'. If this is seen as a need to consume to be part of life, then we can append another behaviour of the pig, 'wallowing', to link in the tendency to sentimentality and the generosity of the patient.

Keynotes and Characteristics

- **Grief** — **Exciting cause**. These types are very emotional and sensitive.
- **< disappointed love** — **Exciting cause**. Too idealistic in love.
- **Sentimental** — They are romantic dreamers. Naive in some respects.
- **Overcome by mellow lights** — Their moods are changed by atmosphere, especially those which affect their sentiments.
- **Sympathetic** — They are so sensitive and can put themselves in others' shoes.
- **Write poetry** — To express their feelings. They will even talk in rhymes or verses.
- Melodramatic — Indulge their romanticism.
- **Suicidal** — They want to drown themselves.
- **Loathing of life** — Because they are so disappointed. They are besides themselves and cannot cope.
- Weep at slightest cause — They indulge their passions.
- **Easily startled** — Because they are so sensitive, < slightest noise.
- **Stubborn** — Like Calcarea carbonica to protect themselves.
- **Do not want to be spoken to** — They are surly, do not want to be noticed.
- **Dislike to be touched or looked at** — Reserved persons.
- **Angry at any little attention**
- **Sulky** — Any refusal strikes deep as a rejection.
- **Peevish and fretful** — They really want to be loved – think of the child.
- **Cross** — Often they are defending their vulnerable core.

180

- **Quarrelsome** — Nothing satisfies them. They want the moon!
- **Overeat** — When emotions are disturbed.
- **Obesity** — A natural result of the symptom above.
- Distended abdomen even after a little food — There may be the sensation of a lump.
- **Belch constantly** — And don't we call them 'pigs'?
- **Nausea at the sight and smell of food** — Not at rights with their world.
- **Loathing of food** — Is a strong revulsion of life.
- Child vomits milk in curds — The acid stomach turns the milk.
- **Crave pickles and acid food** — Which do not agree with them.
- Tongue coated white and thick — Showing disordered digestion.
- Diarrhoea < night with thirst for cold water — Compare with Phosphorus and Arsenicum
- **Stool lumpy with much mucus** — It is described in various ways including stool covered in mucus, or little lumps joined by mucus.
- Suppressed menses — From emotional trauma or cold bathing.
- Lumps in throat — With continual desire to swallow.
- **Lumpy** — Lumpy stool, lumpy leucorrhoea.
- **Acrid, excoriating discharges** — Can be seen in sweaty feet, leucorrhoea, mucus from anus, curdled vomit.
- Cracked, sore commissures — At corner of mouth and nostrils.
- Cracked soles of feet — So sensitive, can't walk on them.
- Suppurating eruptions — Pustular acne, smallpox, crusty impetigo.
- **Eruptions alternate with gastric symptoms** — Both with plenty of mucus or pus.
- **Skin thickens** — e.g. on palms and soles.
- Split fingernails — Like pig's trotters.
- **Horn-like excrescences** — And 'abnormal organizations of the skin' – von Lippe.
- Corns and callouses — Wherever the part is in touch with the outside world. See also on ME level!
- Symptoms change location — Often from one side to another.
- Chronic catarrh — Sycotic remedy.

Modalities

- < **left side**
- < **cold bathing**
- < **getting wet**
- < **overheated**
- < radiant heat
- < acids
- < pork
- < bread and pastry

> open air

ACTIVITY 1

In the essence, Antimonium crudum was noted to vary between 'hard' and 'soft'. List those symptoms that correspond to hardness and softness.

ACTIVITY 2

Antimonium crudum is a remedy of suppuration and over-function (sycosis). Make a list of symptoms that illustrate this character.

Wallowing in Emotions

Mentally, when healthy they may be happy youngsters who easily melt into smiles, and want to be beneficent and share friendship warmly. They are *sympathetic* and happily fit in, but if they are *disappointed or hurt*, they become *stubborn* and *will not communicate*. They shut themselves off, like Natrum muriaticum patients, and become *grumpy* and *argumentative – nothing satisfies them*. They just feel hurt.

Children become *sulky* and *cross* and even *quarrelsome* (very like the Nux vomica patient) and they *do not want to be spoken to* or, another keynote is *cannot bear to be touched or looked at*. The child may then become angry at any little attention that is given to it. They are warm affectionate little souls who take things personally and become *peevish and fretful* like Pulsatilla. They live in a *romantic world* becoming disillusioned and hurt when the real world impinges. This is where the *sentimentality* fits in. The adult can appear as a little *naive*.

Antimonium crudum is one of the remedies of *sentimental love* easily recognizable as they 'moon around' a lot (think of Ignatia) and would even *write poetry* to romanticize their loss (like Ignatia) but this patient *eats for comfort* (like Pulsatilla). They can be *melodramatic*, a bit like Pulsatilla, but will go further and become depressed to such an extent that they become *suicidal* and *want to drown themselves*. Pulsatilla will never get this far.

The sentimental Antimonium crudum patient tends to be *dreamy and sad*, *weeping at the slightest cause*. A keynote is that they are *overcome by mellow lights*. Moonlight fits into this category. Moonlight can lead to ecstasy or exaltation of their romantic tendencies and outbursts of affection! Some of the earlier homoeopaths described this remedy as hysterical. Living in such an unreal world it is easy to see how open they are to hurt. Then they are *edgy* and *easily startled by slight noises*. They withdraw into themselves to protect themselves and a bitterness or *loathing of life* develops. Even then the bitterness is not hard like that of Natrum muriaticum but melts easily like Pulsatilla when the right note is sounded.

ACTIVITY 3   Her favourite pop star has just had an accident. Describe the behaviour of the Antimonium crudum teenager at tea-time.

Disordered Digestion

The stomach is easily disordered as all the emotional symptoms centre on the stomach. There is a tendency towards *nausea* and *vomiting*, *diarrhoea* and *overeating*.

They tend to overeat considerably when the emotions are affected. They will eat anything that gets in their way but will *react badly to bread, pastry, rich foods, pork and acid foods like vinegar*.

The stomach is often *distended*, even when very little has been eaten. There may be the *sensation of a lump*. There is much *belching that tastes of food eaten*. The abdomen *rumbles* fiercely. Heartburn is common. Sometimes there is such a severe *burning in the epigastric area* that the patient despairs and is driven to suicide. At such a time we would expect to see the *thickly coated white tongue* showing *over-acidity*.

The digestive symptoms are a powerful repulsion of the life energies. The *loathing of food* parallels the loathing of life in the mental realm. It often arises from emotional disturbance, so may not be accompanied by the over-acidity symptoms above. Here the patient goes to the opposite extreme to reject food because of *nausea at the sight and smell* of it. They swing to the other pole of the magnet or cannot select a pole when they *vomit without gaining any relief* or even *vomit without nausea* – what is the vital force trying to achieve? The vomit often contains much mucus as in Ipecacuanha but that of Antimonium crudum is recognizable as lumpy. This is clearly seen in the *curdled, lumpy milk* vomited by the child. There is much *mucus in the stool* which may alternate from lumpy mucus-covered knots in constipation to watery diarrhoea which also has lumps and much mucus. Copious excoriating mucus oozes out with the piles. These excretory symptoms are especially found in old people.

ACTIVITY 4   Explain how the genital symptoms of Antimonium crudum show the sensation and appearance of lumpiness, copious mucus and 'burning'.

The Skin

The skin symptoms alternate with the gastric symptoms showing once again the tendency to swing between two poles of the magnet. The lumpiness now becomes hard growths. *Warts*, *calluses* and *corns* are described as *horny*. The burning is present in *dryness*, so the *horn hardens and cracks*. The *nails distort* or pull apart into two *like a pig's trotter*. The feet are tough and hard, but *crack open* so they are sensitive. The corners of the mouth, nose, the eyes, dry and crack. The nipples crack. *Hard, thick scabs* form in the skin eruptions. The copious mucus becomes *pus* under the scabs or in impetigo. *Pustules* are produced as easily for the dreamy teenager's *acne* as for *smallpox* or *chickenpox*.

ACTIVITY 5 Compare the skin symptoms of Antimonium crudum and Graphites.

ACTIVITY 6 Compare the effect of heat on the Antimonium crudum patient and on the Sulphur patient.

ACTIVITY 7 What is the characteristic presentation of symptoms in the following minor ailments?

Sore throat
Headache
Earache.

ACTIVITY 8 Describe how the striving for connectedness shows in mental and physical symptoms. Use keynotes and characteristic symptoms to illustrate your answer.

Similar Remedies

Rhus toxicodendron produces pustular eruptions that itch – as in chickenpox. These eruptions are also red with a white top.

Ipecacuanha has copious mucus in gastric symptoms. It vomits without relieving because the pneumo-gastric nerve is affected. The Ipecacuanha patient is just as dissatisfied but tends to be more capricious.

Graphites produces hard, thickened skin that burns but is less likely to crack. The Graphites patient is also sentimental and much moved by music.

Antimonium Tartaricum

Pentasulphide of antimony [K(Sb O), $C_4H_4O_6$]2 + [H_2O]

Origin

The remedy was prepared from the potassium deposit found on the sides of wine casks, tartar emetic. It was proved by Hahnemann amongst others. Tyler reminds us that it contains the pentasulphide which is the same red-orange colour that is found in the lungs of dogs who have been poisoned.

Essence

This remedy has many similarities to Antimonium crudum but it strikes deeper. It is used for 'broken down catarrhal constitutions' usually in older patients. Where Antimonium crudum affects skin and mucous membrane, Antimonium tartaricum affects the lungs – where the life-giving oxygen enters.

183

Keynotes and Characteristics

• Pale and cyanosed	Blood is stagnant, not oxygenated.
• **Hippocratic countenance**	Dark rings around sunken eyes.
• Nostrils dilate and flap	As in Lycopodium.
• **Cold sweat**	Exudes because skin and mucous membrane is so relaxed.
• **Prostration**	There is much weakness.
• **Pallor**	Life has withdrawn from the extremities.
• **Blueness of the face**	Because low in oxygen.
• Irregular pulse and breath	It is a remedy of the last stages of disease.
• **Coarse rattling in chest**	Much mucus, but little is raised.
• Cannot lie down as they suffocate	There is so much mucus in the lungs.
• **Thick, ropey mucus**	Compared to Kali bichromium which is yellow, this is white.
• **Rattling cough**	< 3–4 a.m. Old people get this every cold spell of winter. < anger.
• Pit of stomach sensitive to touch	The pneumo-gastric nerve is affected.
• Cough ends in vomit	Especially after eating.
• **Violent retching with sinking at stomach**	Yet great effort to expel, so sleep afterwards.
• **Thickly coated white tongue**	Sometimes red at the edges and centre where dry.
• **Nausea comes in waves**	As in Ipecacuanha.
• **Loathing of all food**	Even vomit water.
• Milk aggravates all symptoms	Usually they are averse to milk.
• Desire acid food such as apples	Which make them ill.
• **Thirstless**	But can have the opposite too.
• **Abdomen feels full of stones**	
• Violent, cutting colic	'As if the bowels would be cut to pieces'.
• Diarrhoea alternates with eruptions	A difficult symptom to find from the patient as they do not notice the alteration.
• Painful urge to urinate	Stitching and burning of parts.
• Pustular eruptions with sacro-lumbar pain	**Strange, Rare and Peculiar** symptom.
• **Extreme irritability**	They hate to be disturbed.
• **Averse consolation**	It makes them more irritable.
• **Does not want to be touched**	Mentally, or physically.
• Fear of being alone	Despite the despondency they hang on to the threads of life.
• **Apathetic and despondent**	They are so low they don't have the energy to take an interest.
• Whining and peevish	They moan all the time.
• **Child wants to be carried**	This resembles Pulsatilla and Chamomilla.
• **Very drowsy**	Because so little energy.

Modalities

< warmth	> open air
< anger	> sitting upright
< **milk**	> bringing up expectoration
< **cold, damp weather**	
< change of weather	

ACTIVITY 9   List those symptoms which are similar to Antimonium crudum.

ACTIVITY 10

Study the following terms in a medical textbook:

Pulmonary oedema
Right ventricular failure
Pneumonia.

How do the symptoms relate to Antimonium tartaricum?

Lack of Life

Antimonium tartaricum is a step further on from Antimonium crudum. It is a deep remedy of final stages or serious illness having its action on the lungs.

Mentally the patient *does not want to be bothered* because there is so little energy and everything is a burden. The patient is extremely *irritable* and *hates to be disturbed*. They may be so ill they just *want to be left alone*. They may not even have the energy to be frightened when they are alone. Their energy is so low there is little left for interaction. There is much *drowsiness*. When there is more energy you will find the *peevish* picture we saw in Antimonium crudum. They whine and moan all the time but they are too *apathetic* to do anything about it. We usually say this patient feels sorry for him/herself. As the crisis deepens we may find the patient anxious and *fearful for his/her condition*. As with Antimonium crudum they *do not want to be touched or looked at*.

The vital energy is low so there is a tendency to *take colds on the slightest exposure to cold, damp conditions*. The cold goes rapidly to the chest, producing much mucus. The *rattly cough* indicates the presence of mucus. As the symptoms deepen there is difficulty bringing some of the mucus up. They become *breathless*. Inhalers and decongestants do not help. Postural drainage does help. As they get to the end, the lungs are so filled with fluid they drown. They cannot lie down in bed because they *fear they will suffocate*. The effort of trying to *bring up mucus exhausts them* so they fall asleep, or so violent is the retching the pneumo-gastric nerve causes them to *vomit violently* and of course it is mucus that is brought up.

In the most serious cases of pneumonia in old people they will be found propped up on pillows with a *hippocratic expression*, dark sunken eyes and lean pale face. They may be wrapped in a rug because they are so cold. That may not help much because there is *not enough energy to generate their own heat*. There cannot be too much heat in the room because they cannot breathe. There is a *pallor* with *blueness and cold, clammy sweat*. It is the collapse state of the end of life. This is why Antimonium tartaricum has such a reputation, like Carbo vegetalis as a corpse reviver. It gives the body energy to create heat and life.

Not all patients go to the end though. There is a middle stage when you might see the *white-coated tongue*. As the symptoms enter the digestive system this dries up so you see *red, dry patches* along the *edge of tongue* and in the centre. There may be a *tenderness in the pit of the stomach* especially if there is *violent retching*. The burning pains will be present in the stomach and if there is much mucus the patient will *crave acids*, particularly *apples* to 'perk' it up. In the long run this may create more mucus because acid food is mucus-forming. Full of mucus the patient will *lose the appetite*. They may even have a *loathing for food*. This is a rejection of the life sustaining forces we came across in Antimonium crudum.

In the healthier Antimonium tartaricum patient you can see the life enhanced in the digestive symptom with the *wave motion of the nausea*. This is enhanced action of the digestive system even if it brings exhaustion after it. Further down the digestive system this same liveliness is seen in the *cutting, colic pains* and in the *urge to urinate* with inflammatory burning and stitching of bladder and urethra. When there is even more energy in the system the vital force can express itself through *pustular skin eruptions* – it will then resemble Antimonium crudum even more.

ACTIVITY 11

Compare the skin symptoms of Antimonium crudum and Antimonium tartaricum.

ACTIVITY 12 — Compare the digestive system of Antimonium crudum and Antimonium tartaricum. Are there exciting causes? What are the modalities? What level of disorder do the symptoms belong to – sensation, dysfunction, pathology?

Relaxation

There is much about *relaxation of tissue* in the Antimonium tartaricum symptom picture. In the final stages this is similar to Mercurius in that the patient *dribbles* so much but whereas Mercurius acts on excreting glands the action of Antimonium tartaricum is on mucous membrane and skin. Hence the *copious secretion of mucus*, even from the stomach, as the symptom picture builds up. On a healthier level this is represented by the pustular spots.

In the final stages, as the life withdraws, the *copious expectoration* is accompanied by *sweat*. As pallor and shock increase a *cold sweat oozes from the extremities*. There is not enough activity to bring the blood back so fluid stagnates in pools all over the body – *dropsy*.

The muscles are so weak they are relaxed, so there is not enough action to cough efficiently to clear expectoration. They *drown in fluid* – hydrothorax.

ACTIVITY 13 — Describe the rheumatism of Antimonium tartaricum. Include the keynotes and characteristic symptoms where appropriate.

Similar Remedies

Lycopodium in its final stages may resemble Antimonium tartaricum. Then we will see Lycopodium affect the fluid balance through the kidneys and lungs. The hippocratic expression may also be present, the nostrils may flap and have sooty deposits. The Lycopodium patient will also feel sorry for themselves and go from peevishness to indifference.

Pulsatilla does not go to the depths of Antimonium tartaricum but may produce a similar symptom picture of oedema and peevishness, at one stage. At another level, pustular acne and eruptions are common in the Pulsatilla patient as are catarrhal discharges.

Carbo vegetalis is another remedy for the final stages which produces much cyanosis because of poor oxygen supply. It is also a remedy of relaxed tissues producing varicose veins and oedema in the extremities.

Review Sulphur

Both the Antimonies contain a good deal of Sulphur and so we might expect similarities. Sulphur is one of the most egocentric remedies in the Materia Medica. They are not always selfish, though this is usually the case, but they are always independent and less affected by others. Many a marriage comes a cropper because of lack of affection from the Sulphur spouse! So, how can we say that Sulphur resembles the Antimonies? It would appear the antimonies seek to relate; the Sulphur patient has no need to relate.

Self-indulgence

When we speak of self-indulgence we usually mean food. Antimonium crudum shares the appetite of Sulphur – they will eat anything. Sulphur is a volcano that is forever pushing outwards oblivious to those around it. It needs food to fuel its irregular heating mechanism which is wasteful. Both Antimonies ultimately align themselves, but as the disorder is taken within the disturbance goes deeper so they have a loathing for food. They turn against the life pole which Sulphur devours rapidly.

Even the sentimentality is a self-indulgence. There is a difference in its expression in that Sulphur is a very mental patient whilst the Antimonium crudum patient is more emotional, like the Pulsatilla. Antimonium crudum will write poetry and howl at the moon. Both are dreamers but Sulphur is practical, planning and theorizing, whilst Antimonium crudum and Antimonium tartaricum are romantic and sentimental. Both Sulphur and the Antimonies spend much time in this inner world.

Areas Affected

Sulphur and the Antimonies both have a strong action on the skin. The Antimonies are more sycotic producing pustular eruptions. Sulphur certainly can produce these but its skin problems tend to burn and excoriate and swell in inflammation.

When the skin is suppressed there is a similar movement to the digestive system with burning pains and colic. Once again Sulphur is less likely to produce the slimy vomit of the sycotic miasm but all affect the epigastric area. In Sulphur there is emptiness, in Antimonium tartaricum there is tenderness. Antimonium crudum feels there is a need to keep stuffing food into this area.

When the disease moves even deeper Sulphur is a major lung remedy of disorders such as tuberculosis and pneumonia. It affects the deepest lobe of the left lung. Only Antimonium tartaricum goes deep enough into the lungs. Instead of Sulphur's inflammation, it produces suppuration. It has much lower energy than the other two, so problems arise because it cannot expel the mucus – can't lie down, can't breathe well enough.

Sulphur and Antimonium tartaricum can be seen as extremes. Sulphur is fiery and explosive – it has so much energy. In later stages the rheumatism is inflammatory in an overactive metabolism. Sulphur is choleric. Antimonium tartaricum is phlegmatic. Antimonium tartaricum cools down drastically and is even cyanosed because of lack of flow. The cold, clammy sweat and pallor is a chilling of the body and life force. Antimonium crudum is in between. It has Sulphur's fiery feet. They tend to sweat because they are hot, not as in Antimonium tartaricum because they are cold.

Review
Pulsatilla

Pulsatilla contains a great deal of Sulphur as Kali sulphuricum. Also it is remarkably similar to Antimonium crudum in its sentimentality and emotions. Both can be seen to express and need a great deal of affection and suffer when this is withdrawn. The soft centre of both can be easily influenced. Both are locked inside in shyness so demonstrate sullenness and mood swings. It can be difficult to tell these remedies apart. Their food cravings and aversions are similar. They both eat for comfort, and wallow in their emotions.

Both remedies have pustular and glandular problems. Pulsatilla affects the gut's ability to absorb iron so can become anaemic with LBP. In its end stages Pulsatilla can resemble Antimonium tartaricum although it never really affects the lungs. It has the same laxity of tissue, giving rise to varicose veins and oedema. The fluid imbalance of Pulsatilla is more likely to affect the kidneys than the lungs. The energy does not appear to drop as low as in Antimonium tartaricum. Pulsatilla retains the ability to throw out an inflammatory illness. When too relaxed, gentle exercise will stimulate circulation and organs in the Pulsatilla patient. The Antimonium tartaricum patient would not have the energy.

ACTIVITY 14

Create a table of comparison for Antimonium crudum, Antimonium tartaricum, Sulphur and Pulsatilla listing the following:

Exciting causes	Digestion
Zones of body affected	Lungs
Inflammatory symptoms	Kidney
Suppuratory symptoms	Personality
Skin	Modalities.

SELF-TEST QUESTIONS

You will find the answers in the text when you review it. Check these in the answer section.

1. What will the Antimonium crudum child do if you look at it?
2. How would you describe the skin symptoms of Antimonium crudum?

3. What does the cough of Antimonium tartaricum sound like?
4. How does Antimonium crudum's loathing of life show in the digestive system?
5. Describe the nostrils of the Antimonium tartaricum patient.
6. What accompanies the cold sweat of the Antimonium tartaricum patient?
7. Compare the modalities of Antimonium crudum and Antimonium tartaricum.
8. What kind of food does Antimonium crudum crave?
9. Which remedy desires apples?
10. Describe how the mucus of Antimonium tartaricum resembles that of Kali bichromium.
11. How does the self-indulgence of Sulphur differ from that of Antimonium crudum?
12. In what way is Antimonium crudum sentimental?
13. The nausea comes in waves and there is much mucus. Which remedy?
14. Describe the discharges of Antimonium crudum.
15. How does the oedema of Pulsatilla differ and resemble Antimonium tartaricum?
16. Describe the sensation in the epigastric area of Antimonium tartaricum.
17. Which symptom is accompanied by backache in the Antimonium tartaricum patient?
18. Describe the exciting cause of Antimonium crudum.
19. What happens after the Antimonium tartaricum coughing fit?
20. Give examples of the lump symptoms of Antimonium crudum.
21. Which two of the remedies studied in this lesson are thirstless?
22. Describe the Antimonium tartaricum child.
23. How do lights affect the Antimonium crudum patient?
24. What happens when you console the Antimonium tartaricum patient?
25. Which food symptoms of Antimonium crudum are the same as Pulsatilla?
26. Why does the Antimonium tartaricum patient fear suffocation?
27. Describe the colic of the Antimonium tartaricum patient.
28. Which attributes of Antimonium crudum are similar to a pig?
29. How do the stomach problems of Sulphur compare with Antimonium crudum?
30. What effect does cold bathing have on the menstrual cycle of Antimonium crudum?

Further Studies

Antimonium Crudum

1. Antimonium crudum has a rush of blood to the head. What other remedies you have studied have this symptom? Note other similarities between these remedies and Antimonium crudum. What types of pathology produce a rush of blood to the head?
2. Compare Antimonium crudum and Sulphur with particular reference to skin and digestion. How do these two remedies show you the link between the inner and the outer tube?
3. Compare Antimonium crudum and Pulsatilla in a case of rheumatism.
4. Describe the behaviour of the Antimonium crudum child with measles. Pay particular attention to differentiating your picture from that of Pulsatilla which is regarded as a very common remedy in measles.
5. State how the gastric symptoms compare in the Antimonium crudum and Arsenicum patients.

Antimonium Tartaricum

1. Compare the respiratory symptoms of Antimonium tartaricum and Lycopodium.
2. Compare the collapse state of Antimonium tartaricum to that of Camphor and Veratrum.
3. Compare the rheumatism of Antimonium tartaricum, Antimonium crudum, Sulphur and Pulsatilla.
4. List the Strange, Rare and Peculiars of Antimonium tartaricum.
5. In what symptoms does the relaxed state of Antimonium tartaricum resemble Mercurius?
6. Label the exciting causes of Antimonium tartaricum.
7. Define how Antimonium tartaricum is similar to Arsenicum.

Two Psoric Remedies

Baryta Carbonica, Graphites

Aim: To explore the quality of the psoric miasm in remedies.

Objective: To identify the nature of psora in the symptoms of Baryta carbonica and Graphites.

Headings: INTRODUCTION
BARYTA CARBONICA: Origin; Nature of the Mineral; Essence; Keynotes and Characteristics; Modalities; Lack of Growth; Lack of Rational Thought; Glandular Affections; Discharge; Similar Remedies
GRAPHITES: Origin; Nature of the Mineral; Essence; Keynotes and Characteristics; Modalities; Slow and Thick; Lack of Security; The Graphites Child; Similar Remedies
SELF-TEST QUESTIONS
FURTHER STUDIES

Introduction

Psora is the first of Hahnemann's miasms. He claimed all of us have this.

He first became aware of the miasm when he realized homoeopathic medicines could remove symptoms very effectively, but did not always improve health. When the patient came with sore throats, he did not expect the patient to develop bronchial problems 1–2 years later. If eczema is cured, asthma should not result. Similarly, effective treatment of rheumatism as a circulatory disease should not be followed at any point by heart problems. All of these examples show a deepening crisis adverse to the Laws of Cure. Hahnemann expected each homoeopathic medicine to improve health.

He became aware of a difference between acute and chronic illnesses. Chronic illness is an underlying weakness, predisposition, which is not necessarily manifest. It may be latent until acted upon by a trigger factor such as an exciting cause. Even then, if vitality is strong, there may be no manifest illness. We inherit these patterns of weakness from our parents. It is possible to acquire them in life through exposure to powerful morbific agents, such as disease, drugs, emotional trauma, serious accidents, continuing environmental pollution and stress. It is also possible to pass this damaged vital force on to our children.

To accommodate such deep damage the vital force alters its centre of gravity. It cannot overcome the trauma, but it will survive. When the new point of balance is reached it is not the centre, so there is wear and tear on parts which take the strain. Thus the system is not perfect and has a built-in decay. As time goes on, this strain shows as the weak parts function less efficiently. Hahnemann said of the miasms that the afflicted vital force becomes more disturbed as the symptoms steadily get worse until death occurs. You could call it the aging process. Each of us has a family pattern which is more or less manifest, depending on our vitality and the vicissitudes of our life. Each has psora because of thousands of years of suppressive treatment for skin disorders. The healthy vital force dispels disease as far as possible to the outside. If this action is suppressed, the vital force must find other outlets to express disease or it holds onto part of the disease and has to re-balance to survive.

Psora is the tendency of the vital force to underfunction.

Baryta Carbonica

Barium carbonate

Origin

Hahnemann proved the remedy from a trituration of barium carbonate.

Nature of the Mineral

The mineral is very poisonous, but can be used in barium meals and enemas because it is absorbed very slowly. It shows opaque when X-rayed.

Its main action in the body is on muscular tissue where it increases the contraction. Eventually it slows down muscles, through paralysis, because of its effect on the central nervous system. Combined in the carbonate, we see the worn down, deficiency character of Barium enhanced.

Essence

The main characteristic of the remedy is an inability to reach potential. Although this can be applied to most people in an imperfect world, it is taken to extreme in the Baryta carbonica patient. *Dwarfishness* describes the essence of this psoric remedy.

Keynotes and Characteristics

• **Young people stunted and wrinkled**	Like the stereotype of a dwarf.
• **Slow learners**	So painfully slow they appear imbecilic.
• **Childlike of mind**	Grown-ups playing with toys. Simple thoughts.
• **Lack of interest**	There is none of the natural curiosity of the child. The child does not play.
• **Bashful**	Not able to extend the self.
• **Lack of confidence**	As above.
• **Lack of courage**	
• **Averse to strangers**	Hides behind furniture, etc. like Calcarea carbonica.
• **Sensitive**	Can feel mocked and laughed at.
• **Indecisive**	Little will.
• **Weak memory**	There is little retentive will.
• **Lack of rational thought**	Because of weak memory.
• **Thoughtless**	There is not enough activity of mind to think of others.
• **Lack of concentration**	They have no will to stay in one place.
• **Imbecility**	They appear a bit thick.
• Grief at little things	Little things mean a lot to these simple souls.
• **Tendency to catch colds**	The body puts up little defence.
• **Copious catarrh**	The mucous membrane yields easily too.
• Catarrhal deafness	As the eustachian tube is blocked.
• **Glandular swellings**	Usually accompanied by catarrh.
• **Induration of glands**	As in Calcarea carbonica and Silicea.
• **Enlarged tonsils**	< right side. Chronically swollen.
• Noises reverberate in ears on blowing nose	The catarrh changes the ear into an echo chamber.
• Cough after getting feet wet	As in Pulsatilla.
• As if the lungs were filled with smoke	Comes mainly with a cough.
• No strength to bring up expectoration	This is weakness again.
• **Indurated testicles**	Especially the right.
• Undescended testes	They have not matured.
• **Impotency**	A lack of sex hormone enhances the childlikeness.

• **Enlarged prostate**	As the old man again becomes a child!
• **Offensive foot sweat**	Soles sore with sweat. If suppressed it becomes glandular problems in throat.
• Muscles tense and shorten	As in Causticum.
• **Muscles weak**	Constantly wanting to lie down or sit down.
• Arteriosclerosis	Is fatty degeneration of the muscles in the arteries – they are lined with fat.
• Weak digestion > cold food	In old people especially.
• **Sudden disgust of food whilst eating**	These patients do not grasp life lustily.
• **Warts**	
• **Fatty tumours**	

Modalities

< slight exposure to cold   > **warmth**
< cold to feet or head   > cold food
< **suppressed foot sweat**
< company of others
< heat
< eating
< right side

 ACTIVITY 1   List those symptoms that show weakness.

 ACTIVITY 2   Which symptoms show *dwarfishness?* List them.

 ACTIVITY 3   Where would you expect to find Baryta carbonica in the *Mind* section of Kent's Repertory? List the rubrics.

Lack of Growth

It is said of Baryta carbonica that the young patient looks old and the old are young, meaning childish. The young are *stunted* and *wrinkled*. It is as if they have not grown enough to fill out their skin! There is little activity, so there they sit like a wizened old man, lacking the curiosity and vivacity of the child. This is different from the Calcarea carbonica child who is placid and receptive and too shy to venture forth. The little Calcarea carbonica mind is slow, but active, and the wheels turn within – you can see the bright little eyes light up when he/she eventually produces the synthesis of all that experience. The Baryta carbonica child simply does not reach the flowering stage – he/she remains a simpleton.

He reminds me of *Bashful*, the dwarf in 'Snow White'. This is different from the Pulsatilla shyness which is coyness, ensnaring you in their world with their charm. What is there in the Baryta carbonica's world? The mentality often remains at the primitive autos level, which has learned to say 'me' but not to distinguish 'me' from the rest of the outside world. Thus this individual can appear very *selfish*, or *self-indulgent*. The adult indulges in pastimes which do not ask responsibility or interaction from them – trains in the attic is a good example. She/he will often annoy others in company when they do not interact at the same level, but interject unrelated trivia into the conversation. The trivia is often personified because the level of consciousness still very much surrounds self in an immature and personal way. Unlike other selfish remedies Baryta carbonica is not egotistical. They are harmless and simple – *childish*. And, like the child, or Bashful the dwarf, they are *vulnerable* and *sensitive* if exposed as out of step, especially since they do not always understand why they do not fit in. They react emotionally, or on an animal level, rather than rationally.

191

ACTIVITY 4   Sketch a scenario that shows the behaviour of the Baryta carbonica patient when approached for a date as a teenager. Which symptoms describe their reaction?

Lack of Rational Thought

Lack of rational thought arises from the *weakness of memory* which cannot hold thoughts and this, in turn, is related to an *inability to focus attention*. The mind is like a butterfly. If we keep this in mind, we will see how it becomes a most useful remedy in old age, when the mind starts to wander and cannot focus.

The remedy is also used for 'old drunkards'. When alcohol starts to affect the brain it weakens the synapses, so the patient cannot connect. Memory is weak and *thought is slow*.

Glandular Affections

The mental symptoms clearly suggest psora or underfunction, whereas the physical symptoms suggest sycosis because they centre on glandular function. This dilemma can be solved if psora is understood as underfunction. There is insufficient development of the wave pattern for the disturbance to reach the surface in the Baryta carbonica patient, so it stays in the great sea of the body which is drained by the lymphatic system. The disturbance concentrates at the exits, discharging catarrh and swelling glands such as tonsils and adenoids. The three major remedies of this miasm, Calcarea carbonica, Silicea and Graphites each have a strong skin picture, but as the disease process goes deeper, there are many acute problems in the lymphatic glands. Calcarea carbonica, Silicea and Baryta carbonica are also major anti-scrofulous remedies and it may come as no surprise to you that the tuberculoid miasm is seen by many homoeopaths as a deeper psoric state (where there is not enough energy to reach the surface) than as a separate miasm. This deeper psoric state concentrates less on the skin than on the lymphatic drainage system and beyond that on the respiratory system.

The lymphatic system is not given the same importance in orthodox medical science.

In this context the most common symptom that arises from it is the disposition to *catch colds easily* (Bar. c., Calc. c., Sil., Tub.). Like Pulsatilla and Dulcamara, the Baryta carbonica patient may take colds easily *after the feet are soaked*. In the Baryta carbonica patient, colds usually go to the *tonsils* which can be *permanently enlarged*, especially on the *right side*. All other glands may also be enlarged including those of the groin and abdomen. Only Calcarea carbonica shares the common involvement of the mesenteric glands. When the child complains of sore tummies he/she is not always feigning illness to avoid school, though the involvement of these glands can be brought on by nervousness. The neck of the Baryta carbonica patient is often stiff because the cervical glands swell. This is common also in the Pulsatilla patient. In serious cases the *glands suppurate* so often the tonsils are removed causing more serious problems in the abdomen. Copious catarrh from the glands bungs up the upper respiratory tract causing headaches and deafness. One Strange, Rare and Peculiar symptom that arises out of this is the *echoing reverberation when blowing the nose*. The child is more likely to find this frightening than fascinating. When the cough develops in the chest there is another Strange, Rare and Peculiar symptom – *it is as if the lungs were filled with smoke*. The cough is difficult because there is not enough activity to clear out the lungs which feel blocked.

When the sex glands are involved, there are problems of *undescended testes*, as in Calcarea carbonica, and *early impotency*. Lack of sex hormone in both of these cases enhances the childishness of the adult by taking away the drive and determination of the normal adult male! The remedy comes in use for *prostate problems* when that gland enlarges. One of the associated problems of this in the Baryta carbonica patient is cystitis – *burning pains on urination*.

ACTIVITY 5   Describe in detail the cold symptoms of the Baryta carbonica patient. Use keynotes and characteristic symptoms and pay particular attention to include general and particular symptoms.

Discharge

Most discharge is catarrhal, from the glands or the mucous membrane. There is a relationship between these and sweat. Both arise from the lymphatic system as the great sea of the body. Lymph nodes are the gates to the lymphatic system. Other glands follow the same pattern but are more separated. Remedies with a strong effect on the glands are usually also catarrhal remedies. Baryta carbonica, Calcarea carbonica and Silicea all fit into this picture. All are remedies of *hardened glands* and of significant sweats.

The sweat glands are a direct outlet from the great sea, in which all the body cells float. They perform excretion by secreting sweat. The *foul, smelly foot sweats* of Baryta carbonica, Calcarea carbonica and Silicea act to excrete and detoxify the body. Wet, cold feet, or any other form of suppression, may block this route putting pressure elsewhere. In Baryta carbonica the tonsils may enlarge and catarrhal throat problems develop when foot sweat is suppressed. It is possible that colds may develop.

The other side of the discharge coin is absorption. Absorption is one of the purposes of the inner tube, the gastrointestinal tract. In the Baryta carbonica patient the intestinal wall may be so swollen and engorged that *food cannot be absorbed*. Remember, the wall of the intestine is full of secretory cells. The end-product of such digestive problems is *malnutrition* and resultant emaciation. A *bloated face* is a strange concomitant symptom of the swollen intestines in the Baryta carbonica patient. This symptom is often seen in old people.

ACTIVITY 6

Outline the appearance of the old gent (Baryta carbonica patient) at the bowling club AGM. Use as many keynotes and characteristics as appropriate.

Similar Remedies

Calcarea carbonica like Baryta carbonica, is delayed in development of mind and body. Both have a strong effect on the glands and muscles. Calcarea carbonica also has an effect on the bones. Whilst Calcarea carbonica is lazy because of lack of stamina, Baryta carbonica is deficient and cannot try. Both are shy people who do not like to be exposed.

Silicea is a remedy which does not fulfil its potential because of fear of failure and lack of energy. The Silicea patient differs from the Baryta carbonica patient in that Silicea has the structure to work from. However, in another type of Silicea patient there is backwardness of mentality like Baryta carbonica. It shows the glandular affections and catarrh of Baryta carbonica. Silicea goes deeper to ulceration.

Graphites

Black lead

Origin

Hahnemann prepared the remedy from a trituration of 'the purest black lead taken from a fine English pencil'.

Nature of the Mineral

Graphite is an isotope of carbon which is one of the most common elements forming many isotopes, amorphous and crystalline. Carbon is one of the fundaments of organic chemistry.

In its natural state graphite is insoluble and inert. This preparation contains an impurity of iron so the remedy has similarities to Ferrum metallicum and Pulsatilla.

Essence

The inertia of the mineral can be seen in the *blandness* of the symptom picture of Graphites. It is one of the *fair, fat* and *forty* remedies which gathers bloatage as time passes. The skin dries, thickens, indurates and then cracks.

Keynotes and Characteristics

- **Overweight** — Metabolism is slow.
- **Skin dry and flaky** — The energy withdraws to the inside.
- **Lack of sweat** — As above. Weakness.
- **Excoriation of skin in folds** — A typical site of eczema.
- **Excoriation at muco-cutaneous junctions** — As in Natrum muriaticum.
- **Fissures** — Because of dryness.
- **Cracks** — As above.
- **Skin hardens** — And thickens before cracking.
- **Scratches eruptions until they are raw and bleed**
- **Eruptions < heat** — As in Sulphur.
- **Thick, sticky exudate, dries to yellow crusts** — These are found in eye problems and in the nose colds.
- **Burning in many places** — Even in varicose veins.
- Nails thickened and distorted — You will see this in skin disease.
- Thickened eyelids — Where the skin joins the mucous membrane, lining tissue.

- **Intense photophobia**
- See double — The muscles do not co-ordinate.
- Fiery zig-zags outside field of vision
- **Recurrent styes** — As in Staphysagria.
- **Contraction of tendons** — Especially behind knees.
- **Constriction of many parts** — e.g. throat, compels to swallow. This is because of drying and thickening.
- **Offensive discharges** — Smell sour.
- **Burning in stomach** — Antimonium crudum has this with skin problems.

- Averse sweets < sweets — Gives rise to nausea.
- **Voice lacks control of modulation** — Like Phosphorus.
- **Deafness – hears > in a noise** — **Strange, Rare and Peculiar**.
- **Flushes upwards** — This is a remedy of menopause.
- **Craves air** — Like many of the carbons.
- **Chilly** — In the carbons the heat mechanism is upset.
- **Disposition to catch cold** — Poor vitality.
- **Anxiety** — Low in confidence.
- **Foreboding that something will happen** — Concerned about their salvation.
- **Irresolute** — They cannot quite make up their mind. Too weak.
- **Moods change constantly** — As impressed by events.
- **Timid and hesitant** — Poor self-esteem.
- **Weeps easily from music** — This patient is sentimental.
- **Slow of thought** — Fidgety trying to concentrate.
- **Mistakes reading and writing** — Because mind is weak.
- **Remembers the past only** — Forgets more recent events.
- **Impudent child** — This is a sign of inner insecurity. The child acts out with those most familiar to it.
- **Laughs at reprimand** — 'Come and catch me'.
- Head pain, one sided > cool air — Once again, the carbon modality.
- Pains in uterus, reaching high — This occurs when the dryness and contraction reach this organ.
- Bearing down pains — There is heaviness and congestion at period time.
- Leucorrhoea instead of menses — Occurs in gushes.
- Aversion to coition — There is too much movement for this slow remedy.
- Large, knotty stools covered in mucus — Once again, dryness and contraction, yet the excess secretion of mucus.

194

Modalities

< change of weather   > open air
< during and after menstruation
< suppressed menses
< suppressed eruptions
< **cold**
< wet feet

ACTIVITY 7   List the symptoms of dryness and contraction. Can you see this on the mental level as well as the physical?

ACTIVITY 8   Which symptoms of Graphites show a lack of oxygen and life?

Slow and Thick

Slowness and *thickness* characterize the symptom picture. The symptoms are slow to develop and are usually of a more chronic nature. It is as if the mind works through treacle; the skin builds thick layers, often calloused, which make it difficult for the patient to feel the outside world; slowness of assimilation leads to obesity which further slows down the physical and mental spheres. I see them as 'Michelin men'. As in the advertisements for Michelin tyres it is as if they are ensheathed in rubber.

Apart from *anxiety*, little registers in the mind, so *short-term memory is very poor*. As in the Baryta carbonica patient, this is the reason that thinking is such an effort. Long term memory is fine in the Graphites patient, because this material has already got through the thick screening process. This process is further illustrated by another symptom. The Graphites patient *makes mistakes in reading and writing because attention is not properly focused*.

The slowness and thickness can be seen throughout the remedy, but especially on the skin. Skin problems are common, but usually of a deep, chronic nature, as in eczema. *Burning, itching* and *dryness* characterize the first stage. The main areas attacked are around *folds and flexures*. The dry skin *flakes and cracks* around the nose, eyes, ears, anus, nipples and fingertips. Where scabbiness develops there are *thick deposits*. The eczema has thick deposits. Where the skin cracks there is a *thick honey-like fluid* that flows forth and *dries into yellow crusts*. This helps us to distinguish the Graphites eczema from others. There are also herpetic eruptions with thick yellow crusts and it is not uncommon to find a *thick crustiness at the back of the head* which does not really fit into the definition of cradle cap (as in Calcarea carbonica).

When the skin is injured it heals poorly in the Graphites patient. *Scars are thick and hard* and often there are *burning sensations* under these.

Burning and hardness are found around ulcers. Thickening is found on the eyelids as are *cystic tumours*. Graphites is a remedy of cancer especially of the breast. The nails are characteristically affected so badly that they are *thick* and *distorted*.

The glands and tendons are affected. *Glands* are *enlarged* and *hard*, e.g. tonsils and ovaries. *Tendons contract*, especially behind the knee. Weakness is similar to Calcarea carbonica, but in the Graphites patient it is of the tendons like Rhus toxicodendron, whereas the Calcarea carbonica patient has weak muscles. As in the Rhus toxicodendron patient, the Graphites patient is *sensitive to over-lifting* and *easily strains tendons*. In the throat, constriction means a constant desire to swallow. If the vocal cords are affected, the *voice lacks modulation*.

ACTIVITY 9   Describe how slowness and thickness are reflected in the cold symptoms of Graphites. Use keynotes and characteristics where appropriate.

Lack of Security

The mental picture is one of dullness and a lethargy that *dreads all mental work* though there is a marked difference between the morning and the evening pictures. The mental faculties are *weak in the morning* and so *exhilarated in the evening* that he/she may not be able to sleep. In the morning he/she cannot think because of sluggishness, so is poorly equipped to come to decisions. *Irresolution* and *anxiety* predominate in the symptom picture. Although anxiety is described in the Materia Medica as *a foreboding of something about to happen*, it could also be described as *a lack of security*. The Graphites patient is *hesitant* and *cautious*. There is a fear of committing themselves for others to be in control. Thus during the interview little may be said of their condition. They will not give themselves away. There is a fear for the consequences when the mind is active enough to register this situation. At other times they may simply be unable to reach the information because memory is so poor. If we compare this with other remedies we will find that Silicea do not commit themselves because they fear failure, because they do not have enough energy to carry out whatever; Calcarea carbonica is lazy and may not look for the energy to commit themselves; Lycopodium holds self away from others because they fear they will be belittled; Natrum muriaticum protects their private and very vulnerable emotions because they do not have control over them; Thuja gives only the information asked for because they may be functioning 'logically' and anything else is out of sync. The Graphites patient often appears *timid*. This is not bashfulness as in Baryta carbonica. It is a *fear to commit themselves* for fear of what the consequences might be. The insecurity gives rise to *moodiness* which is an inability to express emotions. On the one hand they may be very depressed and miserable, but on the other hand they may be *irritable* and *easily take offence*.

This is one of the remedies that are *worse for music*. Music brings out the worst in the Graphite patient – they cry and become very depressed. A sad play or film may have the same effect. Many people cry at sad films so note that this has to be out of proportion.

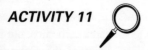

ACTIVITY 10 How would the Graphites patient behave at the office Christmas dinner? Use keynotes and characteristic symptoms as appropriate.

The Graphites Child

The Graphites child is described as *impudent, teasing* and *laughing at reprimands*. This would seem quite a contradiction from the description above of the adult. It should remind us not to take things at face value. These characteristics do not need to belong to an extrovert. Someone lacking in confidence and unwilling, or unable, to fit in socially often makes a joke out of a situation, especially if it implies negative criticism that would devastate him/her. The child, and perhaps some adults, have enough energy to attempt to deflect rather than become passive and let things bounce off their thick skin.

ACTIVITY 11 Draw a sketch of the Graphites child in nursery school. In his excitement he dropped all the milk. Use keynotes and characteristic symptoms as appropriate.

Similar Remedies

Baryta carbonica. Both are glandular remedies. They are difficult to tell apart in children. Both are timid. The Baryta carbonica patient is undeveloped, whilst the Graphites is thick. The skin is strongly affected in the Graphites patient.

Silicea. Both are glandular remedies, chilly and with a tendency to take a cold. Both are timid and lack courage. The Graphites patient is rounded and bland, whilst the Silicea patient is thin, angular with a tendency to ulcerate.

Antimonium crudum. Both of these remedies have copious bland discharges. When the skin is affected it is dry, thickens and cracks.

196

ACTIVITY 12 Construct a table of comparison between the following remedies (all are psoric except Antimonium crudum): Calcarea carbonica, Silicea, Graphites, Baryta carbonica, Antimonium crudum. Compare:

Essence
Modalities
Mental picture
Effects on skin
Effects on mucous membrane
Effects on digestion
Peculiarities.

 SELF-TEST QUESTIONS

You will find the information in the text, perhaps not in this lesson. Answers can be found in the answer section.

1. Name two remedies which look old and wrinkled.
2. Compare the chilliness of Graphites and Calcarea carbonica.
3. List the modalities of Baryta carbonica.
4. Describe the skin of the Calcarea carbonica child.
5. Which remedies you have studied produce fissures?
6. How do the moods of Graphites resemble those of Pulsatilla and Silicea?
7. List the indecisive remedies you have studied.
8. Which remedy describes the lungs as full of smoke?
9. How does music affect the Graphites patient?
10. Describe the problem that might develop in the testicles of the Baryta carbonica child.
11. Describe the stool of the Graphites patient.
12. Name two remedies in which the muscles tense and shorten.
13. How is the mind of the Graphites patient affected?
14. List those remedies you have studied which have a tendency to take a cold.
15. Name three remedies you have studied which are averse to coition.
16. Why is Baryta carbonica a remedy of arterio sclerosis?
17. Name three remedies of imbecility.
18. Describe the tonsils of the Baryta carbonica patient.
19. How do the stomach symptoms of Antimonium crudum compare with those of Graphites?
20. Which remedies you have studied have offensive foot sweat?
21. Describe the leucorrhoea of the Graphites patient.
22. How do the nails of Graphites resemble those of Silicea?
23. Describe the Graphites child.
24. Name one remedy which has pains in the uterus reaching up.
25. Name the left-sided remedies you have studied.
26. Describe the eyelids of the Graphites patient.
27. Compare the feet of Baryta carbonica, Graphites, Silicea and Calcarea carbonica and Antimonium crudum.
28. How does contraction affect the throat of the Graphites patient?
29. What remedy has nausea after eating sweets?
30. List the remedies you have studied which flush upwards.

Further Studies

Baryta carbonica

1. How does the appearance of the Baryta carbonica child resemble that of the Lycopodium child?
2. Compare Baryta carbonica, Graphites, Calcarea carbonica and Silicea in the classroom.
3. Compare the tonsillitis symptom picture of Baryta carbonica, Calcarea carbonica and Silicea.
4. Describe the use of Baryta carbonica in diseases of old age.
5. Compare Baryta carbonica and Baryta muriaticum.
6. List five Strange, Rare and Peculiar symptoms of Baryta carbonica.
7. Describe the digestive symptoms of Baryta carbonica.
8. Find out how you can suppress foot sweat.

Graphites

1. Compare the healing capacity of Graphites and Silicea.
2. Why is Graphites a remedy in common use at menopause?
3. Compare the skin symptoms of Graphites, Petroleum and Antimonium crudum.
4. In which symptoms does Graphites resemble Sulphur?
5. Which other remedies have mucus-covered stools?
6. Describe how the Mercurius child resembles the Graphites child.
7. Distinguish between the Graphites symptom picture and that of Pulsatilla.
8. List the rubrics in the *Mind* section of Kent's Repertory that contain Graphites.

Two Major Miasmic Remedies

Thuja, Mercurius Solubilis

Aim: To introduce two major polycrests with a strong miasmic taint.

Objectives: To define the miasmic taint in the essence of Thuja and Mercurius.
To outline the over-function in the symptoms of Thuja.
To identify the mutation in the symptoms of Mercurius.

Headings: INTRODUCTION
THUJA: Origin; Characteristics of the Tree; Essence; Keynotes and
   Characteristics; Modalities; Growths; Dampness; Dryness; Fixity
   – The Mind, Never Been Well Since ..., Suppressed Acute
   Symptoms; Paralysis; Similar Remedies
MERCURIUS SOLUBILIS: Origin; Characteristics of the Metal; Essence;
   Keynotes and Characteristics; Modalities; Excretion; Suppuration;
   Bones; Mental and Emotional Symptoms; Similar Remedies
SELF-TEST QUESTIONS
FURTHER STUDIES

Introduction

Even when people survive disease, they may continue to be debilitated. When this happens we say the disease has entered a deeper, more chronic stage. The disease is still curable if the treatment can bring it back into a more acute form that can reach a crisis.

Some diseases, especially those which affect the reproductive system, transmit disorders to the offspring. Usually it is only lowered vitality that is transmitted to the offspring. For example, when a child is conceived to someone who has chronic bronchitis and a long history of debilitating drugs, such as antibiotics, the child may have a lot of snuffles and colds, and a tendency itself to respiratory complaints. With good feeding, etc. the child's health may improve. When the diseased parent had gonorrhoea or syphilis, this may also be transmitted to the child, in a form that is curable. However, if the parent was treated, the disease may have entered another phase. The homoeopath recognizes that the child may not be able to bring the disease back into its acute form in which it can be resolved. The whole economy of the organism of the child is now affected. When the disease was gonorrhoea this will produce the over-functioning pattern of the sycotic miasm, as in the Thuja symptom picture. When the disease was syphilis, the destructive pattern of the syphilitic miasm is present in the symptom picture of remedies like Mercurius.

Thuja

Latin name:	Thuja occidentalis
Common name:	Arbor vitae, the tree of life, white cedar
Botanical family:	Coniferae
Habitat:	A native of North America, it grows in swampy areas along the banks of rivers

Origin

Hahnemann proved the remedy from a tincture of the fresh green twigs.

Characteristics of the Tree

The botanical nature of this tree is interesting in relation to the symptoms produced in the

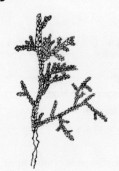
Thuja occidentalis

199

proving. The tree grows in swamps and in waterlogged zones along the side of rivers. The bark is covered in calluses and exudes a sticky, yellow resin. The tree is not a true cedar, but resembles one in appearance. It is related to the junipers and the cypresses.

Essence

The essence of Thuja is *fixidity*. It is a waterlogged remedy that moves into a dry phase which becomes static and dead.

Keynotes and Characteristics		
	• **Warts and condylomata**	Of all kinds. They grow anything.
	• **Smell of old cheese**	Like Silicea.
	• < suppressed warts	
	• **Polypi**	
	• Waxy, shiny face	As if smeared with grease. May look transparent.
	• **Thickened, distorted nails**	As in Silicea. Cheesy-smelling deposits beneath.
	• **Growth of hair on parts not normally covered by hair**	e.g. hair growing out of moles.
	• **Lank, greasy hair or dry, fly-away hair**	This polar opposite occurs in different stages of the disease process or in different Thuja types.
	• **Scurfy skin**	The skin may flake all over.
	• Dandruff	Scurfy skin on the head.
	• **Sweat on uncovered parts**	As in Aconite. **Strange, Rare and Peculiar.**
	• Pustular eruptions only on uncovered parts	This may be seen in acne.
	• **Fastidious**	Scrupulous in small details.
	• Anticipatory fears	As in Lycopodium.
	• **Haste**	In eating, speech and walking. As in Lycopodium.
	• Sensitive to music	Can weep.
	• Prolonged thoughtfulness over trifles	'Why on earth are they taking so long to give a simple answer?'
	• **Slow in speech**	They have trouble finding words.
	• **Split personality**	This is a deep pathological state.
	• **Delusions**	
	– of another person by their side	
	– under a superior intelligence	
	– sensation of an animal inside the abdomen	So used in false pregnancies.
	• **Averse to touch**	Especially their hair.
	• **Irritable**	
	• **Quarrelsome**	They can be picky and insistent on details.
	• < vaccination	Especially smallpox which produces pus.
	• **Left-sided**	Like Silicea.
	• **Dreams of falling**	There is a marked degree of disorientation from their body.
	• **Dreams of flying**	
	• **Dreams of dead people**	There is both decay and other-worldliness in this remedy.
	• **Sweats only when sleeps**	Stops when wakes up.
	• Sweats on side not lain on	Because this is the uncovered side.
	• **Vertigo on closing the eyes**	They are easily disoriented.
	• Head pain as if nail driven in	Usually this is in the temples.
	• **Pain in small spots**	As in Ignatia.
	• **Thick, green mucus**	The yellow-green coloration is common in sycosis.

- Suppressed discharges — e.g. in gonorrhoea.
- Profound action on glands — Stitching, tearing pains.
- Chill begins in thighs — Unusual.
- **< onions** — As in Lycopodium and Pulsatilla. They cause wind.

- < tea, potatoes, fats
- Drinks fall audibly into the stomach — An odd noise.
- Receding stool — As in Silicea.
- Teeth decay at roots
- **Dream of teeth breaking off** — Or of damage occurring to their teeth.
- Geographical tongue — As in Natrum muriaticum.
- Scalding pains on urinating — Like Cantharis it is a remedy of the urinary system and of fluid balance.

- **Split stream of urine** — Often because of warts.
- Feeling as if urine moves along the urethra — Especially where suppressed gonorrhoea.
- **Menses very short** — May only last one day.
- **Vagina very sensitive so averse coition** — Ignatia can also have this symptom.

Modalities

< 3 a.m. and 3 p.m.	Warmth
< cold and damp	open air
< vaccination	
< tea, narcotics, tobacco	

ACTIVITY 1 List the symptoms of overproduction or of excessive function.

ACTIVITY 2 Research the symptoms of gonorrhoea. How do these fit the symptoms of the Thuja patient?

Growths

The appearance of the Thuja patient takes two forms. One of them has a yellow, *waxy face* with *lank greasy hair* and *many warts* on the face and fingers. It is often called the 'witches remedy' or may be described as the figwart remedy. There are many different types of warts, and the Thuja patient may have hundreds of them. One of the peculiar traits of this patient is to miss out symptoms, unless specifically asked for, so you may never know about the warts if your questions are too vague, or you do not examine the patient physically.

The back may be covered by brown *pedunculated* warts that rise out of the skin with an oily sheen, like the bark of the tree. These are often accompanied by *blood-filled vesicles*. Sometimes the warts are *flat*, without any colour. They may be *horny* or *look like cauliflowers*.

The genitals are a favourite spot for warts. When they grow in the urethra they give rise to one of Thuja's keynotes – *forked stream of urine*.

The growths may be of *moles*, usually the outsized freckle type, but sometimes a large, brown, raised patch. Thuja should be considered as a remedy especially if there is hair growing out of the moles.

There is much disturbance of the hair in the Thuja patient. Pubic hairs grow out of place. The female of the species may have a well-endowed moustache and beard, or grow hair around the nipples. Since this is a hormonal problem, there are usually *scant periods* and *lowered sex desire*. In teenage acne, the pimple often contains an inverted hair. Cysts containing hair may be found at the base of the spine.

ACTIVITY 3   Use your Repertory to find out the variety of growths and types of warts produced by Thuja. Look up the skin section, breasts, face, extremities, etc. Make a list of these.

Dampness

The Thuja patient may not sweat, but simply exude grease. At other times there may be a sweet smell like *honey around the genitals* when they sweat, and a *garlic smell* in the *axillae*. The sweat *stains yellow*. These symptoms are keynotes. The most remarkable keynote symptom is seen on few patients, i.e. *sweat on uncovered parts*. This can be seen on the arms as the sleeves are rolled up. Gradually each freshly exposed part takes on a sweaty sheen.

In dark, dank places, fungus grows. Athlete's foot is the most common fungal growth. There are many more, including candida. If we look at the disease process, it is possible to recognize a general breakdown of health after continued stress, antibiotics, etc. producing a metabolism that suits fungal invasions. This problem is common these days, but does not necessarily respond to Thuja unless the symptom picture of Thuja is also present. Thuja is one of the major remedies in cancer, another growth, which may be preceded in the uterus by fibroids, yet another type of growth.

The Thuja patient is much worse for damp. This is most obvious when applied to diet. Food containing a lot of water may aggravate the Thuja patient, or he/she may be averse to it, e.g. mushrooms. The most noted dietary symptom is a strong aversion to onions which are watery and generate heat. The last creates the opposite, dryness, which aggravates Thuja because, being a homoeopathic remedy, Thuja may become the opposite – too dry.

Dryness

The other type of Thuja patient arises out of a dry symptom picture. The dryness is under-function, lack of lubrication, but it is not psoric. It is the ultimate result of excessive oiliness as the oils dry up. The *skin dries and flakes* all over, especially on the scalp. The hair is *dry and frizzy*, unmanageable. They *hate their hair touched*. Thuja does not like to be touched at all. This would bring them too much into communication with the real world. The lifelessness may be seen in the hair which may be so dried and lifeless, it falls out. Thuja patients suffer from *premature baldness* with a greasy pate. The oil may be there, but it is as if it does not go far enough.

If the nails are greasy, they are often *distorted*. When they are dry they become *brittle and break easily*.

ACTIVITY 4   What kind of eruption does Thuja produce? Study these in terms of dampness and dryness.

Fixidity

The oil on the skin and the growths represent (as with the Natrum muriaticum patient) an inability to control appropriateness – they are out of phase. We will speak more of this when we come to the mental and emotional level. The opposite trend to growth is to fix things rigidly. A major keynote of the remedy is *fixed ideas*, a wooden thought process or *obsessiveness*.

The Mind

There is a great deal of fixidity in the mind symptoms of Thuja. The keynote *fixed ideas* refers to obsessive ideas and *dogmatism*. It refers equally to the child who sits and rocks rhythmically, to the child who crawls around the floor seeking out feet to cuddle, and to the rigid dogmatist whose ideas do not bode questioning. The dogmatism is not necessarily stubbornness. If you look closely, you will find this patient has very carefully considered all aspects of the problem and come to a rational conclusion. In argument, you will not have much impact on the Thuja patient, unless you can show you have done your spadework well, too. They are *perfectionists*, like Arsenicum and know when they are right.

There is a coldness, or alienation about the Thuja patient, who will not tell you their symptoms if you do not ask. You are supposed to know your job, he/she will tell you. Once again the behavioural pattern is similar to Natrum muriaticum, but the reasons behind it differ.

The Thuja patient comes across as very sly and greasy. He/she knows what is wanted and goes about getting it, but awkwardly, because inside he/she is shy. They are frequently misrepresented as sly, or dogmatic, because not all the action is visible. There is a lot of thought and feeling going on, but it is fixed inside. You will need to cultivate the children (like mushrooms) to allow them to balance. They can be fragile people. One of the Strange, Rare and Peculiar symptoms is *as if made of glass*. Conversely, the head may feel so solid that it is described as *made of wood*. The shyness is a lack of flexibility which means they can't get out of themselves.

There is a *duality* developing – what is within and what is without. Unlike the Natrum muriaticum which has a horizontal polarity, the Thuja patient splits vertically. In the *paralysing dream* the mind is still active. It is the body that ceases. The *flying dreams* and the *falling dreams* are a plague to the psychic, as she/he slips out of control of the body. Even the *boring pains* are similar to a description of 'elementals feeding off the psychic body'. The patient projects the sensations and feelings outside their own being. The keynote symptom *movement as if a living thing, especially within the abdomen* is an example of this. The dead feelings of numbness when the part has been lain on represent a separation of the physical part and nerve experience of it.

The next step is the separation within consciousness. There are *dreams of the dead*. There are sensations *as if a man were walking by their side*. When it reaches the psychotic state, the obsessiveness becomes the keynote *as if under the control of a superior being*, who talks to them and tells them what to do. Psychosis is a mental state of isolation from the normal process of the social animal; it is isolation of a most extreme kind. The obsessiveness often takes the form of *religious mania*. Even in health, this individual stands on the outside looking in, totally detached and objective, like a visitor from outer space.

The remedy can be difficult to recognize, because of the psychism because there is no language to express much of their experience. It is primitive, like a species left over from a past phase of existence.

Never Been Well Since...

The remedy is most commonly used for two physical conditions:

- never been well since vaccination
- never been well since gonorrhoea.

I have phrased both of these symptoms carefully. They could have been worded 'history of gonorrhoea' or 'after-effects of vaccination' which are common terms. I have not used these terms because homoeopathy is very precise and we do not give remedies simply for 'a history of ...' When symptoms have appeared after a particular incident, or exciting cause, these become prescribing symptoms, as does the exciting cause. The remedy selected will then depend on matching the patient's symptom picture to the symptom picture of a remedy. Thuja is often indicated for the after-effects of vaccination and gonorrhoea. Both vaccination and gonorrhoea have a powerful effect on the vital force. Gonorrhoea is usually suppressed by antibiotics which only take away the acute symptoms. If the body cannot express its symptoms acutely, deeper chronic symptoms develop with which the body cannot heal without producing the acute. When the acute symptom is suppressed again and again, the chronic symptoms become 'fixed'. Similarly, vaccination works because it prevents the expression of the acute disease by introducing it then locking it in, in the form of more disguised chronic symptoms. Thuja is particularly useful for smallpox vaccination because the acute presentation of this disease is through pus-filled spots. The pus, like the gonorrhoeal discharge, is a sticky, greeny-yellow substance, similar to the sticky resin on the bark of the tree. Thuja cures both of these rigid patterns because it has the same symptom picture at acute and chronic levels, so can change from one to the other.

Suppressed Acute Symptoms

Suppressed discharge will go to the next level, or a parallel level, if it cannot break out again. When smallpox vaccination was rife, so were snotty-nosed kids – greeny-yellow, thick nasal discharge. These people could take colds easily, or even bronchitis with thick yellowish expectoration. In some types, otitis media became a common complaint after smallpox vaccination, and as this was suppressed, kidney problems developed. Once we pass the stage of discharge, and the epithelial tissue dries, allergies develop. The gooey discharges change to watery discharges and puffiness. There is excessive itchy activity or a fieriness. Arsenicum, the acute remedy to Thuja, is needed to help the patient cope with the acute phenomenon, but Arsenicum cannot reach the 'fixidity' erected by the exciting cause.

The suppressed growth becomes polypi in the nose or anal area. Cysts occur where the disease is driven into the lymph system. Cysts on the left breast are common when antiperspirants suppress the flow of sweat. Fibrosis and even cancer are the end of the line of suppressing growth, showing the ability of tissue to change levels (from epithelial to connective tissue in fibroid, i.e. endoderm/epiderm to mesoderm). Similarly, cancer is a change of level of organization.

ACTIVITY 5 Read *Vaccinosis* by Crompton Burnett, Jain, New Delhi. He details about 50 cases showing the many varied symptoms that arise out of vaccination that can be treated with Thuja.

ACTIVITY 6 Describe the symptom picture of Thuja in the ear, throat and urogenital system. Use keynotes and characteristic symptoms.

Paralysis

Extreme fixidity in Thuja becomes paralysis. This may affect the bladder muscle so he/she either *waits to urinate*, or if the sphincter is paralysed open, he/she *dribbles urine constantly*. Thuja has many symptoms associated with nerves although it is not usually seen as a remedy strongly connected with the nerves. The symptoms most commonly show overactivity. A keynote is *pain in spots* (Ignatia). It may be random as if the nerves just fire off. When the patient is low in vitality, the whole of the nervous system is affected by disorientation shown in another keynote, *paralysing dreams*. The patient wakes up but cannot move at all and there is no control over the nerves. Even in danger, he/she cannot move. The opposite is found in another keynote, *dreams of falling*. Here there is too much movement and no control but it is still disorientation. The remedy begins to resemble Natrum muriaticum which is known as a remedy that holds on to the past and has problems with no flow or too easy flow across boundaries.

ACTIVITY 7 Find more examples of Thuja's effect on menses. Are the nerves involved? The menstrual cycle has two poles. How is each of these affected independently by Thuja?

ACTIVITY 8 Where have you seen behaviour similar to this? Make a few notes of your observations – remember to be objective. Which symptoms do you recognize as keynotes and characteristics?

Similar Remedies

Natrum muriaticum resembles Thuja in its isolation and ability to rationalize. Natrum muriaticum also dreams of the dead, after grief. It is fixed too with its tormenting or persistent thoughts.

Arsenicum is closely related to Thuja as its main acute remedy. Both are correct and fastidious. Both suffer waterlogged tissues and tend towards dryness. Whilst Thuja, the chronic remedy, presents mainly suppurative symptoms as yellow-green discharges Arsenicum, the acute remedy, produces inflammation, heat and dryness.

Mercurius Solubilis

Black oxide of mercury

There are several Mercurius preparations. Mercurius solubilis and Mercurius vivus are often put together with no attempt to differentiate. Mercurius solubilis is the preparation from mercury, nitric acid and caustic ammonia. The solubilis is more commonly used because of its milder action.

Origin

Mercurius solubilis was potentized and proved by Hahnemann. Other symptoms arise from poisoning cases of the metal and from the side effects of medical use of Mercurius solubilis to treat syphilis.

Characteristics of the Metal

The metal mercury has some interesting properties which are reflected in the symptom picture. As a metal it is very sensitive to atmosphere and thus is used in barometers and thermometers.

It is one of the few metals that remain liquid at normal temperatures and this is seen in the symptom picture in the tendency to have few boundaries. Mercurius patients fit in. Sometimes it is difficult to distinguish the mental and emotional symptom picture of Mercurius because it so fits into its surroundings.

Mercury is very scattered – the metal flies to pieces when touched and just as easily unites with other mercury balls again. Hence an important part of the curative action of Mercurius is to rebuild integrity and unite split-off parts.

Essence

Instability and sensitivity will characterize this remedy, tying in with the destructive nature of the syphilitic miasm. The Mercurius patient just dissolves away. The nervous system and the brain are destroyed. Every part of the body is affected as mercury combines with sulphur, so acting on all proteins in the body, stimulating excretory glands in particular.

Keynotes and Characteristics

• **Offensive**	These form the three main characteristics in all ailments.
• **< night**	
• **Excess salivation**	
• **Profuse sweat**	The sweat glands are excretory organs.
• **Scattered in all directions**	So difficult to get a core when taking the case.
• **Flies to pieces**	This is more exaggerated and distressing than the above.
• **Up and down people**	Moody, because strongly affected by changes.
• **Sensitive to atmospheric change**	They sense the slightest change.
• **Dissatisfied**	Everything is felt so intensely and they can be quite negative.
• **Hurried nervous**	
• **Stammer**	Because in such a hurry.
• **No staying power**	So keep moving, or changing.
• **Weak memory**	Mainly short-term. Forget names, etc. if sycotic.
• Precocious children	Forget past if syphilitic.
• **Fear of insanity**	They can see disturbance in the mind so fear the worse.
• **Fear of their own violence**	Strong impulses to do harm, sudden desire to kill.
• **Desire to catch passing strangers by the nose**	You will see children grasping for the nose.
• Judge people by their noses	Syphilis attacks and destroys bones, especially of the nose.

• **Amoral**	Though they can appear nice and ashamed of their vices.
• **Disgusting, filthy habits**	e.g. pick their nose and eat it!
• **Alcoholism**	It is an escape.
• **Tendency to take cold**	Corrosive discharges or yellow-green purulent catarrh. Colds settle in eyes.
• **Mouth ulcers**	Offensive smell.
• Profuse, slimy saliva	Dribbles on to the pillow at night.
• **Metallic taste**	This may come with the ulcers, tonsil problems even digestive problems.
• **Flabby tongue shows the imprint of teeth**	Mercurius patients are impressionable.
• Bleeding gums	And gum disease.
• **Crown of teeth decay, roots remain**	All syphilitic remedies have a strong effect on bones producing caries and necrosis.
• **Abscesses slow to suppurate**	There is little energy to heal.
• **Glands suppurate**	Producing foul discharges.
• Burning, stinging pains	
• **Chilliness creeps < evening and night**	The cold goes through to the bones gradually.
• **Chilliness of single parts**	If general chilliness has not advanced far.
• **Profuse sweat brings no relief**	Excretory organs are stimulated.
• **Sweat stains clothes**	Yellow.
• **Sweat with pain**	As in Chamomilla.
• **Milk at menses or instead of menses**	The mamma is a gland and can excrete.
• **Milk in the breasts of virgins or young boys**	The mamma are specialized glands. Here the rhythm of the body has changed.
• Raw, corrosive leucorrhoea burns the parts touched	Most discharges are excoriating.
• **Moist, crusty eruptions that bleed easily**	
• **Ulceration**	Is a general state in a syphilitic remedy.
• **Ravenous hunger, or complete loss of appetite**	They may swing from one to the other when ill.
• **Desires cold drinks and beer**	
• **Feel as if made of sugar**	Can crave sugar too.
• **< milk**	It can produce diarrhoea.
• **Diarrhoea offensive with blood and slimy pus**	It occurs in dysentery, ulcerative colitis and many diseases with diarrhoea.
• Chilliness after stool	**Strange, Rare and Peculiar** symptom.
• **Tenesmus continues after stool**	Even with diarrhoea.
• **Rectal spasm**	Even after the rectum emptied.
• Can faint after stool	It takes so much out of them.
• **Burning urine – must wash parts to prevent pain**	They wash to get rid of the discharge.
• **Inflammatory rheumatism with lot of sweat and < heat of bed**	May then have chilliness in single parts or excoriation where two parts meet.
• **Nightly tearing pains with perspiration**	Usually these affect bones.
• **Bone pains < night**	The children will show this as they grow.
• **Tremor and great weakness**	Trembling at least exertion e.g,. of tongue when put out.
• **Cannot lie on right side**	This is the opposite of Phosphorus.

Modalities

< night

< damp weather   > rest

< autumn, when warm days and cold nights

< lying on right side
< perspiring
< milk
< heat of bed
< wet feet

ACTIVITY 9 List those symptoms which illustrate sensitivity.

ACTIVITY 10 List those symptoms which demonstrate increased excretion.

ACTIVITY 11 Which symptoms show you the destructive aspect of the syphilitic miasm?

Excretion

The Mercurius is *very sweaty*. A keynote is *sweats with pain*. The sweat is profuse, very offensive, < at night, and *stains the clothes* an unhealthy yellow. Whenever the patient is ill the sweat increases.

The salivary glands are next most notable for excessive flow. This can be so bad that it *dribbles out of the corners of the mouth at night and soaks the pillow*. It is *slimy* and *acrid*. The mouth may have a *metallic taste*. There are frequently *ulcers*. The mouth of the Mercurius patient shows many of its symptoms, starting with excessive secretion and progressing to ulcerative breakdown. The teeth rot easily and there is a tendency to abscesses which are slow to suppurate. The gums frequently bleed. The tongue is *flabby* and *shows the imprint of the teeth*.

Mercurius has a strong effect on the bowel and on the urinary system. It is often indicated in diseases that respond with *diarrhoea* which is *offensiveness*, *bloodiness* and *slimy*. Despite the looseness of the stool, there is a marked *tenesmus* which continues afterwards. The patient then may become *chilly*, then weak and sweaty as they return to bed.

As the urinary system becomes disordered, the acidity of the urine increases, so the *parts may burn* or become raw. The adult will *wash the parts to stop the pain*. Where there is cystitis there may be a lot of blood and even pus. The discharge has a most *offensive smell*. Mercurius may be found in gonorrhoea because it can produce the yellow-green discharge and grow warts on the parts.

ACTIVITY 12 Compare the urinary symptom of Mercurius, a syphilitic remedy, and Pulsatilla, a sycotic remedy.

Suppuration

There are *abscesses* and *glandular swellings* that are *cold* and *inclined to suppurate*. This is a useful remedy for mumps when there is *offensiveness*. Breasts and ovaries are also glands, so they are affected by Mercurius. The swelling stage will have *burning, stinging pains*. The discharge stage will be foul, acrid and *bloody*. The bloodiness is to be expected in a syphilitic remedy which emphasizes the final stage of disease, i.e. ulceration. In the sore throat, eventually we will see ulcers on the tonsils after the foul, slimy catarrh. The patient is prone to catarrhal colds which settle in the eyes.

Chilliness precedes the suppuration stage, even if it is a local abscess. In a more generalized state of the disease, such as flu, it *creeps* from the site of the 'cold', e.g. from the sore throat to other parts of the body.

ACTIVITY 13   Compare the cold symptom picture of the Mercurius and the Sulphur patient. Sulphur is a psoric remedy.

Bones

The final disease stages of syphilis, and of Mercurius, is destruction of the bones. This is not often visible today, except in the mouth, where there is considerable *decay of the teeth*, from the crown down. It could be argued that this is aided by the presence of mercury in the amalgam used to fill teeth. The remnants of ancestral use (in the treatment of syphilis), or of the syphilitic miasm, is to be seen in the absence of a bridge to the nose. Such patients may have a turned-up nose! The disease and the remedy both attack the nose of the victim, dissolving the cartilage, then the bone, until there is no nose. The nose fixation comes through the remedy in a strange Mental and Emotional symptom – *desires to catch passing strangers by the nose.* Their whole life may be devoted to noses(!) so that they judge the character of others from the nose.

Mercurius may be a useful remedy in rheumatism and arthritis. The *pains are tearing* on the nerves, causing *sweating* and followed by *chill*. Where sweaty parts meet there will be excoriation. There will be a *foul smell* and a *peevish, dissatisfied* patient, who may become depressive. There will be *weakness* and *trembling* of the limb. Because the remedy is Mercurius, the bones will be affected. There will be tearing pains, especially at night, on the *right side*, so they will *not be able to lie on the right side*. The bones may even 'crumble'.

Mental and Emotional Symptoms

Whilst there are clear characteristic symptoms, it is often difficult to recognize this remedy because it takes on the character of the surrounding environment. If you seek for the essential components of a case rather than descriptively listing a lot of unprocessed data, then you should find that this patient is *sensitive to atmospheres;* emotionally, is *moody,* and *dissatisfied with life.* It is difficult for them to hold things together as there is a perpetual tendency to '*fly to pieces*' or to *scatter their energy.* This is a cross between Pulsatilla and Phosphorus. Like Pulsatilla, *lack of confidence* and *shyness* destroy their energy. Like Phosphorus, there is a tendency to use their energy to be *restless, nervous and hurried.* They move on so quickly that often things are dealt with only on the surface. There is a weakness of the mind that prevents them from going too deeply into life. The *memory is weak.* The will is weak, so they sink into situations like *alcoholism.* The laziness resembles Sulphur and the Mercurius patient can be *lax in his/her habits* like the Sulphur patient. The child is known to have *disgusting habits*, like *picking the nose and eating it.* Often the Mercurius patient is described as having *a nice exterior, but rotting away inside.* There may be *amorality* and secret vices! As they retreat into this inner world, *they start to fear for their sanity.* There are such strong impulses from within that they *fear the violence they may be capable of.* Usually the weakness prevents them doing much about the impulses, which is just as well, as there is *an impulse to harm people, to throw the baby on the fire.* This comes out of frustration regarding their weakness and inability to project an identity. It is not a pleasant situation because, being syphilitic, it is very destructive, and they do not pick up some of the positiveness and support that others may find in counselling.

ACTIVITY 14   Read up on the usual presentation of psychosis from a textbook on Psychiatry. Which aspects fit the Mercurius symptom picture?

Similar Remedies

Pulsatilla has none of the offensiveness or excoriation of Mercurius but has great similarity in its ability to *change* all the time and on its action on the glands. Both pick up their moods from the surrounding atmosphere.

Phosphorus has the lack of stability of Mercurius. Both find it difficult to concentrate or to stick to one subject. Both are bloody remedies that show a lot of degeneration. Phosphorus is more easy-going and desires to please. Mercurius is dissatisfied and despondent. Mercurius has little capacity to recoil like the Phosphorus patient.

Silicea has a deep pathology affecting the glands. There is offensive pus and catarrh, even ulceration. Both are mild and yielding. One of the few differences is the Silicea patient is easy-going whereas the Mercurius patient is dissatisfied.

ACTIVITY 15   Create a table of comparison for Calcarea carbonica (psoric), Thuja and Mercurius, showing:

Exciting causes
Modalities
Symptoms of a cold
Weather reaction
Mental/Emotional
Mode of action

   SELF-TEST QUESTIONS

Answers can be found in the answer section.

1. Where do warts occur on the Thuja patient?
2. Which remedies are aggravated by onions?
3. What happens in the mouth of the Mercurius patient?
4. What happens when the Thuja patient drinks cold water?
5. Name a disgusting habit of the Mercurius patient.
6. How does Mercurius resemble Pulsatilla in breast symptoms?
7. How is the hair of Thuja affected?
8. Which remedy has chilliness after the stool?
9. In what way does Thuja resemble Aconite?
10. Where does the chill begin in the Thuja patient?
11. Why does the Mercurius patient stammer?
12. Of what is Mercurius afraid?
13. Compare the fastidiousness of Thuja, Arsenicum and Sepia.
14. Which remedy feels made of sugar?
15. How does the headache of Thuja resemble that of Ignatia?
16. How does Mercurius show an energy similar to the diffusion of Phosphorus?
17. How does the stool of Thuja resemble that of Silicea?
18. Describe the tenesmus of the Mercurius patient.
19. How do the delusions of Thuja resemble those of Lachesis?
20. Which remedy dribbles on the pillow all night?
21. In which pain symptom does Mercurius resemble Chamomilla?
22. Compare haste in Thuja and Lycopodium.
23. Describe the chilliness of Mercurius.
24. Name two remedies that have a split stream of urine.
25. Describe the dreams of the Thuja patient.
26. Give four key characteristics of Mercurius that accompany all ailments.
27. Give a Strange, Rare and Peculiar symptom of the urogenital system of Thuja.
28. Describe the sweat pattern of the Mercurius patient.

Further Studies

Thuja

1. Describe the two types of Thuja patient.
2. Why is Thuja of use in antidoting the smallpox vaccination?
3. Compare the duality of Thuja and Lachesis.
4. Why is Thuja a well-indicated remedy in many sycotic cases?
5. In which symptoms does the headache of Thuja resemble that of Ignatia and Arsenicum?
6. Compare Thuja with Lycopodium and Natrum muriaticum.
7. List ten Strange, Rare and Peculiar symptoms of Thuja.
8. How does Thuja affect the sexuality of the patient?
9. Describe the development of cancer in the Thuja patient.

Mercurius

1. Compare Mercurius solubilis, Mercurius corrosivus and Mercurius vivus.
2. What are the distinctive characteristics of Kent's *six* mercury salts?
3. Mercurius is the syphilitic Pulsatilla – would you agree with this?
4. Name three distinctive characteristics of Mercurius solubilis and give examples as to how each of these may be present in a case.
5. Compare Mercurius solubilis, Silicea and Pulsatilla in the ear problems of children.
6. Describe a Mercurius solubilis case of flu.
7. Describe the skin problems of Mercurius solubilis.
8. Compare Mercurius solubilis, Rhus toxicodendron and Arsenicum in rheumatism.
9. Comment on the mischievous, precocious Mercurius child.
10. What effect does Mercurius solubilis have on the digestive system? How does this differ from Mercurius corrosivus?

Answers and Test-cases

Answers to Activities

LESSON ONE

Activity 1

Strange, Rare and Peculiar
Sweats on uncovered parts; everything tastes bitter except water.

Mental/Emotional
Fear; convinced he will die at a specific hour; restlessness.

General
< fright; tearing pains; sensation of a tingle; full, bounding pulse; copious drenching sweats; thirst for bitter things; < cold, dry; < midnight; left-sided.

Particular
Pupils contract to pinpoints; paralysis after fright; retention of urine in the newborn; hot, swollen redness; redness, deathly pale on sitting up; convulsions with jerking and twitching of single parts; < apex left lung; dry, hard cough on expiration; < trigeminal nerve on left side.

Activity 2

Symptoms of sensation
1. Tearing pain.
2. Sensation of a tingle.
3. Everything tastes bitter except water.
4. Pains like knives.
5. Heaviness in inner parts.
6. Pains worse touch.
7. Anxiety in the stomach.
8. Burning on skin.
9. Tightness in muscles.
10. Prickling, crawling sensations.

Activity 3

Symptoms of causation
1. < fright.
2. < cold, dry conditions.

Activity 4

Earache
Step 1. Heat < cold, dry.
Step 2. Swelling, redness. Tingle.
Step 3. Pain – neuralgic. Anxiety, Restlessness < midnight. Sensitive to noise. As of a drop of water in the ear.
Step 4. Fever, bounding pulse. Red face pale on sitting up. Drenching sweats. Convulsions. Everything tastes bitter. Thirst. Sweats on uncovered parts.

Throat Pain
Step 1. Heat < cold, dry.
Step 2. Swelling, redness. As if constricted. Dryness.
Step 3. Tearing pain. Cannot swallow, chokes. Cough on expiration. Anxiety. Restlessness < midnight.
Step 4. As above.

Neuralgia
Step 1. Heat. Tingle < cold, dry.
Step 2. Prickling. Redness.
Step 3. Numbness. Heavy feeling. Pain tearing. Anxiety. Restlessness < midnight.

Step 4. Trembling. Jerking. Paralysis of muscle + above.

Note: Although it is useful to separate out steps to gain a deeper understanding of levels of severity and therefore of potency, the edges are never as clearly defined in the patient.

If you have read your philosophy you will recognize that these stages go from local to General and Mental/Emotional. Many Strange, Rare and Peculiar symptoms occur in Step 3 when the disturbance is fully developed and the remedy's characteristic pattern clear. Step 4 occurs when the vital force has failed to keep the disturbance at the local level – in this instance it is generalized fever. In another example Step 1 and 2 might represent sensation, Step 3 dysfunction and Step 4 pathology. Homoeopathy is truly preventive medicine because it does not need to wait until the disturbance reaches the level of pathological change to recognize it and take curative action.

Activity 5

Symptoms of modality

Aggravation
1. Fright, cold dry conditions, shock, vexation. Menses. Chilled especially after sweating.
2. Evening and night, rising up, lying on affected side, pressure, touch, light, noise, music.
3. Inspiration.

Amelioration
1. Rest, sweating.
2. Open air.

Note: I may have tried to be a little too clever here but I have tried to make some sense of the lists of modalities by putting them into three groups. Group 1 are causative. Group 2 are modalities proper, i.e. once you have it what makes it better or worse. Group 3 represents modalities that only occur in special situations or to specific parts, e.g. No one is worse for breathing in but in some situations the lung symptoms might be aggravated by inspiration.

Activity 6

Symptoms of Turmoil in Circulation
Mental
Anxiety. Delirium.

General
Full, bounding pulse. Sudden sinking of strength. Fevers > rest < excitement. Palpitations.

Local disturbance
Hot, swollen, redness. Redness of face deathly pale on sitting up. Pulsating pains. Congestion to the head – apoplexy – and chest. Haemorrhages – bright red. Swelling, redness, heat. Parts feel enlarged. Bruised, heavy feelings.

Activity 7

Fear overwhelms so he/she is oblivious to all else. They tend to hold so the breath is held, there is tension in muscles. The stomach holds fear. In terror the pupils are contracted. They may freeze with terror or when the terror continues the relaxation stage may cause them to wet themselves. Cold drenching sweats belong to this stage. The bounding pulse and palpitations, even hypertension in the adult, are caused by 'tension' in the arteries. This last may be accompanied by the red face which will become apoplexy in severe cases. The fear is irrational, of the unknown. It disappears once they have dived off the side of the swimming pool for the first time, etc.

Activity 8

Strange, Rare and Peculiar
Radiating heat; visible throbbing of carotid.

Mental/Emotional
Sensitive to noise; delirium; outbursts of wild laughter; bites and strikes; rips pillows; rage; fear of dogs; fear of water.

General
Bright redness; dryness; throbbing pains; shooting pains; < heat; < sun; upwards movement to the head; right-sided; red streaks along lymph nodes; < jar; violent spasm; convulsions; sensitivity to getting head wet; < 3 p.m.

Particular
Dilated pupils; aversion to strong light; wild staring look.

Activity 9

Symptoms of sensation

1. Throbbing pains.
2. Shooting pains.
3. Upward movement to head.
4. Discharges feel hot.
5. Fullness in parts, as if would burst.
6. Burning in inner parts.
7. As if a mouse were running in the muscles.
8. Prickling in muscles or bones.
9. Pain shoots from one ear to the next.
10. Heavy breasts.

Activity 10

Major causations are sun, getting the hair wet or chill to the head, rage. Epilepsy will have a clear exciting cause such as sun, light, or rage. The main sensation or aura will be as if a mouse were running over the muscles. Heat may rise from the stomach. The face will look bloated and red, the veins swollen, the pulse full. One side may be in spasm, the other paralysed. Spasms may start in the limbs and throw the body forwards and backwards. The spasms recur with the slightest touch. Involuntary micturition and defecation.

Activity 11

Aggravation
1. Sun, draughts to the head, looking at shining objects, suppressed sweat.
2. 3 p.m., touch, light, noise, motion, jar, lying down.
3. Hanging down affected parts, swallowing liquids.

Amelioration
1. –
2. Bending backwards, standing, warm room.
3. Leaning the head against something.

Activity 12

Bee Sting
Step 1.
Step 2. Swollen, red, hot, throbbing < heat < touch.

Step 3. Red streaks along the lymph vessels.
Step 4. Heat to the head. Fever, red face. Sensitivity to light. Convulsions. Delirium, sees monsters. Rage. Bites and strikes. Opisthotonos. Fear of water, dogs.

Note: Step 4 will be seen in the most allergic types.

Sunstroke
Step 1. Heat. Redness.
Step 2. Throbbing. Radiating heat. Dryness. Sensitivity to touch.
Step 3. Visible throbbing of carotid. Sensitivity to light, jar, noise.
Step 4. Dilated pupils. Delirium, sees monsters. Convulsions. Wild staring look. Heat to head.

Throat pain
Step 1. < after chilling.
Step 2. Hot. Dry. Right sided. Bright red.
Step 3. Pain, throbbing or shooting upwards. Swollen tonsils. Chokes when swallowing, because throat constricted. < 3 p.m.
Step 4. Fever. Heat to head. Delirium, sees monsters. Sensitivity to noise, jar, light, touch. Visible throbbing of carotids.

Activity 13

Mental
Delirium; outbursts of wild laughter; bites and strikes; rips pillow; rage; fear of dogs; fear of water; restless; desires to escape.

General
Upward movement of heat to head; violent spasm; convulsions; oversensitivity of all senses; vertigo with vanishing sight, stupefaction and debility; fever with loss of consciousness.

Local disturbance
Visible throbbing of carotids; dilated pupils; < jar; wild staring look; things look red; opisthotonos.

Activity 14

The Belladonna child is hot-headed so flies into rage when its ego is challenged. He/she may stamp and fume, almost spitting out words of hate, depending on the age. If you come within range he/she may sink his teeth into you. When things are thrown they are meant to hit you although sometimes they will simply be tossed away violently. As the rage nears mania the eyes will have a staring, wild look.

Activity 15

Strange, Rare and Peculiar
Sweats with pain; one side of the face hot and red; face sweats after eating and drinking; teeth feel long.

Mental/Emotional
Rage; throws things; nothing satisfies; capricious; contrary; quarrelsome; rude; sends doctor from the room; rocks to and fro; restlessness.

General
< teething; < carried; < vexation; < chagrin; < humiliation; < bad news; intolerable pains; oversensitive to pain; numbness with

pain; nerves over-stimulated; cutting tearing pains; > warmth; thirst.

Particular

Twitching calves; lienteric stools; stool green; stools smell of rotten eggs; colic pain in umbilicus; copious salivation; > pressure abdomen; > warm drinks.

Activity 16

Symptoms of sensation

1. Intolerable pains.
2. Numbness with pains.
3. Cutting, tearing pains.
4. Pulsating pains.
5. Throbbing half of brain.
6. Labour pains pass upwards.

Activity 17

Symptoms of modality

Aggravation

1. Vexation; dentition; coffee; being looked at; suppressed sweat.
2. 9 a.m. and 9 p.m.; getting warm in bed; cold damp air; warm food; touch; open air.
3. Eructations.

Ameliorations

1. Being carried; fasting.
2. Sweating; cold applications; warm, wet weather.
3. Pressure in abdomen.

Activity 18

Earache

Step 1. Exposure to cold winds.
Step 2. Intolerable, tearing pains. Restless. Rocks back and forth. > warmth. < 9 a.m. and 9 p.m.

Step 3. Numbness. Sweating. As if full. As if hot water running out of.
Step 4. One side of face hot and red. Capricious, contrary. Quarrelsome. Sends doctor from the room.

Toothache

Step 1. May start after a warm drink, or coffee.
Step 2. Rocks back and forth. Intolerable pain. < warmth. One side of face hot and red. Restless. Copious salivation.
Step 3. Diarrhoea with green or lienteric stool. Smells of rotten eggs.
Step 4. As above.

Headache

Step 1. May start after vexation, chagrin, humiliation, etc.
Step 2. Throbbing one side. Intolerable pain. Sensitive to noise, etc. Open air.
Step 3. Numbness. Sweats with pain.
Step 4. As above + convulsions. Diarrhoea, with sour slimy stool.

Activity 19

She dominates the scene, making demands on the whole family as a unit. Nothing pleases her. She asks for 'X' and creates a scene, screaming and writhing uncontrollably. She gets herself into such a state that she loses contact with reason. She is so out of proportion she can no longer accept what was asked for originally. She will dash it away from her. Mum knows she has to take control of the situation because the child cannot connect. More screams ensue as mum enforces her will. Then she picks up the child and rocks her, which soothes eventually.

Activity 20

Textbook research.

LESSON TWO

Activity 1

Mental/Emotional

Leave me alone, I'm alright; fear of being approached; wakes suddenly with thoughts of accidents; dreams of an accident or of being harmed; asks questions when in a coma then falls off again; quickly forget what is said to them.

General

Pains bruised, as if beaten; parts lain on feel bruised; haemorrhagic tendency; shock; cold extremities.

Particular

The bed feels hard; as if hit by a blunt instrument; bruising.

Note: Four of the General symptoms refer to the parts. Why not put these symptoms under the *Particular* heading? Any individual occurrence may indeed be put under the *Particular* heading but here I have put the general tendency under *General*. 'Bruising' and 'as if hit by a blunt instrument' could also be put under the *General* heading using this same rationale. This problem will occur repeatedly. When treating cases we may be led to different conclusions depending on how some symptoms are interpreted.

Activity 2

Symptoms of sensation

1. Parts feel bruised or as if beaten.
2. Parts lain on feel bruised.
3. The bed feels hard.
4. As if hit by a blunt instrument.
5. Cold extremities.

Activity 3

Aggravations

1. Shock, physical trauma such as a fall or injury, poisonings from organic derived gases, alcohol, overexertion, jet lag.
2. Touch, motion, noise, lying down, after sleep, lying on the left side, jarring.

Ameliorations

1. –
2. Motion, lying down with head low.

Activity 4

Symptoms showing lack of integrity

1. Leave me alone, I'm all right.
2. Haemorrhagic tendency.
3. Shock.
4. Fear of being approached or touched.
5. Sleep disturbed by thoughts of accident.
6. Forget quickly what is said to them.
7. Answers questions then relapses into coma.

Activity 5

Self-research question.

Activity 6

They are stunned and numbed, keep themselves to themselves in order to reintegrate. They will even deny any harm or will ask a helper to go away.

Activity 7

Strange, Rare and Peculiar
Bone pains after a fracture has healed; sensation as if the lid passed over a lump when closed.

Mental/Emotional
Cannot bear to be approached.

General
Prickling pains in the bones.

Particular
Irritability at the point of the fracture; spasmodic jerkings of the affected part; pain in the eye as if from a blunt instrument; eyelid closes spontaneously of its own accord; eyelid appears to droop; as if the ears were stopped up; back pain from sexual excesses.

Activity 8

Reading exercise.

Activity 9

Reading exercise.

Activity 10

Experiment.

Activity 11

Self-research question.

Activity 12

There are different degrees of burns. In a simple burn there may be redness, swelling and throbbing pains, or pains may tingle or feel numb. If more of the part is exposed or the burn is more severe there may still be redness and swelling but now the pain is more severe. It may burn or shoot upward towards the spinal cord if touched. These pains may be described as lacerating. Where sepsis occurs there may be a local yellow discharge. Where this proceeds to a systematic level delirium will occur, as if the brain is loose. Overall there will be much stupor and heaviness but you should note the nervous involvement of Hypericum so jerkings and convulsions will be part of this deeper picture.

Activity 13

Reading exercise.

Activity 14

Aggravations

1. Injury, burns, shock, concussion of head or nerves, after forceps delivery.
2. Motion, touch, pressure, change of weather, fogs, cold damp.
3. Touch, cold applications.

Ameliorations

1. –
2. Lying quietly.
3. Rubbing, bending back, lying on face.

Activity 15

Strange, Rare and Peculiar
Coldness of part, > more coldness; ecchymosis green-yellow.

General
Blueness; numbness; twitching around the wound; left to right side; symptoms start below and travel upwards; lack of vital heat; desires alcohol.

Particular
Swollen, hot joints; << heat; boils; stiff muscles; bruised feelings in muscles; intense itching feet and ankles.

Activity 16

Symptoms of sensation

1. Coldness, better more coldness.
2. Numbness.
3. Twitching around the wound.
4. Swollen joints, worse heat.
5. Stiffness of muscles.
6. Bruised feelings in muscles.
7. Intense itching of feet and ankles.

Activity 17

Aggravations

1. Alcohol, injury.
2. Heat, walking, night, alcohol.
3. Motion, spitting.

Ameliorations

1. –
2. Cool air, cold applications, rest.

Activity 18

The temperament is distinct. They avoid company and tend to despise and scorn others. They are very irritable.

The causes and modalities are clear. The gout comes on after a bout of alcohol especially wine (red). Rich food may cause it. Once there the part needs cool air. It is markedly aggravated by heat or motion.

The part will swell greatly. There is much stiffness and pain of a tearing kind. The part is cold and may be purple or blotchy.

Activity 19

Research exercise.

Activity 20

General

Venous stasis; bruised sensation; effects of blows to soft tissue; < sudden soaking; < cold drinks when overheated; left-sided; tired, desires to lie down; sleeplessness at 3 a.m.; wakes early and can't sleep again.

Particular

Stitches in spleen; head pain from occiput to sinciput.

Activity 21

Reading exercise.

Activity 22

Research exercise.

LESSON THREE

Activity 1

Strange, Rare and Peculiar

As if a dry spot in the throat; consciousness in fits.

Mental/Emotional

< fright; prattles; hands pick at bedclothes; jealous; < disappointed love; < rage; bite and strike; incoherent speech; paranoia; fear poisoning; fear of being alone; fear of running water; starts awake again; suddenly sits up in the middle of the night; restless in sleep; cruelty; imbecility; expose themselves; sing lewd songs; make gestures; cunningly deceitful; sees dead loved one sitting in a chair or standing in the room.

General

Spasm; sleepless.

Particular

Eyes stare; jaw drops.

Activity 2

Symptoms of spasm

1. Dry hacking cough as if a dry spot in the throat.
2. Start awake in sleep.
3. Suddenly sit up in the middle of the night.
4. The opposite of spasm is seen in symptoms such as jaw drops and incoherent speech.
5. On the mental level the equivalent might be prattle, hands constantly on the move.
6. Picking at the bedclothes, even paranoia is a tension that won't let go!

Activity 3

Exciting causes

Fright, disappointed love, rage, jealousy.

Aggravations

1. Fright, disappointed love, rage, jealousy, emotions.
2. Eating, drinking, before and during menses, touch, lying down, sleep, cold.

Ameliorations

1. –
2. Sitting up, stooping, motion, warmth.

Note: I have organized the aggravations into three groups, so group 1 is causative, group 2 general modalities and group 3 modalities of specific parts.

Activity 4

Self-directed research.

Activity 5

Self-directed research.

Activity 6

The attack begins with a gnawing hunger at the pit of the stomach or sparks may appear in front of the eyes. During the attack the eyes protrude, the face is purplish, urine is voided, the teeth may be grated. Convulsions are long-lasting and shake the whole body. There may be great anguish then loss of consciousness. After the attack the patient will be sleepy. The causes may be grief, disappointed love or jealousy. More immediately convulsive movements may occur at the slightest attempt to swallow liquid (see Sivaraman P 1980 *Epilepsy cured with Homoeopathic Remedies,* Jain).

Activity 7

Reading exercise.

Activity 8

Strange, Rare and Peculiar

< looking at glistening objects; small objects look large; painlessness where pain to be expected.

Mental/Emotional

Terror; < fright; dread of the dark; see animals jumping about in the dark; scream in nightmares; rave; desire to escape; cannot bear to be alone; want their hand held; talk incessantly; struck speechless; call things by the wrong name; speech incoherent with headache; consciousness during convulsions; moods swing between joy and sadness; pray all the time; sing all the time; obsessive; lewd; fumble genitals.

General

Rigid with fear on waking; cold sweat; << alcohol; hot red face; cold hands and feet; cannot bear to be uncovered in a sweat; spasm; spasm in top half of body only; voluntary muscles more mobile, involuntarily slow; < suppressed eruptions.

Particular

Eyes stare.

Activity 9

Exciting causes

Fright, looking at glistening objects, suppressed eruptions.

Aggravations

1. Fright, looking at glistening things, suppressed eruptions or discharges, intemperance.
2. Dark, after sleep, touch, when alone, touch, cloudy days.
3. Swallowing, especially liquids.

Ameliorations
1. Light.
2. Company, warmth.
3. Cold water.

Activity 10

Symptoms of disturbance in sensorium
1. See animals jumping about.
2. < looking at glistening objects.
3. Painlessness.
4. Consciousness in convulsions.

Activity 11

Self-directed research. Use above as an example.

Activity 12

Measles — Fiery red spots that burn and itch as if something crawling there. Or as the spots fail to appear the mental picture arises – fits with consciousness, screaming in the night through nightmares and wake as if still in sleep or with body rigid. The eyes may be very sensitive to shining objects, light in general.

Sore throat — The throat is very red and dry. Whilst they may have a great thirst and wish to drink they cannot swallow. There is no pain. The larynx may appear to move up and down as if they are swallowing. They are worse in the morning or after sleep, on touch of any kind. The throat may be better for warmth.

Fright — If the fright is severe there may be paralysis, e.g. of speech. More commonly the adult or child may relive it at night as nightmare from which they may wake screaming. They may want to talk about the subject continually and excitedly, they may laugh at their reaction. In severe states there may be convulsions or mania.

Activity 13

Strange, Rare and Peculiar
Nausea as if the abdomen were hanging down; nausea > uncovering the abdomen; vision < looking at white things; as if looking through a veil.

Mental/Emotional
Loquacity; apathy; despondency; paranoid.

General
Nausea; vertigo on opening the eyes; vertigo increases to loss of consciousness; deathlike pallor; nervous tremor; debility; weak irregular pulse; spasm; constriction muscles of hollow organs; paralysis; periodicity.

Particular
Vomit < movement of any kind; weak sinking in the stomach; icy coldness of skin with cold sweat; icy coldness from the knees down; sensitive to noise and light*; palpitations from tobacco*; paroxysms of sneezing lasting weeks; cramps in calves; renal colic; spasm of anal sphincter; hiccough; dry tearing cough > cold water; prolapse ani; seminal emissions involuntarily at night; blindness through atrophy of the optic nerve.

*These symptoms could belong to the organ in particular or the person in general.

Activity 14

Symptoms of spasm	*Symptoms of relaxation*
Vomiting worse movement of any kind.	Nausea as if the stomach were hanging down.
Palpitations.	Vertigo on opening the eyes.
Paroxysms of sneezing, lasting weeks.	Vertigo increases to loss of consciousness.
Constriction of muscles of hollow organs.	Death-like pallor.
Cramps in calves.	Nervous tremor.
Renal colic.	Debility.
Spasms of anal sphincter.	Weak irregular pulse.
Hiccough.	Icy coldness of skin with cold sweat.
Dry teasing cough > cold water.	Apathy. Despondency.

Activity 15

Exciting Causes
Motion particularly of a boat, or riding in a carriage or some modern cars depending on the suspension.

Aggravations
1. Motion particularly of a boat, riding in a swaying vehicle.
2. Extremes of heat or cold, heat, walking, evening.
3. Lying on the left side, opening the eyes.

Ameliorations
1. Twilight.
2. Fresh open air, cold applications, weeping.
3. Uncovering abdomen, vomiting, vinegar.

Activity 16

Self-directed research.

Activity 17

Travel sickness on a bus — Motion and constantly changing the focus brings on nausea so patient is worse opening the eyes, and on movement of any kind. There is a deathly pallor. The stomach feels as if it is hanging down. Fresh air helps so the window is open. All improves when they get off the bus.

Cholera — There is much weakness with deathly pallor and violent colic. The abdomen will feel hard as the muscles contract. In some patients the navel may be retracted. Amelioration on uncovering the abdomen will be noticeable. The patient will be worse in heat. Stools will be watery or curdled like sour milk.

Constipation — Much tenesmus although stool soft. Violent pain in the small of the back.

Activity 18

Self-directed research. Look up neurasthenia and ME and compare with the symptoms of Tabacum.

Activity 19

Strange, Rare and Peculiar
Crusts red-rimmed.

Mental/Emotional
Depressed; can't concentrate; confused – can't find the right word.

General
< cold; damp; < getting soaked; < chilled after overheating; < suppressed sweat; sour smell; one-sided paralysis with speechlessness; restlessness*; spasms and twitching; restless in sleep; offensive sweat all over body; rheumatic dropsy; paralysis from lying on the damp grass**; dry red crusty eruptions**; menses suppressed.

Particular
Cutting pain at the navel; green slimy stools; yellow, watery stool < damp weather; excessive urination; milky deposit in urine; perspiration on palms; tearing pains in limbs; head feels large; eyes discharge; eyes twitch.

*Restlessness could be of the body or the mind. When of the body, it is put under *General*.
**This symptom may refer to an individual part, or it may be a characteristic symptom and therefore a *General*.

Activity 20

Exciting causes
Suppressed menses, suppressed eruptions, hot days and cold nights, getting soaked.

Aggravations
1. Suppressed eruptions, suppressed menses, hot days and cold nights, sudden changes in temperature, exposure to cold wet conditions, autumn.
2. Cold air, wet weather, night, resting, cold drinks, ice cream, damp ground, before storm.
3. Uncovering, cold to feet.

Ameliorations
1. Dry weather.
2. Warmth, walking, motion.
3. Moving affected part.

Activity 21

Laryngitis Starts after exposure to cold, wet conditions, perhaps after suppressed menstruation or suppressed sweat. The latter is usually caused anyway by chilling after overheating. These conditions will predominate in the autumn! Someone living in a damp environment may be more prone to frequent throat affections.

The throat will be better for warm drinks but worse for cold ones. There may be few other individualistic symptoms except the sensation as if the uvula were elongated.

Headache Exciting causes and modalities as above. May be prominent before a storm. There may be a pressing pain on the forehead. The enlarged sensation this time is at the occiput. Amelioration from motion is here seen in the SR&P modality better for conversation.

Cystitis Exciting causes and modalities as above. Pressing pain during and after urination. There may be retention of urine after chilling, this may be due to slight paralysis.

Activity 22

All three are irritable, Rhus toxicodendron the more so. It is active and restless. Bryonia tends to fall into a dopey stage and exhibits touchiness when disturbed. Unlike Rhus toxicodendron it dislikes motion which it resists aggressively. Rhus toxicodendron's irritability comes from a need to move, here it is as if there is not enough movement so the mind follows the physical restlessness. Dulcamara is very similar to Rhus toxicodendron in finding ease in movement and warmth. It is much more likely to go into paralysis. Dulcamara will resemble Bryonia in temperament when the 'paralysis' theme enters the mind as confusion and lack of ability to concentrate. The Dulcamara patient is lost for words in this stage. Before they reach this level, or on some of their brighter days(!), they may be more critical of others and out of tune with the world, not quite knowing what they want. This last is similar to Rhus toxicodendron though without the vehemence.

Activity 23

This is a summary of your work in this lesson. Do it for yourself.

LESSON FOUR

Activity 1

Symptoms of anxiety
1. Restlessness.
2. Anxiety about health.
3. Great fear of death.
4. Fear of suffocation.
5. Despair of recovery.
6. < alone.
7. Fear of the unknown.
8. Suicidal.
9. Fastidious.
10. Well organized.

Activity 2

Aggravations
1. Periodicity, milk, ice cream, cold food and drink, rotten food, alcohol, suppressed eruptions.
2. Midnight, 1–2 a.m., cold and damp, watery fruit and vegetables, rapid walking, lying on the affected side especially with head low, tobacco.
3. On entering a cold place.

Ameliorations
1. Heat, company.
2. Warm applications, warm food and drink, lying with head elevated, moving about, open air, sweating.

Activity 3

Active integration/control	*Broken down integrity of whole*
Ambitious.	Sudden prostration out of all proportion.
Fastidious.	Chilly.
Tidy, well-organized.	Restlessness.
Diarrhoea as a reaction to food poisoning.	Anxiety about health.
	Fear of death or suffocation, or of the unknown.
	Suicidal.
	Watery diarrhoea smells rotten, excoriates.
	Nausea at the sight and smell of food.

Activity 4

Self-directed research.

Activity 5

There are many watery symptoms. Watery coryza, much lachrymation, watery diarrhoea, eruptions are herpetic with moist discharge after scratching. In later stages there may be much dropsy of extremities with cardiac problems in particular. Duodenal ulcers show internal oversecretion.

Activity 6

There is a great heat in Arsenicum which dries skin and mucous membrane. Also secretions are very acrid, burning parts touched. This gives rise to some of the burning pains and, when it reaches a deeper level, to ulceration, decay, even necrosis. This is one of the remedies of gangrene. Hence, when you see the dryness of Arsenicum look carefully for the wet exudate which will then burn and rot the part, e.g. in the skin eruption, in coryza the dry nose will run watery excoriating discharge, the burning dry eyes of conjunctivitis will run copious fluid. This is not a contradiction but a study of the unique pattern in each homoeopathic remedy.

Activity 7

General symptoms of Apis

Similar to Arsenicum	*Different from Arsenicum*
Bright red swellings.	Apis swellings are shiny.
Burning pains.	Apis pains are also stinging.
Oedema.	Apis pits on pressure though.
Both right sided.	Apis is thirstless whilst Arsenicum drinks small quantities.

Activity 8

Modalities of Apis compared with Arsenicum

Similar	*Different*
Both < getting wet.	Apis > cold, Arsenicum > heat.
Both > in the open air.	Apis < 4 p.m., Arsenicum
Both better sitting erect.	< midnight, 1–2 a.m.
Both < pressure.	
Both < suppressed eruptions.	

Activity 9

Self-directed research.

Activity 10

The throat is much swollen with red fiery tonsils. It is markedly better for cold drinks although it may be so swollen and oedematous that it is painful to swallow. It is sensitive to pressure and touch of any kind. It often accompanies other illnesses such as measles or may arise from suppressed skin eruptions. The swelling may occur separately in allergic situations.

Activity 11

Reading exercise.
Apis is useful in anaphylactic shock because it swells the mucous membrane so rapidly and dramatically.

Activity 12

Self-directed research.

Activity 13

Self-directed research.

Activity 14

This is related to Activity 13. The build-up of lactic acid in the tissues causes stiffness and soreness. To avoid this you need to keep the muscles slowly active or use massage and heat to passively stimulate circulation. Rhus toxicodendron's main keynote applies here, viz worse first movement, better continued motion. The modalities also fit clearly, viz better heat, better rubbing, worse cold damp, worse rest. The type of pains that appear in the Rhus toxicodendron patient are sore, bruised. They even dream of overexertion!

Activity 15

Reading exercise.
To answer second part of the activity look at Rhus toxicodendron in inflammatory conditions, in fever and in its effect on connective tissue.

Activity 16

Self-directed research. Study the symptoms of congestive heart disease then compare these to the Rhus toxicodendron symptoms.

Activity 17

Symptoms of irritability
1. < slightest draught of air.
2. < slightest touch of clothing.
3. Volatile temper.
4. Nothing pleases.
5. Everything disturbs.
6. Haste.
7. Splinter-like sticking pains.
8. Quarrelsome.
9. Desire constant change.

Activity 18

Aggravations
1. Slightest draught of cold air.
2. Cold dry air, becoming cold, uncovering, night especially nightly chill, noise, cold food and drink, exertion.
3. Lying on the painful part, touching affected part.

Ameliorations
1. Moist heat.
2. Warm applications, heat, in general.

Activity 19

These people may be well in themselves until they meet and have to recognize outside stimuli. This irritates. They may become quarrelsome and irksome. Nothing you do will help. In fact the more you try to do, the more impossible it will be to please them. They will become more irritable as they have to leave their nice cosy bed to venture into the cold world, as they go from one room to another which has not yet been heated up. And so they keep on the go, moaning their dissatisfaction and erupting into temper if you cross their path – you won't need to disagree, just being there might be enough.

Activity 20

The Hepar sulphuris patient desires strongly stimulating food which is highly seasoned or strongly stimulates the mucous membrane to secrete, such as acid foods.

Activity 21

Sore ear Exposure to cold air brings on the complaint. The remedy is particularly right sided so you may see the right ear red and inflamed, stitching, darting pains appear. Excessive secretion producing catarrh in the middle ear which may cause perforation then a dirty yellow, foetid discharge. Heat will give amelioration to the pain and if applied early enough may prevent the middle ear activity.

Sore throat Once again exposure to cold is often a clear exciting cause. The tonsils and the glands may swell producing the typical sticking pain as if there were a splinter in the throat. On yawning or opening the mouth wide the pain will shoot up to the ear (usually right). Catarrh will be produced which may block the ear causing deafness. It gives the sensation as if there were a plug in the throat.

Headache Exposure to cold started the headache then it is sensitive to any little movement. It appears in the right temple, a boring pain. This is one of the few remedies that also affects the root of the nose so you may recognize it here. It might be described as a sinus headache worse on stooping.

Activity 22

Create a table.

LESSON FIVE

Activity 1

Over-stimulation
Impulsive.
Impatient.
Spasm.
Dissatisfaction.
Fastidious.
Fault-finding and critical.
Desires alcohol.
Desires highly seasoned foods.
Desires fats.
Jerking limbs.
Tetanic spasm.

Exhaustion
< slightest noise.
< overheating.
< rich foods.
Ineffective urge to stool.
As if part of the stool remains.
Paralysis.

Activity 2

Self-directed research.

Activity 3

Self-directed research.

Activity 4

Self-directed research.

Activity 5

Self-directed research.

Activity 6

After overeating, rich foods, alcohol, or after overstimulated nerves especially as in anger, the headache arises. That relating to overindulgence is more likely to be a congestive headache with pressing on the vertex. The head is pulled into the shoulders as if the patient wants to escape the weight on top. The slightest stimulation, especially noise will aggravate the pain causing greater irritability in the patient. The tension headache often comes from the shoulders which are held tightly. The head is often retracted into these like a tortoise. The patient often describes this as a migraine although it is not one sided because it is accompanied by nausea of such intensity that 'if only I could be sick' but of course being Nux vomica the patient does not vomit. Noise, touch, music and overheating all aggravate. The patient is relieved in the cold resting.

Activity 7

Self-directed research.

Activity 8

Self-directed research.

Activity 9

Symptoms of spasm
1. These are similar to those of overstimulation in Nux vomica.
2. Globus hystericus.
3. Sighing respiration.
4. Internal trembling.
5. Hiccoughs.
6. Yawns spasmodically.

7. Convulsive twitches.
8. Tonic spasms.

9 Jerks on going to sleep
10. Throat pain better on swallowing.

Activity 10

1. Laughs when should cry.
2. Emptiness not relieved by eating.
3. Headache < or > by stooping.
4. Roaring in the ears > hearing music.

5. Lump in throat cannot be swallowed better eating solids.
6. Boring pains in spots > pressure.

Activity 11

Self-directed research.

Activity 12

Self-directed research.

Activity 13

The symptom pain in small spots appears in the headache as a boring pain or as if a nail were driven into the temples. There is often an emotional cause such as disappointment. This patient has strong ideals and when thwarted tenses when these are violated, e.g. rudeness. By dwelling on any situation she will make the tension worse and bring on the headache. Worry, shock, tobacco will also bring on the headache. Pressure, deep breathing, even eating acid foods will relieve it. If it continues she will often yawn then go off to sleep – yawning of course is deep breathing, or the scene may end in vomiting especially if caused by tobacco or other odours.

Activity 14

Self-directed research.

Activity 15

Symptoms of 'Over the top'
1. Indignation.
2. Mind dwells on sex.
3. Violent outbursts of passion.
4. Violent itching.
5. Crawling as from insects.
6. Crumbling black teeth.

7. Ravenous appetite for days after a fever starts.
8. Constant urging for only a few drops of urine.
9. One-sided paralysis from anger.

Activity 16

Keynotes showing the effect on nerves
1. Trembling.
2. Prickling sensation.
3. As if the stomach hangs

down and flabby.
4. One-sided paralysis.

You'll find more in the text books.

Activity 17

Self-directed research.

Activity 18

Self-directed research.

Activity 19

Throat problem The most likely exciting cause is emotional indulgence or outrage. Tobacco smoke or cold drinks may irritate the throat. Once there, it will be sensitive to touch and will produce a coughing spasm. It will be dry and sore stabbing into the ear on swallowing or perhaps even on talking if the situation is severe.

LESSON SIX

Activity 1

Strange, Rare and Peculiar
Catarrh flows better at night lying down; sweats on the front of body only; as though a hair hung over the eye; as if sand in the eye.

General
> lying down; frequent yawning walking in the open air; chilliness; heat descends the body; menses very short; amenorrhoea with catarrh in the eyes.

Particular
Profuse lachrymation; acid lachrymation; red swelling of the eyes; burning sensation in the eyes; photosensitive eyes; copious fluid discharge from the nose; violent cough; hawks catarrh in the morning; pressing pain beneath the sternum; eyes agglutinated in the morning; dimness of vision.
1. Lachrymation and runny nose in cold.
2. Red swollen eyes with lachrymation.

Activity 2

Symptoms of sensation
1. Burning sensation in the eyes.
2. Chilliness.
3. Heat descends the body.
4. Pressing pain beneath the sternum.

5. As though a hair hung over the eye.
6. As if sand in the eye.

Symptoms of pathology
1. Profuse lachrymation.
2. Burning sensation in the eyes.
3. Eyes agglutinated in the morning.

4. As though a hair hung over the eye.
5. As if sand in the eye.

These symptoms point to various kinds of eye disease. The sensation of a hair in the eye may involve the nervous system, the other symptoms are more local referring to the eye. A homoeopathic remedy may appear in any condition. You must look for the symptoms which are unique and individual to this patient in order to select the best homoeopathic remedy. Study diseases such as glaucoma and look up the symptoms in your repertory. How often does Euphrasia appear?

Activity 3
Self-directed research.

Activity 4
Reading exercise.

Activity 5

Euphrasia
Profuse acrid lachrymation, with red rimmed eyes and burning sensation. Agglutination in the morning. < light, warmth, touch. May start after exposure to warmth.

Arnica
Tired heavy eyes after overuse. Bloodshot and photophobic. Feel bruised or as if hit. Objects looked at may appear to fall.

Ledum
Bruised feeling. Bloodshot. After injuries to the eye. Acrid tears.

Symphytum
As if lump in the eye. Eye closes spasmodically. After injuries to the eye.

Activity 6

Symptoms of Euphrasia – I've translated these into the language of the Materia Medica.
1. Chilliness.
2. Heat descends.
3. Perspiration on the front of the body only.
4. Violent cough.
5. Hawks catarrh in the morning (not necessarily the same as gags).
6. Profuse lachrymation.
7. Eyes agglutinated in the morning.
8. > lying down.

Activity 7

Modalities in the case.
1. > lying down.
2. Catarrh worse in the morning.

Activity 8

Strange, Rare and Peculiar
Vicarious menstruation.

Mental/Emotional
Child dislikes to be carried; fear of poverty; wants to go home; talks anxiously about business; touchy

General
Slow onset; < cold damp; affects epithelial lining tissue; copious white catarrh*; thirst for great quantities; < slightest movement; lies on the painful side; grasps painful part to stop it from moving; sticking, stitching pains; < heat; sensation of stuffiness; < before menses; < 9 p.m.–3 a.m.

Particular
Cannot breathe deeply enough; bursting headache; vomits bile; dry hard stools look burnt; constipation when abroad; stone hard breasts.

*Once again some symptoms could easily belong to either *General* or *Particular*, depending on whether they refer to one part in particular or the type of symptom produced in general.

Activity 9

The head feels full to bursting and is worse when stooping, or for heat or motion. It often comes before the menses when all is congested but it may be part of the general congested picture, in which case it is often called a migraine and is accompanied by constipation. After exposure to cold damp the head sinus may be so full of mucus that a head cold and sinusitis are present. This gives the same sensation of fullness worse when stooping, or with heat. The sensation may also be described as heavy, worse moving the eyes or even coughing.

Activity 10
Self-directed research.

Activity 11
Self-directed research.

Activity 12
Self-directed research.

Activity 13

Aggravations
1. Cold damp conditions, vexation, financial loss.
2. Motion, 9 p.m.–3 a.m., heat, exertion, eating.
3. Stooping, coughing, deep inspiration, touch, lying on the painless side.

Ameliorations
1. Being held tightly, i.e. security.
2. Pressure, rest, cold food and drink, open air, cloudy damp days, descending.
3. Lying on the painful part, bandaging, drawing the knees up.

The aggravation from inspiration makes sense when we realize the mucous membrane lining the air passages is very dry and worse for any movement. The aggravation of motion in general worsens those parts which are dry, as does the aggravation to heat although this also affects the congested parts as it increases circulation and therefore movement. Congestion is worse for pressure, coughing, stooping, eating and exertion. When full and congested this patient prefers to lie low unmoving and very still.

Activity 14

Strange, Rare and Peculiar
Shivers up and down the spine; as if water trickles down the spine; as if the heart would stop beating if they cease to move; headache better urinating.

Mental/Emotional
Apathy and indifference; wants to be left alone; answers slowly; cannot grasp thoughts; fear of falling; < bad news; < disappointment; < fright;

General
Trembling; heaviness; relaxation and prostration; numbness; lack of co-ordination; thirstlessness; yellowness; < anticipation; paralysis; diarrhoea; vertigo; never been well since flu.

Particular

Sensation of emptiness in the epigastric area.

Activity 15

Aggravations
1. Bad news; disappointment, shocks; fright; anticipation; damp; sun; dentition; thunderstorms.
2. Thinking of symptoms; cold damp; tobacco; periodicity; spring; foggy weather; motion.

Ameliorations
1. –
2. Urination; sweating; afternoon; reclining with head high.
3. Shaking; bending forwards; continued motion.

Activity 16

Reading exercise.

Activity 17

During chest problems such as flu.

Activity 18

He/she may tremble or have heavy leaden limbs with dullness of consciousness. They may even be apathetic and want to be left alone. They may answer slowly. All these symptoms show a lowered vitality.

Where the disease penetrates more deeply into the CNS you may find the patient lacks co-ordination, cannot gather any thoughts. They may be disturbed in such a way that they fear they will fall down, so little control do they have.

Activity 19

Strange, Rare and Peculiar

Chilly in the daytime only; sense of duality; one limb speaks to another; one part is in conflict with another; parts feel scattered about the bed; can only swallow liquids; painless ulcers.

Mental/Emotional

Besotted; drowsy; falls back to sleep half way through a sentence; mutters in delirium; < bad news.

General

Rapid prostration; feels bruised and sore all over, especially parts lain on; the bed feels too hard; offensive discharges; < after 2 a.m.; < after first waking; < fog and damp; < sewers, swamps, inhaling foul vapours; < night watching.

Particular

Dull red face; burning heat on the face; eyeball sore when moved; phagedenic ulcers; dry tongue with brown streak down the middle; bitter taste in the mouth.

Activity 20

Symptoms of sensation
1. Feel bruised and sore all over, especially parts lain on.
2. The bed feels too hard.
3. Burning heat on the face.
4. Painless ulcers.

Activity 21

Self-directed research.

Activity 22

Self-directed research.

Activity 23

Aggravations
1. Fog and damp, sewers, swamps, inhaling foul vapours, night watching, bad news.
2. Humid heat, pressure, after first waking, open air, autumn.

Ameliorations
1. Open air.
2. Drinking liquids, movements.

Activity 24

The throat is dark red, the breath foul. There may be spasms so only liquids can be swallowed. The patient is more liable to these quinsy throats in the autumn when the weather is foggy, or humid. It will cause them to become dopey as their vitality drops.

Activity 25

Both patients have much soreness and may feel the bed hard. Arnica is slightly worse lying on the left side. Both are very tired and inclined to drop off between conversations, Baptisia in the middle of a sentence. In Arnica, the pains may shift from joint to joint or may only be stiff in rest and ameliorated if the patient keeps moving. Both have foul discharges and suppurating glands. Arnica is worse for cold and damp whilst Baptisia is worse for humid heat conditions.

LESSON SEVEN

Activity 1

Symptoms of contrariness
1. Grey hair in early life.
2. Fear of being on their own but hate crowds.
3. Hate to be contradicted but full of contradictions.
4. Hungry but full after a few mouthfuls.
5. Emptiness in the stomach not relieved by eating.
6. Burning pains better heat.

Activity 2

Symptoms of inferiority complex
1. Fear of failure.
2. Anticipatory fear.
3. Arrogant.
4. Traditionalist.
5. Avoid responsibility.

Activity 3

Symptoms of inertia
1. Cowardice.
2. Traditionalist.
3. Constipation.
4. Lack of vital heat.
5. Numbness in spots.
6. Impotence.
7. Kidney stones.

Activity 4

He/she has been thinking of this coming event for days. Now they are constantly in the toilet. They fear they will forget, that they will fail and not be able to face anyone. The stomach gnaws in the epigastric area producing wind. They may take it out on their family, bossing them around. Once in the driving seat they may tremble but after a short while will calm down and perform well because ultimately they have faith in their ability – anyway, they dare not fail.

Activity 5

Self-directed research.

Activity 6

Basically the digestive system slows down so wind and constipation are produced. The aggravation from onions worsens the wind. The pressure of clothes increases the pressure of flatulence. The tympanic abdomen is a symptom of the flatulence.

Activity 7

It causes an allergic reaction which may be visible at first as nausea and diarrhoea. Much wind again accompanies symptoms, if disturbance.

Activity 8

Symptoms of psora, insufficiency
1. Emaciated from the neck down.
2. Baldness in spots. Grey hair.
3. Fear of failure.
4. Fear of the future.
5. Cowardice.
6. Fear of being on their own.
7. Avoid responsibility.
8. Dread lest they forget.
9. Flatulence even after a few mouthfuls.
10. Constipation.
11. Lack of vital heat.
12. Numbness in spots.
13. Impotence.
14. Gout.
15. Kidney stones.
16. Brick red deposit in the urine.

Activity 9

Symptoms of imbalanced heating mechanism
1. Redness of orifices.
2. Sudden hot flushes.
3. Hot hands and face, cold feet.
4. Burning feet at night, stick out of bed.
5. Heat.
6. Burning pains on the vertex.
7. Burning, itching, smarting skin.

Activity 10

Symptoms showing need for stimulation
1. Inquisitive.
2. Enthusiastic for all causes but do nothing.
3. Imagines nasty smells.
4. Need to nibble food constantly.
5. Crave spicy, highly seasoned food.
6. Crave alcohol and stimulants.

Activity 11

Symptoms of self-centredness
1. Indulge in philosophical obscurities.
2. Absent-minded philosophers.
3. Lazy.
4. Bullies.
5. Impatient.
6. No one does anything to please them.

Activity 12

Self-directed research.

Activity 13

Basically untidy and disorganized, full of weird trophies or attachments which make little sense to others, i.e. everyday objects seem beautiful.

Activity 14

Earache   A cold may develop after a change in the temperature. This may settle in the ears which may be red at the time of exposure. Catarrh will fill up the middle ear causing deafness. There may be a sensation of water swishing around inside the ear. Although the patient is much worse for heat, the part may benefit from warm applications.

Activity 15

Symptoms showing lack of assimilation
1. Imperfect ossification.
2. Pot belly.
3. Thoughts vanish.
4. Repeat themselves over and over.
5. Easily tired.
6. Crave indigestible foods.
7. Desire farinaceous foods.
8. Curvature of bones.
9. Easy strained muscles and ligaments.

Activity 16

Symptoms of a slow metabolism
1. Imperfect ossification.
2. Bloated appearance.
3. Damp, cold, boneless handshake.
4. Lethargic and slow.
5. Poor concentration.
6. Chilly.
7. Feet sweat as if wet stockings on.
8. Offensive foot sweat.
9. Easily tired.
10. < ascending.
11. Feel better constipated.
12. Kidney and gall stones.

Activity 17

< exertion, < ascending – muscles are slow to recover from exertion.
< dentition – the bones are slow and painful to form.
< milk – adds to the calcium imbalance. The body cannot cope with such an influx.

Activity 18

Menses are early and protracted, and often heavy. The breasts are tender and engorged. There may be congestive headaches.

Activity 19

Self-directed research.

Activity 20

Calcarea carbonica is cold in spots, Lycopodium numb in spots and Sulphur hot in spots.

Activity 21

Create a table.

LESSON EIGHT

Activity 1

Symptoms associated with lax tissue

General	Particular
1. < becoming heated.	4. Varicose veins.
2. > continual movement.	5. Haemorrhoids.
3. Pains wander.	6. Copious bland green catarrh.
	7. Throbbing pains.
	8. Involuntary urination on coughing.

Activity 2

Symptoms showing response to change

Worse change	Better change
Indecisive.	Crave fresh air.
< becoming heated.	Continued motion.
< rich foods.	
< puberty.	
< before menses.	

Activity 3

Shy. Does not want to leave Mum to enter an unfamiliar situation. Weeps. In class withdraws coyly. Responds to sympathy and warmth. Fine once has a special friend, often becomes teacher's pet.

Activity 4

There are different kinds of Pulsatilla grandmas! One may sulk sullenly with some anger. Another will be so hurt she may weep openly. Another may go on and on telling you how awful you are.

Activity 5

Tonsillitis — Right sided swelling. There may be copious white or green catarrh that then becomes stuffy yet the patient is thirstless. They will want to be warm but may desire fresh air to breathe. They may want cool ice cream or other comforting foods. It may have come on because they were susceptible before the menses to getting their feet soaked.

Sinusitis — This may present as a stuffy dry head that may ache when in warm air or if there is any cause for the catarrh to shift, e.g. bending down. In the cooler air the catarrh may become looser and flow. There may be sneezing then. If the situation were worse they may have a pounding headache above the right eye and in the cheek and down the side of the head.

Activity 6

The rhythm of the period may be irregular. The flow may vary. The period may be absent.

Activity 7

Like gran above she may react in different ways. Pulsatilla is one of the remedies of silent grief who cannot express their feelings so they become sad and despondent. They are unable to do much for themselves. Another will weep and moan all the time, inconsolably, no matter how much love and attention they receive and this may go on for years with no change. Another may take comfort from the family if it is close and able to demonstrate affection openly. This one may hold many fond memories of the spouse, somewhat romanticized. The first may think only of her loneliness and be bitter that they are left behind.

Activity 8

Space	Time
Dryness of vagina.	< grief, disappointed love.
Greasy face.	Clumsy before menses.
Cold sore on lips where skin joins mucous membrane.	< going without meals.
Eruptions on the hairline.	Averse coition.
	Starts awake on going off to sleep.
	Headaches after work or at weekends.

Activity 9

1. Craves salt or averse to salt.
2. First part of stool very hard then more liquid.
3. Watery leucorrhoea, dry vagina.
4. Herpetic eruptions dry then break down and weep.

Activity 10

Symptoms of polarity

1. Want attention but consolation aggravates.
2. Clumsy and lack of flow as period starts to flow.
3. Emaciate whilst eating well.
4. Craving or aversion for salt.
5. Worse or better by the seaside.
6. Stool hard and dry then soft and flowing.
7. Greasy face, dry vagina.

Activity 11

Excessive fluid discharge, much sneezing, becomes drier. May develop cold sores at the junction of lips and skin. May become dry and stuffy with severe pounding headache. Want to be alone. In dry state, unlike Pulsatilla, will want fluid. Better open air, occupying the mind. They will get on with their work.

Activity 12

It will occur along the hair line particularly at the back of the head. It will go through phases of being dry and scaly then will break and weep thin exudate.

Activity 13

Self-directed research.

Activity 14

Self-directed research.

Activity 15

Symptoms of sag

Mental
1. Causeless weeping.
2. Total indifference.
3. Indolent.
4. Postnatal depression.

Physical
5. Bearing down pains.
6. As if all would fall out.
7. Prolapse uterus.
8. Tendency to abort 5–7th month.
9. Back pain worse standing.
10. Desires vinegar.
11. Piles.
12. Varicose veins.
13. Better violent exertion.

Activity 16

Self-directed research.

Activity 17

Self-directed research.

Activity 18

Your own observations.

Activity 19

Effects of sag on the digestive system
1. Nausea at the thought or smell of food.
2. Desires vinegar and acid foods.
3. Empty sinking feeling in the epigastrium.

Activity 20

Common cold

Catarrh starts thin, then thickens to green and drips down back of the nose. Worse before menses. Able to hold all together, so only ill after ordeal. Better exertion, better occupation.

Activity 21

Create a table.

LESSON NINE

Activity 1

Symptoms of dryness

Physical
1. Dry skin. Cracks around the mouth, nose, eyes, anus, bends in the fingers.
2. Limbs dry and shorten causing deformities.
3. Shrivelled appearance. Skin tightens and shrinks.
4. Dry throat producing hoarseness. Dry hollow cough.
5. Retention of urine with burning pains.
6. Worse cold, dry conditions.

Mental
7. Censorious – in a dry sarcastic manner.
8. Dry wit.

Activity 2

The cold may start after exposure to cold dry conditions. There may be copious flow at the start, as in a runny nose with sneezing. As the cold settles in the cough is the most prominent feature. This may be excitable spasm at the beginning but it becomes hollow as it dries. The voice may become increasingly hoarse as the throat dries. When the voice is lost the vocal cords may be paralysed. In sensitive individuals this last may occur soon after onset displacing the cough as the most prominent feature. In some, the cough may be associated with involuntary urination and/or retention of urine as paralysis affects the bladder muscles.

Activity 3

Your personal observations.

Activity 4

Aconite	Causticum
Pupils contract.	
Palpitations.	
Raised Blood Pressure.	
Tension in muscles.	Tension in extensor muscles.
Cold sweat.	
Hold their breath.	
Involuntary urination.	Involuntary urination.
Retention of urine.	Retention of urine.
Restlessness.	
Toss and turn at night.	
Nightmares.	
Dread of death.	Foreboding of doom.
	Depression.
Trembling.	Exhaustion.
	Paralysis of single parts.
	Loss of voice, speechlessness.
	Numbness of parts.

Activity 5

Self-directed research. Symptoms similar to the Causticum

symptoms picture include paralytic trembling, jerking and spasms.

Activity 6

Symptoms of sciatica

1. Tearing pains better for warmth.
2. Numbness.
3. Trembling weakness.
4. Depressive, gloomy, mistrustful.
5. Worse right side.
6. Worse morning.
7. Sour perspiration.

Activity 7

A prophet of doom looks on the black side. Reminds others of their less favourable habits and features. Distrustful and suspicious. Censorious.

May shake and tremble or have tics, or paralysis of a single part such as an arm.

Dry cracked skin. Warts on nose, fingers and elsewhere.

Dry shortened tendons distort shape.

Hoarse dry voice could become a cackle!

Activity 8

Mental	*Physical*
Excited, effusive persons.	Easy haemorrhage.
Day dreaming.	Blood streaked sputum.
Lascivious.	Bleeding piles.
Vivid dreams.	Bleeding moles.
Imaginative.	Epistaxis especially after excitement.
	Nocturnal emissions.
	Easily flush and blush.
	Coryza flows easily, and copiously.

Activity 9

1. Clairvoyance.
2. Oversensitivity of sense organs.
3. Wants to be magnetized.
4. Worse twilight.
5. Easily catches cold.
6. Easily influenced by others.
7. Imaginative. Vomits as soon as water becomes warm in the stomach.
8. Nausea placing the hands in warm water.

Activity 10

Hyperactive digestive symptoms of Phosphorus

1. Vomits water as soon as it is warm in the stomach.
2. Mucus in stool.
3. Diarrhoea pours out as from a hydrant.

Activity 11

Self-directed research.

Activity 12

The lungs are sensitive to cold wet conditions. Colds easily go into the chest. Often the Phosphorus patient produces pneumonia after a growth spurt at puberty or after excessive excitement that drains the system. The older Phosphorus patient may be very worn down and apathetic, easily affected by slight causes.

The patient will be prostrated. Copious expectoration may become blood streaked as the condition deepens. The exhaustive cough may be excited by slight changes in air temperature, and may be worse lying on the left side. He/she may describe a tickling sensation behind the sternum provoking the cough. There may be a sensation of a weight on the sternum or severe pain in that area.

The lower right lobe is most profoundly affected.

Activity 13

The mind is so active, the excitement keeps them awake. Their fantasies are so enjoyable.

Sometimes the overactive imagination surrounds them with monsters that frighten them preventing sleep.

Activity 14

1. Tendency to catch cold.
2. Emaciation.
3. Profuse perspiration on head and feet.
4. Lack of vital heat.
5. Lack of healing ability.
6. Catarrhal states.
7. Fearful.
8. Cannot concentrate.
9. Easily exhausted.
10. Starts easily.
11. Oversensitivity especially to noise.
12. Mild, yielding personality.

Activity 15

A scrofulous constitution is one in which the glands are strongly affected and catarrhs persist.

The Silicea patient has many glandular problems. Glands are chronically enlarged and/or indurated. Catarrhs are produced with each cold and persist long after the colds 'finish'. Minor organs such as the ear are also affected by catarrhs as in 'glue ear'. Tonsillitis is common.

Tuberculosis work is self-directed research.

Activity 16

Observation exercise.

Activity 17

The Silicea child is very timid. It is locked in its own world and may not even attempt to come out so it sits in a corner reading a book. It may look from behind its protection at the other children enjoying themselves and not quite have the courage to come out and play with them. When invited it may not be able to reach over the barricade – you will need to be very patient. Sometimes attention will cause them to remain even more entrenched behind their barricade. You almost need to keep on inviting and keep on stepping back to allow them to come out in their own time. They may do this when you least expect it. They will then be very sensitive and easily startled back in if you come too close. Given plenty of support and understanding at an early age they may be more able to share their very rich inner world and appear a bit exhibitionist like the Phosphorus patient. Any criticism will seriously injure them emotionally. The other children will not be able to cope well with them because their world is so different and more sensitive.

Activity 18

The earache will be left-sided and begin after exposure to cold winds. It may appear red but that is unlikely. Pains will be severe, often throbbing. As the acute progresses you will see the bulging eardrum showing catarrh is present in the middle ear. The child or adult will hold the ear, lie on it even, to keep it warm.

Activity 19

The Silicea patient easily catches cold after exposure to cold conditions especially if these are also wet. Catarrh flows copiously with little encouragement. Although this may start clear it will rapidly colour so it is white then green as the situation deepens. The glands are quickly affected. The tonsils swell on the left side. The catarrh continues as the glands become indurated and throb violently. The patient is often recognizable from the hat they wear on their head! As the situation deepens even further there may be copious sweats around the head, with or without the hat. The lung symptoms are characterized by much green catarrh and debility. The cough brings up much expectoration almost choking them.

Silicea has the profuse night sweats of Tuberculosis. It also has the scrofulous constitution. They are lean and emaciated types which produce copious purulent catarrh and a fatiguing cough.

Activity 20

Create a table.

LESSON TEN

Activity 1

Symptoms of sluggish circulation
1. Worse after sleep.
2. Worse heat.
3. Better discharge. Better commencement of menses.
4. Constipation.
5. Venous congestion.
6. Blue mottled skin.
7. Varicose veins.
8. Thrombosis.
9. Haemorrhoids with hammering pains.
10. Black blood soon coagulates.

Yes it is different from congestion which has more throbbing, bursting sensations and engorgement. See Bryonia.

Activity 2

Symptoms of decay and perversion of function or structure
1. Black blood soon coagulates.
2. Ulceration.
3. Sepsis.
4. Foul discharges.
5. Stop breathing as soon as falls asleep.
6. Cynical and mocking.
7. Malicious.
8. Project poison into the atmosphere.
9. Delusions.

Activity 3

Self-directed research.

Activity 4

Overactivity of mind
Excitable.
Easily startled.
Touchy.
Suspicious.
Cynical and mocking.
Jealous.
Malicious.
Project poison into the atmosphere.
Loquacious.
Flicks from one subject to another.
Fear of being poisoned.
Delusions.

Sluggishness of mind
Indifferent.
Averse to talking.
Time passes slowly.

Fear damnation.
Guilt.
Voluptuous thoughts.
Vivid dreams.

Activity 5

Earache Usually comes from sore throat. Extends to left ear. Pulsating pain. Much wax causes deafness. Worse slightest touch, better firm pressure. May be locally better from heat.

Activity 6

Diphtheria Begins on the left side and goes to the right. Pain is excessive on swallowing yet could swallow solids more easily. They have a sensation as if a lump. There may be a sore spot at the back of the throat. Membrane is present.

Activity 7

Both have flushes of heat that move upwards, palpitations, prolonged heavy periods. Both have burning pains and may suffer fibroids. Sepia has bearing down pains as if the contents would be expelled.

Activity 8

Symptoms of restlessness
1. Fidgety.
2. Hurried motion.
3. Constant motion though worse motion.
4. Restless legs want to walk.
5. Chorea.
6. Impulsive.
7. Moods suddenly alternate.
8. Hysteria.
9. Rhythmic movements.

Activity 9

Cough is the main respiratory symptom. There are paroxysms that give rise to much excitement and fear. The attack comes on suddenly and deepens rapidly, producing breathlessness. The patient may describe the paroxysms 'as if they were torn to bits'. The rhythmic, jerky movements are seen as they toss from side to side in anguish.

Activity 10

Self-directed research.

Activity 11

There is much restlessness, the patient is constantly moving with jerks and twitches. They will pick at the bedclothes with their hands. They are discontented types who may lash out. Like Belladonna they may tear up the pillows. Unlike Belladonna they will have a thirst. When the chill comes they may describe it as if cold water were poured over them.

Activity 12

1. Aversion to black/red/ yellow and green.
2. Kleptomania.
3. Angular movements.
4. Right pupil only, enlarged.
5. Spine sensitive to touch.
6. Headache better rubbing head on the pillow.
7. Headache with pain in the uterus.
8. Flatus from the vagina.
9. Menstrual flow profuse with erotic spasms.
10. As if cold water were poured on the head.
11. Cough at night better smoking.

Activity 13

Self-directed research.

Activity 14

The pain is burning as if raw. Blisters at the back of the throat turn black, and ooze acrid fluid. They are thirsty but cannot drink without the throat going into spasm. The patient will be irritable and restless. Warmth may help the throat pain.

Activity 15

Hyoscyamus	Stramonium	Cantharis
Flushed dark red.	Painless inflammation.	Skin fiery and inflamed.
Jaw drops.	Fiery red patches.	Burning pains especially affecting cavities.
Convulsions.	Crawling sensations.	
Spasms.		
Constricting pains.		Rawness.
Cannot swallow liquids		
< touch	< touch	Sensitive to touch.
Aversion to water.	Great thirst yet dreads water.	Drinking produces spasms.
Photophobic.	< shining objects.	Objects look yellow.
Lids close spasmodically.	All objects look black.	

Quarrelsome, lascivious.	Terror.	Sings lewd songs.
Laughs and sings.	Prays, sings. Lascivious, wants to kill.	Restless, dissatisfied.
< Emotions	< shining objects. < after sleep, dark.	< bright objects. < sound and sight of water.

Activity 16

Cantharis	Urtica urens	Hypericum
Burns which blister.	Stinging, burning pains.	Lacerating pains show depth affected.
Stinging pains.	Raised blotches.	Sepsis with yellow discharge.
Go into spasm (twitch) if touched.	Vesicles.	< touch.
Fluid loss.	Itches with burns.	

Activity 17

Sepia
This animal produces an ink cloud to hide in in order to escape or to attack. It changes its colour to camouflage and merge with its environment. Most species can change their sex. Keynote symptoms include:

Fastidious re surroundings.
Merges self into environment.
Nags family and is irritable at home.

Re sex change, Vithoulkas sees the remedy as well indicated in homosexuality!

Calcarea
The oyster is mainly a head which attaches itself and seldom moves thereafter. It responds to the tides, opening itself. Irritation over a very long period eventually produces a pearl. In the patient many symptoms surround the head – heat moves upwards; the head is greatly enlarged in the child; many skin complaints start or centre on the head; they sweat primarily on the head; they have a rich inner life before this is projected into the outer world. The patient is very shy, retreats into their shell(!) often stubborn and resistant to movement. The child sits passively absorbing much, is slow to speak then opens its mouth and speaks sentences.

LESSON ELEVEN

Activity 1

As you will read in your Medical Science Textbooks, Hay Fever is an allergic response of the upper respiratory tract producing sneezing, runny nose and lachrymation. In some patients there might be much swelling and redness. In other patients a rash may be produced on the skin. Hay Fever is usually a result of exposure to pollens.

Hay Fever corresponds to the Allium cepa symptom picture which contains copious flow from the nose and eyes. The sneezing is frequent and violent. The eyes itch and burn. Individuality is found in the Allium cepa symptoms of:

Excoriating discharge from nose, bland lachrymation from the eyes.
The left nostril flows more freely.
Sensitivity to the scent of flowers and peaches.

Activity 2

Allium cepa	Arsenicum	Aconite	Pulsatilla	Phosphorus	Euphrasia
Sneezing from scents and warm room	Sneezing	Sneezing	Sneezing coming into a warm room	Sneezing from scents	Sneezing
Copious fluid left nostril	Copious fluid right nostril	Copious fluid	Copious white mucus	Copious fluid	Copious fluid from nose and eyes, acrid from eyes
After exposure to flowers	After cold, wet or anxiety	After cold, dry or fright	After cold, wet or getting feet wet	After cold, wet	After warmth
With headache	Prostration	Neuralgic pains especially left face	Whiney, wants comforting	Nosebleeds	Light sensitive
Goes on to hoarseness with thick catarrh	Inflammation right sided tonsils, ear or chest Green expectoration	Inflammation left sided tonsils, ear or apex left lung	Inflammation right sided going to left tonsil, ear Sinus headache Copious mucus dries Thirstless	Inflammation tonsils, lungs. Blood streaked mucus Frothy green expectoration	Thick yellow catarrh and agglutinated eyes
Worse warmth Better open air	Worse cold including food and drink	Worse warmth, evening Better open air	Worse going into warmth Better open air	Better cold, food and drink, after sleep	Worse light and warmth

Activity 3

Phlegmatic patients have a dominance of lymphatic problems, oversecretion of mucous membranes in particular, drainage of lymph vessels giving rise to sluggish constitution and oedemas. They might also be described mentally and emotionally as self-pitying, whiney, pathetic, lacking in initiative.

Allium cepa has not been sufficiently proved on the mental level to comment on the latter but it could certainly be said the symptom picture is dominated by an abundance of flow from epithelial lining tissue. The deeper lymphatic symptoms involving drainage and oedemas are not associated with the remedy because it has not been proved at that level.

Activity 4

Reading exercise.

Activity 5

The child is often colicky. He/she is so easily agitated it is as if they eat wind. Everything they eat turns to wind which gurgles continuously in their abdomen. He/she has strong desires for sugary food that makes the wind worse. There is much belching after eating – it explodes out.

Further down the gastro-intestinal tract there are strong spasms which restrict the even flow of the wind incurring violent pains. Eventually it explodes out often accompanied by diarrhoea (especially if they have eaten much sugar) which also explodes out with much mucus.

Activity 6

Angina is most often brought on by anxiety particularly anticipation of events. Their usual way to cope with these is agitation and fuss, hurrying to and fro with much tension. The attacks may bring palpitations which are accompanied by digestive symptoms such as nausea. These heart patients are easily misdiagnosed as having digestive problems. Fainting and vertigo may occur from over-stimulation of the autonomic nervous system. Tension may give rise to High Blood Pressure with congested head and throbbing carotids. Angina pain is a violent spasm arising out of the tension and fluster. Any or all of the above symptoms may also be present at some stage in the attack.

Activity 7

The Argentum nitricum patient who is agoraphobic is reflecting the keynote fear of crowds. In the crowd this patient's movements are restricted – another keynote is fear of narrow places. Both of these keynotes reflect the need of the Argentum nitricum patient to relieve anxiety by continual movement. Freedom is important to the Argentum nitricum patient.

In an anxiety attack this patient will show much agitation expressed as physical movement, restlessness. They may also babble constantly and nervously. They will hold themselves tensely with such force their movements are often jerky or uneven.

Activity 8

Self-directed research.

Activity 9

Symptoms of heart pathology

1. Thinking of the future so always anxious.
2. Walks faster and faster until he stops.
3. Gets into a flap and rushes around doing so many things.
4. Excitement gives rise to palpitations.
5. Fear.
6. Thoughts torment.
7. Throbbing throughout the whole body.
8. Palpitation with nausea.
9. Sensation of fullness around the heart.
10. Irregular intermittent pulse.

Activity 10

Self-directed research.

Activity 11

Rhinitis	Violent itching. Coryza comes with lachrymation, and itching. Worse warmth, before and during menses.
Sore throat	Sensation of a splinter, worse swallowing. Has to hawk thick mucus continually. Can have sensation of a hair. Worse sugar, warmth, before and during menses.
Leucorrhoea	Profuse excoriating. Worse before and during menses. Worse when part closed in and too warm.

Activity 12

Copious catarrh. Indurated glands. Sensation as if a red hot ball in the throat which they continually try to swallow. Pain shoots from the throat to the ear. Metallic taste. White spots on the tonsils coalesce. Ash coloured membrane on the tonsils and throat. Ulceration. Worse damp cold, better warmth.

Activity 13

Rheumatism is worse in cold damp weather or change of weather.

There is a bruised sensation all over the body. Pain is drawing in the muscles, or like electric shocks. Sciatic pain shoots down the outside of the thigh. In the upper body there is weakness so the arm cannot be raised or the humerus extended.

Activity 14

Digestive symptoms
Violent retching every few minutes. There may be no nausea. This may be worse at menses and aggravated from warm drinks. Like Lycopodium they are hungry again soon after eating.

Activity 15

Self-directed research.

Activity 16

There is a great deal of stringy saliva, with painful ulcers in the mouth. Vomit is violent with retching every few minutes.

Activity 17

Self-directed research.

Activity 18

Create a table.

LESSON TWELVE

Activity 1

Symptoms of hardness	Symptoms of softness
Loathing of life.	Sentimental.
Stubborn.	Overcome by mellow lights.
Lumpy stool (covered in 'soft' mucus)	Sympathetic.
	Write poetry.
Lumps in throat.	Weeps at slightest cause.
Thick hard skin.	Tender feet(?)
Calluses and corns.	Chronic catarrhs.
Horn-like excrescences.	

Activity 2

Symptoms of suppuration and over-function

1. Sentimental.
2. Overcome by mellow lights.
3. Melodramatic.
4. Weeps at slightest cause.
5. Easily startled.
6. Angry at any little attention.
7. Overeat.
8. Obesity.
9. Skin thickens.
10. Growths.
11. Chronic catarrh.

Activity 3

She is overconcerned for him. What if . . . (and here the imagination might run riot a little). You are expected to show some sympathy too or you will be seen as callous. Break this romantic mood and she may sulk, stomp out where you can't see her or be irritable if you acknowledge her still there. She may now be peevish and fretful when asked to do anything normal.

Activity 4

Discharges are watery and contain lumps. There is a pressure in the uterus 'as if something would come out'. There is a biting, itching of the scrotum.

Activity 5

Skin symptoms

Antimonium crudum	Graphites
Intense itch, < heat of bed.	Burning, worse heat.
Vesicles and pustules.	Moist, crusty and bleed easily.
White with red areola.	Thick sticky exudate. Slow to heal.
Horny warts, and calluses.	Skin thickens.
Crack in creases.	Rawness in folds.
<< suppression of eruption.	Suppression of sweat, or eruption.

Activity 6

Antimonium crudum is uncomfortable when overheated. They may sweat like a pig! All skin symptoms are markedly worse when exposed to radiant heat, i.e. when they are sitting beside a fire.

Sulphur has a defective heating mechanism so is subject to violent surges of heat upwards. This may be brought on by heat, by exertion or emotions. All skin symptoms are markedly worse when the patient overheats. Certain foods, or even the act of eating, may cause overheating. When well, the Sulphur patient is particularly noted for having hot feet especially at night so they stick them out from under the bedclothes.

Activity 7

Sore throat	Eating acid food is often the exciting cause. There is much yellow mucus with a sensation of a lump causing constant desire to swallow. The voice may be hoarse. Cold bathing or getting soaked after overheating may cause a sore throat.
Headache	These may arise after exposure to the heat of the sun, overeating, or cold bathing. It is described as a heaviness about the forehead, worse for touch or on rising up. Often it is accompanied by dizziness or nausea.
Earache	Cold bathing is the most likely cause of this. Much mucus will gather in the middle ear so deafness arises and the patient describes a sensation as if bandaged. There may be ringing.

Activity 8

Connectedness is the underlying desire in sentimental and

sympathetic. This is dramatized by the romanticism. The strength of the need can be seen in two exciting causes, viz < grief and < disappointed love. The loss of connection can be so disharmonious as to make the person ill. They will break off connection then exhibiting such symptoms as:

Quarrelsome
Angry at any little attention
Dislike to be touched or looked at
Do not want to be spoken to
Sulky.

In their distress this may become a suicidal loathing of life. More likely they will connect more emphatically on the next level down, in this case by overeating.

Activity 9

Symptoms of Antimonium tartaricum similar to Antimonium crudum

1. Symptoms in the pit of the stomach.
2. Violent retching with sinking in the stomach.
3. Thickly coated white tongue.
4. Nausea in waves.
5. Loathing of food is one step further on from Antimonium crudum, i.e. a deeper stage, when the patient starts to disconnect on the digestive level.
6. On this same theme the acupuncturist would say the respiratory symptoms of Antimonium tartaricum show a deeper stage as the symptoms move from the large bowel to the lungs. If this were so we should look for the lumpiness of Antimonium crudum in the respiratory symptoms of Antimonium tartaricum.
7. Thick ropey mucus is solidifying but not really lumpy.
8. Cold sweat, hippocratic expression and pallor are all symptoms of disconnection at the respiratory level.
9. Alternating symptoms, in Antimonium crudum case diarrhoea alternating with eruptions, runs through both remedies.
10. Pustular eruptions.
11. Averse consolation is a deeper stage of withdrawal in Antimonium tartaricum.
12. Does not want to be touched.
13. Whining and peevish.

Activity 10

Self-directed research.

Activity 11

Both have pustular eruptions and exudate that forms thick crusts. Antimonium tartaricum, the deeper remedy, tends to have bluer eruptions than Antimonium crudum. In both remedies the eruptions alternate with other symptoms, in Antimonium tartaricum this is usually respiratory though it can be digestive as in Antimonium crudum.

Activity 12

	Antimonium crudum	Antimonium tartaricum
Exciting Cause	Suppressed eruptions. Emotional disappointments. Overheating. Cold bathing. Vinegar, acids. Overeating.	Suppressed eruptions. Anger. Overheating. Cold, wet. Sour things.
Modalities	< heat, cold bathing, vinegar, acids, touch, radiated heat. > lying down.	< heat, sour things, milk, lying down. > sitting erect, vomiting, eructation.
Symptoms	Vomits without nausea < eating or drinking. Vomiting ceaseless, followed by convulsions. Sensitive to touch in epigastrium(*s*). Loathing of all food. Thirstless. Child vomits milk curdled. Feels bloated and always overloaded(*s*)	Nausea in waves with cold sweat. Violent vomiting followed by sleep. Sinking in epigastrium(*s*). Loathing of all food. Sips little and often or thirstless. Aversion to milk.

s = sensation. All others symptoms are dysfunction.

Activity 13

Symptoms of rheumatism

Swollen joints, especially synovial such as knees. Much oedema. Coldness of skin with a tendency to sweat. They cannot get enough heat yet they do not benefit from heat. Cold weather and change of the weather are times when they are much worse. Suppression, e.g. allopathic drugging, will cause gastric symptoms. You will see the thickly coated tongue in the feeble elderly patient. They are extremely peevish and irritable, very negative people whom you cannot make comfortable. The irritability is seen in the restlessness of affected parts. The limbs may jerk up during sleep or, in the deeper stage, they may go dead when lain on.

Activity 14

Create a table of comparison.

LESSON THIRTEEN

Activity 1

Symptoms showing weakness

1. Weak memory.
2. Tendency to catch colds.
3. No strength to bring up expectoration.
4. Muscles weak.
5. Weak digestion better cold food.
6. < slight exposure to cold.

Activity 2

Symptoms of dwarfishness

1. Stunted growth.
2. Slow learners.
3. Childlike of mind.
4. Lack of confidence.*
5. Lack of courage.*
6. Indecisive*
7. Thoughtless*
8. Undescended testes*.
9. Muscles tense and shorten.

*Because this faculty has not yet grown.

Activity 3

Reading exercise.

Activity 4

There is extreme naivety and innocence, so they may happily go along unaware of what is expected of them in an adult world. Thus, they are open to abuse. The more aware teenager may be very bashful and coy, perhaps even unable to accept. If he/she accepts they may be innocently trusting and very easily hurt or may be so exuberant their behaviour is childish and inappropriate.

Activity 5

They easily take cold on least exposure to cold weather. There will be copious catarrh with enlarged glands. So much catarrh may cause deafness and the keynote, as if noises reverbated in the ears on blowing the nose. If the cold progresses to the chest there will be a cough bringing up copious mucus but rapid degeneration to a stage where they do not have the strength to bring up the mucus. They will then be worse for heat.

Activity 6

He is an affable old soul whom you cannot dislike but he may get on your nerves because he never seems to fit in. For example, here he is on his feet at the AGM and what is he saying? He has on his friendly innocent smile and dicky bow tie so you could not bring yourself to say anything harsh to him as you know it would cut him to the quick but ... why on earth is he talking on about how nice it was to see that other club on Sunday and shouldn't we invite them again when in fact we are wrestling with the fact we have a £50 000 deficit in our budget and the newspapers might hear about that shindig last week ...

Activity 7

Symptoms of dryness and contraction

Physical
1. Skin dry and flaky.
2. Lack of sweat.
3. Cracks and fissures.
4. Skin hardens.
5. Thick exudate dries to yellow crusts.
6. Burning in many parts.
7. Contraction of tendons.
8. Constriction of many parts.
9. Burning in the stomach.
10. Chilly.
11. Bearing down pains.

Mental
11. Foreboding that something will happen.
12. Timid and hesitant.
13. Slow of thought, i.e. the mind contracts in its capacity.
14. Mistakes reading and writing.
15. Remembers only the past.

Activity 8

Symptoms showing lack of oxygen and life

1. Skin hardens.
2. Nails thicken and distort.
3. Deafness, hears better in a noise.
4. Contraction of tendons.
5. Craves air.
6. Chilly.
7. Anxiety.
8. Irresolute.
9. Timid and hesitant.
10. Slow of thought.
11. > open air.

Activity 9

Symptoms of slowness and thickness

1. Lack of sweat.
2. Skin hardens and thickens.
3. Thick sticky exudate dries to yellow crusts.
4. Nails thicken and distort.
5. Thickened eyelids.
6. Sees double.
7. Slow of thought.
8. Large knotty stools covered in mucus.

Activity 10

They may be the shy slow type that stands around waiting to be approached, affable but so slow to put thoughts together that you find them a drag. They may be sentimental and slobber over that nice piece of music that is playing and talk a lot of the past. Or, the more lively type may show anxiety changing their mind constantly, well what *do* you want to drink? The more healthy could be mischievous and impudent like the child, perhaps the type that plays practical jokes even! The hesitant type may grapple with their knife and fork and drop half their dinner or pour the wine down your shirt whilst the more exuberant might deliberately stuff custard on your Yorkshire pudding or embarrass you by asking someone at the other end of the table to pass you a third helping of brandy butter.

Activity 11

Basically an affable child he will test your affability to the limit. So when all the milk is on the floor he will draw your attention to this and instead of rushing for a cloth he will persuade his little classmates it would be fun to jump in the milk and see how far they can spread it before you come back with the cloth. When you come back and find this mess he will run away giggling as if it was great fun, which of course it was and boys will be boys, his mum will say.

Activity 12

Create a table of comparison.

LESSON FOURTEEN

Activity 1

Symptoms of overproduction
1. Warts and condylomata.
2. Waxy shiny face.
3. Polyps.
4. Thickened distorted nails.
5. Growth of hair on parts not normally covered.
6. Lank greasy hair.
7. Anticipatory fears.
8. Haste in eating, speech, walking.
9. Prolonged thoughtfulness over trifles.
10. Delusions.
11. Thick green mucus.

Activity 2

Self-directed research.

Activity 3

Self-directed research.

Activity 4

Pustular eruptions are full of yellow pus. Even the warts seem surrounded with moisture or are dry and horny. Herpetic eruptions may start exuding moisture which causes them to itch and smart. There is a great aversion at this stage to washing as cold water increases the burning. Later the eruptions are dry and scaly but this is much less characteristic than the wet stage.

Activity 5

Self-directed research.

Activity 6

Ear symptoms	Dry scurf on the outside of the ear. Much wax is produced and much catarrh during 'infections'. This last produces noises on swallowing as if there were boiling water in the ear.
Throat	There may be copious mucus in the early stages which dries so the mucus is tenacious and difficult to bring up.
Urogenital	Being a deep remedy there are so many symptoms at this level. The parts are surrounded by the greasy sweat and many warts. There may be copious green-yellow leucorrhoea. When the period itself arrives this is short and scanty. From the bladder, the urine burns, cystitis is common with the characteristic symptoms as if a drop is running down the urethra (as in Cantharis). Death enters the symptom picture with paralysis of the bladder.

Activity 7

Self-directed research.

Activity 8

Self-directed research.

Activity 9

Symptoms of sensitivity
1. Scattered in all directions.
2. Up and down people.
3. Sensitive to atmospheric change.
4. Hurried nervous stammer.
5. Precocious children.
6. Tendency to take cold.
7. Eruptions bleed easily.
8. Feels as if made of sugar.

Activity 10

Symptoms of increased secretion
1. Excessive salivation.
2. Bleeding gums.
3. Eruptions easily bleed.
4. Glands suppurate.
5. Profuse sweat.
6. Sweats with pain.
7. Milk at menses.
8. Milk in the breasts of virgins or young boys.
9. Offensive diarrhoea with blood and slime.

Activity 11

Symptoms showing destructive side of syphilitic miasm
1. Fear of insanity.
2. Fear of own violence.
3. Desire to catch passing strangers by the nose.
4. Amoral.
5. Disgusting filthy habits.
6. Alcoholism.
7. Mouth ulcers.
8. Bleeding gums.
9. Crown of teeth decay.
10. Glands suppurate.
11. Sweat stains clothes.
12. Raw corrosive leucorrhoea.
13. Offensive diarrhoea with blood and slime.
14. Burning urine.
15. Bone pains at night.

Activity 12

Mercurius	*Pulsatilla*
Frequent urge – not necessarily much urine.	Frequent urge even after just been.
Itching or burning afterwards.	< lying down.
Blood in urine.	Pressure in bladder after urination.
Pain on urinating during perspiration.	Involuntary on coughing, sudden movement.
	Pain on urinating if menses suppressed.

Activity 13

Mercurius	*Sulphur*
Sneezes < sunshine.	Frequent sneezing < heat.
Eyes red and swollen.	All orifices red, eyes burn.
Rawness of coryza.	Fluent burning coryza < out of doors.
Glands suppurate and ulcerate.	Glands swell, as if a lump.
Much catarrh.	Redness.
Pain extends from throat to ears on swallowing.	Much catarrh.
Catarrhal deafness < heat.	Catarrhal deafness worse after eating or blowing the nose.

Activity 14

Self-directed research.

Activity 15

Table of comparison.

Answers to Self-test Questions

LESSON ONE

1. Chamomilla.
2. Aconite.
3. Aconite.
4. Chamomilla.
5. a) Belladonna.
   b) Aconite.
6. Dogs, water.
7. Sweat, trembling, contracted pupils.
8. a) < cold, dry winds, touch, light, noise, inspiration, > rest, open air.
   b) < heat, sun, draughts to head, light, noise, jar, looking at shining objects. Part hanging down, 3 p.m. > bending backwards.
   c) < anger, dentition, being looked at, coffee, 9 a.m. and 9 p.m., > passive motion – being carried, sweating.
9. Aconite.
10. Aconite.
11. Chamomilla.
12. Belladonna.
13. Aconite.
14. Anger, dentition, bad news, humiliation.
15. Sun, getting head wet or chilled.
16. Fright, cold dry winds.
17. Green slimy, like chopped spinach, sour or smell like rotten eggs.
18. Suddenly appears after fright or shock in single relevant part.
19. Usually occur with high temperature and no sweat. Sees monsters and hideous faces.
20. By dilating involuntary muscle as in coronary arteries in angina. Also for anxiety and fear of death.
21. Nothing pleases. Asks for things then rejects them. Demanding and tyrannical.
22. Pressure on the abdomen, heat.
23. It is dry, i.e. no sweat. It is so intense you can feel it without touching the part.
24. Red lying down, pale on rising up.
25. Right sided, hot, throbbing, red streaks, radiate from the nipples.

LESSON TWO

1. a) Hypericum (or could be Ledum).
   b) Symphytum.
   c) Calendula.
   d) Ledum.
   e) Hypericum.
   f) Hypericum.
   g) Arnica.
   h) Aconite.
   i) Bellis perennis.
   j) Arnica (or Rhus toxicodendron).
   k) Belladonna is better than Hypericum.
   l) Chamomilla.
   m) Ledum.
   n) Hypericum.
   o) Arnica.
2. Belladonna is < heat, Hypericum is < cold.
3. a) Great fear. Much movement or agitation. There is a lot of tensely held muscle as it screams its head off.
   b) Fright less. Does not want comforted or approached. Tolerates no fuss. Holds itself to itself. Bruising develops.
   c) Spasm of the injured part. Later lumps may appear on the bones
4. Wounds to joints or to eye.

   Arnica: Smelly, bruised pains as if beaten < 1st movement > continued movement. Bruising black and blue. Prickling pains inwards. Eyes tired and bruised, bloodshot – as if objects leaning forward and about to fall.

   Ledum: Smelling, green-yellow bruising, tearing pains, cold > cold, numbness, twitching muscles. In eye bloodshot, twitching.

   Symphytum: Prickling, stitching pains. Wounds that penetrate to the bone. Eyes close spasmodically or as if something in them.
5. Shooting, lacerating pains move along the nerves towards the spine. They return at the slightest touch.
6. Both have a very low pain threshold, pain out of all proportion.
7. When the living dermal layer was exposed.

LESSON THREE

1. Belladonna, Hyoscyamus, Stramonium.
2. Stramonium.
3. Deathly sinking feeling, < least motion, < uncovering the abdomen.
4. Dulcamara.
5. Stramonium (Hyoscyamus to a lesser extent).
6. Belladonna.
7. Tabacum.
8. Hyoscyamus.
9. < motion, opening eyes, > uncovering abdomen, fresh air, cold application.
10. Hyoscyamus.
11. Belladonna, Hyoscyamus (Stramonium to a lesser extent).
12. Tabacum.
13. Belladonna, Hyoscyamus, Stramonium.
14. Stramonium.

15. Fright, jealousy, disappointed love, rage.
16. Deathly pallor, icy cold with cold sweat.
17. Belladonna.
18. Chamomilla.
19. Hyoscyamus.
20. Belladonna, Stramonium.
21. Tabacum.
22. Belladonna, Stramonium.
23. Poisoning, being alone, running water.
24. Stramonium.
25. Dulcamara.
26. Belladonna, Stramonium.
27. Dulcamara.
28. Stramonium.
29. Dulcamara.
30. Tabacum.
31. Belladonna, Stramonium.
32. They lie and play games with you.
33. Of animals. They scream out and on waking are rigid or do not appear to be out of it yet.
34. Cold damp, getting soaked, chilled after overheating, suppressed sweat.
35. Belladonna.
36. Stramonium.
37. Tabacum.
38. Chamomilla, Dulcamara.
39. Belladonna, Hyoscyamus, Stramonium.
40. Starts with specific exciting cause, rant and rave, lewd, suspicious and paranoid.

LESSON FOUR

1. Rhus toxicodendron, Apis mellifica.
2. Hepar sulphuris calcareum.
3. Arsenicum album.
4. Arsenicum album.
5. Arsenicum album.
6. Rhus toxicodendron.
7. Apis mellifica.
8. Hepar sulphuris calcareum.
9. *a)* Rhus toxicodendron.
   b) Hepar sulphuris calcareum.
10. Rhus toxicodendron.
11. < cold wet, chilled, especially after sweating, beginning of motion, overexertion, before a storm, side lain on, > heat, continued motion, rubbing.
12. Rotten meat, carrion.
13. Apis mellifica.
14. Rhus toxicodendron, Dulcamara.
15. Splinter-like, sticking pains < slightest draught.
16. < cold dry, slightest draught, uncovering, touch, > heat, hot damp.
17. Burning pains > heat.
18. Poisoning.
19. In hairy parts.
20. Old cheese, sour.
21. < after midnight, 2 a.m., cold food and drink, watery vegetables, cold damp, bad meat and fish, > heat.
22. Fussy, fidgety, on the go needlessly, creates things to worry about.
23. Irritability, overreactive skin, rheumatic diathesis.
24. Puts pictures square, pulls out other people's needs.
25. Stinging.
26. Food poisoning, loss of face, anxiety about health.
27. It pits.
28. They cause an itchy rash.
29. Watery coryza, excoriates the nose. Tears burn the cheeks.
30. Debility. Lack of co-ordination leading to clumsiness.

LESSON FIVE

1. Gelsemium.
2. Dulcamara.
3. Staphysagria.
4. Hyoscyamus.
5. Tabacum.
6. Nux vomica.
7. Stramonium.
8. Staphysagria.
9. Ledum.
10. Belladonna.
11. Symphytum.
12. Rhus toxicodendron.
13. Cantharis.
14. Hepar sulphuris.
15. Arsenicum.
16. Chamomilla.
17. Aconite.
18. Dulcamara.
19. Arnica.
20. Ignatia.

LESSON SIX

1. *a)* Baptisia.
   b) Belladonna.
   c) Bryonia.
   d) Gelsemium.
   e) Aconite.
   f) Arsenicum.
   g) Euphrasia.
   h) Hepar sulphuris.
   i) Apis mellifica.
   j) Chamomilla.
   k) Rhus toxicodendron.

2. *Bryonia*   *Baptisia*   *Gelsemium*
   - < cold, wet   < humid heat   < cold wet
   - < autumn   < autumn   < spring
   - > firm pressure   < pressure.   < motion
   - < motion   < shock, bad news.
   - < deep breathing.
3. Both have a strong effect on the nerves causing trembling. < fright. This can even cause paralysis.
4. Belladonna is inflammatory, causes dryness, heat to rise to the head. Delirium makes them see monsters.
   Baptisia is rapid onset like Belladonna. It produces stupor which is more dopey than active as is Belladonna. Falls asleep answering questions. Belladonna raves, bites and strikes. Belladonna is more inflammatory and will produce the higher temperature.
5. Congestion to head.
   Copious mucus.
   Copious oily sweat.
   Dropsical swellings.
   Gluttony.
   Heavy, full sensation.
6. Each has copious watery discharge. Arsenicum and Euphrasia are acrid. All are < cold conditions but Arsenicum is < dry too.
7. All can enter stupor when heat affects the brain. Stramonium is excitable but gets frightened and then sees animals. Hyoscyamus prattles and picks at the bedclothes, will mutter in their delirium, stupor creeps up so they can't think. Baptisia is more confused. In delirium the brain is affected so they feel parts of their body are split off and they move about the bed trying to collect them.
8. Bryonia and Dulcamara are both remedies of respiratory and rheumatic problems. Both are < cold damp situations. They resemble each other in the initial copious discharge but Bryonia goes into a very dry condition. Dulcamara is > for heat and motion.
9. Gelsemium is benumbed then trembles and feels weak. They wish to be left alone, then become apathetic and depressed. Ignatia may become hysterical, weep and laugh alternately, have a lump in their throat. They may faint. They may want to talk of the event all the time. Staphysagria becomes angry. Why should this be happening? It's not fair. They may storm and throw things.

LESSON SEVEN

1. Lycopodium.
2. Dry scaly eruptions may start on the head only then extend to flexures which sweat. The problem is noticeably < milk. Also < heat.
3. Sulphur.
4. Calcarea carbonica.
5. He wolfs down a whole meal of three courses then looks for more as he is still hungry.
6. Lycopodium.
7. The eyes smart and burn, and are red rimmed.
8. Calcarea carbonica.
9. Lycopodium.
10. They are all sour.
11. There is itching and burning. It swells and/or is sore after scratching. Itch is < heat.
12. Very bloated with gurgling noisy wind > passing it.
13. Sulphur.
14. Profuse and clotty, they come early and are protracted.
15. Lycopodium.
16. Calcarea carbonica.
17. Sulphur.
18. < pressure of clothes on abdomen, red wine, waiting for food, milk, onions, 4–8 p.m, warmth.
    > warm drinks, eructations, urinating.
19. Calcarea carbonica.
20. Hot and restless, especially the feet, kick the bedclothes off.
21. Swollen tonsils are covered in small ulcers, < right side, > hot drinks.
22. Fontanelles are slow to close, dentition is slow, bones are slow to harden, so rickets arise.
23. They feel it ties them down to responsibility.
24. Sulphur.
25. Like rotten eggs.
26. Lycopodium.
27. Calcarea carbonica.
28. Sulphur.
29. Wrinkled forehead with angular shaped head.
30. Calcarea carbonica.

LESSON EIGHT

1. Changeable moods, easily persuaded, < change of weather, change of appetite, menses, bowel.
2. Menstruation, pregnancy, menopause.
3. Natrum muriaticum.
4. Sepia.
5. Pulsatilla.
6. Upwards.
7. Pulsatilla.
8. Robbers.
9. *a)* Natrum muriaticum.
   b) Sepia.
10. Sepia.
11. Pulsatilla. Sepia.
12. Natrum muriaticum.
13. Hormone imbalance or relaxed uterus.
14. She is very shy, prefers the known.
15. Congestion before with migraine, sore breasts, great irritability towards the loved ones. During she has bearing down pains, as if all would fall out, back pain < standing, prolonged, heavy with clots.
16. Pulsatilla.
17. Sun, grief, disappointed love, seaside.

18. Sepia, Natrum muriaticum.
19. Dogs, heights.
20. Natrum muriaticum – as if broken, Sepia < standing < menses.
21. They can avoid emotional demands of others and their own needs.
22. Little balls. Can be hard at first then more soft, loose.
23. Desires sweets, butter, ice cream. Loathes pork and fats.
24. Throbbing above the left eye < before menses. Accompanied by nausea < at sight of food.
25. Changeable and easily persuaded.
26. Natrum muriaticum.
27. Vinegar and pickles.
28. In the morning before the routine of the day occupies them.
29. A thousand hammers pounding in the forehead. < sun. May start 10 a.m., increase and then decrease with the sun.
30. They wilt or become stuffy and dry.

LESSON NINE

1. Silicea shows resistance to situations that cause fear; once frightened the shock 'fixes' so they may have convulsions or paralysis thereafter. Phosphorus is easily frightened because they have such an imagination; they will become excitable and sleepless. Causticum is overshadowed by fright so they are nervous and expect the worst so they become depressed and mistrustful.
2. When they fear failure or that they will not have enough energy to finish things.
3. Nose, face, hands.
4. Fantasy.
5. They go around looking for them and pick them up.
6. Dry cold, fright, suppressed eruptions, getting soaked.
7. On the feet the sweat rots the socks.
8. Causticum.
9. Dark, being alone, ghosts, thunderstorms.
10. Silicea.
11. Phosphorus and Silicea are left-sided. Causticum is right-sided.
12. Silicea.
13. One-sided, or of single parts.
14. Vomits when it becomes warm in the stomach.
15. Can't express themselves properly.
16. Long threads of bright red blood.
17. They look on the dark side all the time, are anxious and think the worst.
18. Causticum.
19. Ice cream, cold food and drinks.
20. Burning pains.
21. Dark.
22. Excitement.
23. It recedes again.
24. They are hot and if placed in hot water cause flushes of heat.
25. Causticum.
26. Large pustules and lumps.
27. < left side, talking, cold air, odours, before thunderstorms, sexual excess, twilight. > sleep, nibbling, cold food and drink.
28. There is bloody discharge.
29. It lacks modulation.
30. Jerk and twitch.

LESSON TEN

1. < after sleep, sun, heat, autumn, eating. > discharge, start of menses.
2. Cantharis.
3. Touch causes pain.
4. To expel any material left behind.
5. Ascending symptoms, left sidedness, throbbings, sensation of balls or emptiness, menopause.
6. Though thirst is burning, they are averse to liquids. Spasms at the sight of water.
7. Under control of another person. That he is dead and preparations being made for his funeral. Hear voices telling them what to do.
8. Cantharis.
9. Jerky and angular.
10. When eyes are inflamed.
11. Very sensitive to slight pressure.
12. Burning cutting pains with constant urge for just a few drops.
13. Tarentula.
14. Because it is generally > discharge.
15. Cantharis.
16. It flicks out and in or is left protruding.
17. Guilt – they fear damnation.
18. Tarentula.
19. The rage is increased.
20. General throbbings and pulsations, varicose veins, thrombosis, < after sleep or eating.
21. Yearly or at the same hour.
22. Of revenge, lust, snakes, quarrels, the dead.
23. Tarentula.
24. Mottled purple and become gangrenous.
25. Disappointed love, bad news, after scolding.
26. Lachesis.
27. When the hands are put in cold water.
28. As if the heart is too big, as if hanging by a thread.

LESSON ELEVEN

1. Watery discharge is blood from the nose, acrid, from the eyes.
2. They are in a constant hurry and need to move in anxiety.
3. Purulent forming thick crusts.
4. Ichorous, foetid discharge.
5. Allium cepa, Phosphorus.

6. They become ever more agitated and scattered as the hour approaches.
7. Mercurius, Phytolacca.
8. Crowds, high buildings, narrow places, of passing a certain point, of dark.
9. Allium cepa comes from the left nostril first, Arsenicum comes from the right.
10. Phytolacca.
11. Aconite, Allium cepa, Bryonia.
12. There is spasm.
13. Sciatica pains move down the outside of the thigh like electric shocks.
14. They move from left to right.
15. Walking, speech, eating.
16. Like electric shocks along the tract of the nerve, or like drawing pains in the muscle.
17. Profuse, bland lachrymation.
18. Phytolacca, Phosphorus.
19. Allium cepa.
20. Indurated especially parotid, testes and breasts.
21. Phytolacca.
22. Palpitations arise.
23. There is an ash-coloured membrane on tonsils and throat.
24. There is excessive mucus.
25. Parotid, submaxillary, testes and breasts.
26. They are in long threads.
27. Argentum nitricum, Natrum muriaticum.
28. Sour, green, splutters with much wind.
29. Argentum nitricum.
30. < cold damp, warm room, stinging,
    > cool open air motion.

LESSON TWELVE

1. Gets angry.
2. Skin thickens so horny, hard or cracked. Eruptions are pustular.
3. A coarse rattling.
4. They have nausea at the sight and smell of food.
5. Sooty deposits, alae nasi fan.
6. Relaxation on skin and mucous membrane.
7. Antimonium crudum < overheating, < certain foods. Antimonium tartaricum > posture that helps bring up mucus.
8. Pickles and acid foods.
9. Antimonium tartaricum, Sulphur.
10. Thick and ropey.
11. Less sentimental and more mental.
12. Romantics.
13. Antimonium crudum, Ipecacuanha.
14. Acrid, excoriating.
15. Pulsatilla affects kidneys, Antimonium tartaricum affects lungs. Pulsatilla congestion responds to gentle exercise.
16. As if full of stones. Sensitive to touch.
17. Pustular eruptions.
18. Disappointed love, grief.
19. They fall asleep or retch and vomit violently.
20. Lumps in throat, stool leucorrhoea, corns and calluses.
21. Pulsatilla, Antimonium tartaricum.
22. Pathetic, whiney with little energy. Do not want to be looked at. Want to be carried.
23. Make them melancholic.
24. They become more irritable.
25. < pork, bread and pastries.
26. There is so much mucus in the lungs.
27. Violent, as if the bowels would be cut to pieces.
28. Greed for food, nails like pig's trotters, wallowing.
29. Huge appetite, emptiness, epigastric.
30. It suppresses the menses.

LESSON THIRTEEN

1. Baryta carbonica, Lycopodium.
2. Graphites is so sensitive it has bone pains. Calcarea carbonica is worse extremes of heat and cold.
3. Worse suppressed foot sweat, slight exposure to cold, heat, company of others. Better warmth, cold food.
4. Dry crusty eruptions (cradle cap) in the child, doughy complexion in the adult.
5. Allium cepa, Arsenicum, Chamomilla, Graphites, Ignatia, Lachesis, Natrum muriaticum, Nux vomica, Phosphorus, Phytolacca, Sepia, Silicea, Sulphur.
6. All three are irresolute and change moods constantly. All are timid.
7. Argentum nitricum, Arsenicum, Baryta carbonica, Calcarea carbonica, Graphites, Ignatia, Lachesis, Lycopodium, Natrum muriaticum, Nux vomica, Phosphorus, Pulsatilla, Sepia, Silicea, Sulphur.
8. Baryta carbonica.
9. Makes them sad.
10. They fail to descend.
11. Large, knotty and covered in mucus.
12. Causticum, Graphites.
13. Slows down and is unable to make decisions.
14. Aconite, Antimonium crudum, Argentum nitricum, Baryta carbonica, Bryonia, Calcarea carbonica, Chamomilla, Dulcamara, Gelsemium, Graphites, Hepar sulphuris, Lycopodium, Natrum muriaticum, Nux vomica, Phosphorus, Pulsatilla, Silicea, Sulphur.
15. Graphites, Natrum muriaticum, Sepia.
16. It increases contraction of muscular tissue.
17. Baryta carbonica, Silicea, Hyoscyamus, Lycopodium.
18. Chronically enlarged.
19. Burning pains. Graphites is better eating, Antimonium crudum is worse eating.
20. Baryta carbonica, Calcarea carbonica, Graphites, Lycopodium, Phosphorus, Pulsatilla, Sepia, Silicea, Sulphur.
21. Profuse, thin, excoriating, flows in gushes.
22. Both may crumble.
23. The Graphites child is mischievous, laughs at reprimands.

24. Graphites.
25. Allium cepa, Antimonium crudum, Antimonium tartaricum, Argentum nitricum, Graphites, Lachesis, Phosphorus, Sepia, Silicea, Sulphur.
26. Red and puffy, sometimes cracks at corners. They may become dry and scaly. Thicken.
27. All have offensive foot sweat. Graphites has burning in the soles and heels. In Baryta carbonica the feet are hot and bruised especially at night. Calcarea may have burning soles that become raw. In Antimonium crudum the feet are tender, wrinkle and crack. In Silicea it is the arch of the foot that aches.
28. There is a constant urge to swallow.
29. Graphites.
30. Calcarea carbonica, Graphites, Lycopodium, Phosphorus, Sepia, Sulphur.

LESSON FOURTEEN

1. Anywhere.
2. Lycopodium, Pulsatilla, Thuja, Nux vomica.
3. Excessive salivation, metallic taste, teeth decay at the crown, gums degenerate.
4. Drinks fall audibly into the stomach.
5. They pick their nose and eat it.
6. The breasts are full of milk at menses.
7. It is either very lank and greasy or dry and flyaway.
8. Mercurius.
9. Sweats on uncovered places.
10. Thighs.
11. Because they are in such a hurry.
12. Insanity, their own violence.
13. Sepia is fastidious about their home and environment. Arsenicum wants to be organized so he/she is less anxious. Thuja has a rigid pattern.
14. Mercurius.
15. Both as if a nail were pushed into a small spot.
16. Mercurius scatters in all directions and does not keep to one theme. They are also very sensitive to atmosphere.
17. It recedes.
18. Tenesmus continues after the stool.
19. Of a superior being or a voice telling them what to do. They both feel someone else is in the room.
20. Mercurius.
21. Sweats with pain.
22. Both have haste in eating, walking, speech.
23. There is a creeping chilliness.
24. Thuja, Mercurius, Causticum.
25. Falling, Flying, Of the Dead.
26. Offensiveness, worse night, profuse sweat, excessive salivation.
27. Forked stream of urine, as if urine moves along the urethra.
28. Profuse sweat brings no relief, it stains clothes yellow. Sweat accompanies pain.

Some Test-cases to Try to Solve

The following are little cases in which I have tried to bring together examples you may come across in practice. I have put them in the language of the patient rather than that of the Materia Medica so you can practise translating the patient's language into meaningful symptoms. Remember, the language of the Materia Medica was that used by the original provers. Some of it is over 100 years old so the idiom is different from today's. It may improve your repertory skills to see how many different ways you might translate the symptoms into rubrics. Note that some choice of rubric may be more accurate than others. Note also the seeming ambiguity of some rubrics.

You will gain much if you use the cases to practise isolating that which is most characteristic and individual to each case. Seek also for the keynotes and exciting causes as these often represent that which is most individual in the case. Do not forget to put the symptoms into hierarchical order. In some cases it might be difficult to separate out only one remedy but I have subtly inserted keynotes to restrict choice – these may not be in the language of the Materia Medica so it may not be too easy to recognize them as the patient speaks in their own language. Good luck! The answers are at the end of this section.

Test 1

1. The common cold starts with a sore throat. There is a sharp pain on swallowing and such an increased flow of saliva that the patient swallows constantly. The breath is very foul. Soon the pain extends to the ear. During the night there are copious sour sweats especially about the head. She is markedly worse when lying on the right side.
2. This is a summer cold brought on by heat. The head is hot and at first there is copious fluid from the nose with itchy, red-rimmed eyes. As the cold continues the eyes dry up and burn, the nose has dry scabs of catarrh and the chest feels heavy. At night there is such burning in the hands and feet. The corners of the mouth become dry and cracked.
3. The cold starts with a tingling in the nose and much sneezing follows with fluid discharge. As it continues the head feels heavy and pain like a tight band is increased if the head is low. As the coryza dries the patient becomes dopey and flushed as if intoxicated. There is some relief from the head symptoms on urinating.
4. The weather has been very wet for weeks and now the child has started with a cough. At first it is dry and starts from a tickle in the throat then it becomes spasmodic as he tries to get up some tenacious mucus. The cough becomes looser as yellow phlegm becomes more copious. At the same time the head is affected. It feels full and each time he coughs it is as if it would explode. He drinks copious amounts of juice.
5. She has been anxious since overhearing a conversation in the office casting doubt on her work. Now her glands are swollen and her throat is tight so it is difficult to swallow.

The slightest touch is very painful yet she has no problems eating. She feels there is something lodged in her throat.
6. In the wet weather her glands swell then a considerable amount of catarrh is produced. As this thickens and becomes green she loses her sense of smell and taste. When the ears are affected there is a loss of hearing on the left side which can disappear with a popping noise.
7. The voice becomes hoarse after exposure to cold but strangely it is better the more he talks. A cough develops which is dry and tickly. It is better when he sips cold water. He wants little to eat. When the disturbance develops into the chest there is a sticking, burning pain. The cough then cannot raise the expectoration – it slips back down. He is anxious and quarrelsome and looks on the black side of everything.
8. After a wet period a cough starts. At first it is an irritating tickle that is worse as soon as she tries to talk. There is rawness and hoarseness. As it goes into the chest there is burning and blood streaked phlegm. She sleeps a great deal and is partial to cold drinks.
9. He went out without a hat this afternoon. Now he has a burning fever. The head is hot and feels very large. There are pains in the eyes. As he goes into delirium there is much anxiety and restlessness. The face is red and the skin is dry.
10. He was out running when he got soaked. The voice became hoarse that evening. During the night he developed a fever with copious sweat. He was very restless during sleep. By morning he had difficulty swallowing. The glands were swollen. The back of the throat was red and itchy.

Test 2

1. Restless in the night, starting at the least noise, after a soaking during the day. The face is covered with profuse sweat. The left ear has smelly wax – the smell is sour. Now there is a stitching pain in the ear on swallowing. The ear is better when warmly covered. The slight deafness disappears when they blow the nose.
2. There is a stitching pain in the right ear. This is also sensitive to the slightest touch and has a smelly discharge. The ear is carefully covered up since the slightest draught increases the pain. This patient is very irritable and cannot bear the slightest disturbance. They are also sweaty in the night.
3. The severe pain in the right ear started after being caught in a cold wind. There is a peculiar redness of the lobe and a

sound of rushing water. They sweat with the pain and are peevish and whiny. The catarrhal deafness appears to disappear when warm clothes are applied to the ear.
4. Shortly after exposure to a cold wind the left ear started to ache. The pains were described as stitching. They were worse when touched but the small patient sat screaming, and holding the ear as it rocked anxiously back and forth. There is fever with profuse sweat.
5. There is a tearing pain in the right ear which is much worse when the patient lies on that side. The pain is very sensitive to draughts but lessens when the patient swallows or blows the nose. The catarrhal deafness is worse when hot. The patient sweats profusely at night. The patient may describe a sensation as if cold water were running out of the ear.

6. There is a discharge of thick yellow, smelly pus from the right ear. The patient describes a sensation as if something were trying to push out of the ear. There is much discomfort when they come into a warm room. In a strange way this patient can actually hear better in the car. Mum describes her as very demanding. She whines all the time and is tearful if you remark on this.

7. The stitching pain and smelly discharge come from the left ear of this patient after exposure in a cold spell. The patient describes a sensation as if water were swishing around inside the ear. There is a marked aversion to heat. In fact it makes the patient irritable. The hearing is very sensitive especially after eating or blowing the nose.

8. Boring pains started in the right ear after the head was soaked. It shoots into the other ear when she hears loud noises or if the right ear is touched in any way. The ear is very hot and throbbing. The patient is so irritable with the pain she says she could tear people apart.

9. There is a throbbing pain in the left ear when he has a burning pain in the throat. The slightest touch increases this pain although firm pressure helps. There is an offensive smell from the ear and you will hear him say he feels full of poison.

10. After exposure to wind there is a roaring in the ears. It is as if a hot blast had reached the right ear. There is a peculiar echo when noises penetrate. The patient comforts himself with hot drinks. The family appear to him to give little sympathy and may in fact avoid him in this state because he is particularly demanding.

Test 3

1. The baby cries all day. It wants fed but takes little. The abdomen is extended with much wind. Its screaming is quietened only after eating a little then it is as if things were much worse. It has a wrinkled little face that makes it look like an old man.

2. The baby has a distended abdomen which feels hot even as you draw your hand near. You do not need to touch it to feel the heat. This is just as well because the baby seems very sensitive to touch although it appears relieved lying on its abdomen. The bulge at the top of the abdomen looks as if the transverse colon were bulging out.

3. The baby has a painfully distended abdomen and colic which causes shortness of breath. It seems to get relief when the abdomen is pressed into the shoulder as the child is carried around. It screams when put down. The accompanying diarrhoea is yellow and smells sour.

4. This baby is so flatulent. Its tummy rumbles all night. The colic seems to come in bursts and the baby is seen to take deep breaths then. The spasms come at the same time every day. The child wants to lie on the abdomen.

5. This baby's swollen abdomen is hard and tender. The child will not eat although you feel it must be hungry. It whines all the time and does not want any pressure on the abdomen. In fact it appears it does not want you around at all. It is a tiny creature.

6. After eating, the abdomen of this baby is distended. In fact it often brings the food back up although it swallowed it without any problem. In fact after a drink of cold milk it appears better for a while, then it brings that back up too. It is soothed from having its tummy rubbed.

7. Even after only a little food the abdomen looks distended and is sensitive to the slightest touch and will only lie on its side. There is very little stool and so much straining it gets angry. The little face goes red and puckers with the strain. He has a slight umbilical hernia with this straining.

8. Each evening the abdomen rumbles and there are spasms of colic. You can feel a pulsation in the pit of the stomach. The baby cries piteously during the attacks. This is worse after mum has eaten onions.

9. Baby has a swollen abdomen with a very smelly stool. It smells as if something has died. The baby seems to shiver yet he is not cold to touch, in fact he feels warm but he needs more heat. He cannot keep any food down. It is difficult to get him to take anything.

10. Baby has a hard swollen abdomen with sour smelling diarrhoea. He has been like this ever since he started to teethe. Yet he is quite a placid baby who never seems to complain.

Test 4

1. This morning there is a redness and swelling of the inner canthi. She did a lot of sewing yesterday. The eyes are relieved a bit when she goes outside but she gets out her sweets and nibbles nervously as she rushes to finish this skirt she's making for the dance tonight.

2. This weak eight-year-old is always producing styes in her left eye. Her feet have a profuse rather offensive sweat. She tends to be quite sleepy during the day. In fact her parents describe her as dull and backward. Her thoughts are certainly a little slow.

3. The student preparing for exams has tired, aching eyes with a twitching of the lower lid. The vision is so poor that distance is a complete blur. If he continues to study a headache develops which he describes as sore all over.

4. Last night he was up all night doing his VAT returns. This morning the eyelids are sore and red-rimmed where affected by the tears which stream constantly. They are very sore when touched. He blinks constantly. He is also very irritable but then he usually is in the morning especially when his writing arm is stiff and sore.

5. The morning after a night out with the lads the eyes are swollen, red rimmed and a dark spot floats before the left eye. As the itch of his skin increased he eventually got out of bed, only to slouch in a chair in his vest and pants, unkempt and thinking about the shed he would build that afternoon.

6. Her eyes are hot and her vision is blurred. She is a sorry sight, restless yet too apathetic to do anything – she shrugs her shoulders at helpful suggestions. It is just before the period again. Her abdomen is enormous and feels as if it is hanging down. Soon the labour-like spasm will start but she knows she could ease the situation if only she could be bothered to get out for a walk.

7. She is so angry that she cries scalding hot tears that leave the

eyes red and very sore. She cannot stand people being so rude to others. It reminds her of how hurtful her mother was and opens up unpleasant memories she would rather forget.

8. He almost expected the throbbing headache after so much brandy last night but he is so cold his joints ache and are stiff. The ankles and feet itch near the fire. His eyes are bloodshot and it is as if the eyeball were being pushed out of its socket.

9. Her eyes are stuck together in the morning. When she washes the crust away they are swollen and tender, red-rimmed. Any

movement or bright light makes them worse so they water profusely. She feels light headed. The headache shoots from the brow into the eyes with every jolt so she walks warily. She is such a gloomy person who thinks the worst all the time. Her husband says she is worried about all the nodules which have appeared under her arm.

10. There is an acute burning pain in the eyes worse with the slightest motion or touch. She says it is as if the eyes were on fire. Strangely, everything she looks at appears yellow.

Test 5

1. The back of the throat is red and swollen, even the glands are swollen and she cannot swallow her saliva. It came on when she caught a chill yesterday after running the cross-country race. She describes the back of the throat as itchy.

2. The throat is dry and burning with swollen tonsils, slightly worse on the left side. There is a dreadful tickle when she tries to talk. Just as well, said her brother, because she is a chatterbox. It all started in the last few days when the air chilled as a cold front passed over. Mind you, she has just finished her exams and she was studying so hard.

3. The pain in the throat extends to the ears when he swallows, especially on the right side. It is as if the throat were scraped. His voice goes in the heat. Maybe he is still in shock after getting news of his mum's death last week?

4. There is a sticking sensation in the throat as if she could not swallow a lump. It goes when she is eating! If she does not keep swallowing she can choke. The pain goes up to the ears but *not* when she is swallowing.

5. This patient has a lump in the throat that appears to rise up although she keeps on swallowing it down again. The throat feels hot. Pain shoots up to the ear on the left side whenever she swallows this lump, but not when she is eating. Her breath is foul. There is so much saliva. Although she grasps her throat firmly to relieve the sensation of the lump she has nothing around her neck because slight pressure aggravates the throat symptoms.

6. The throat is dry, rough and swollen at the back. He drinks a great deal of water. The catarrh is thick and tenacious so comes up with difficulty. He is very irritable and just wants to be left to sit quietly in his chair with a great scarf wrapped tightly around his throat.

7. The throat is so constricted it is difficult to swallow. He says it is as if it were paralysed. He has no power to bring up the catarrh so has to swallow it. Very despondent since stood in that really cold wind yesterday.

8. Swollen tonsils with a sore, dry throat so continually swallowing. When he swallows a pain shoots up to the right ear. He says it is as if water were running out of his ear. His breath is foul. There is a metallic taste in his mouth. He sweats copiously and is very uncomfortable.

9. After falling into the river last week, she developed a great deal of yellow catarrh which appeared to come down the back of the throat from the nose. She coughs as soon as she lies down, or even after eating.

10. The throat is very dry and as if it is on fire. The right tonsil throbs as if it would burst. When she swallows liquids it is as if the throat constricts. She has a strong aversion to water. All this came on so suddenly tonight. We thought she might have caught a chill after the swimming gala – Gran is always telling her about going outside with her hair wet. Mum says it was because she was so excited she won her race.

Test 6

1. She has strange pulsations in the pit of her stomach. She has been like this before an ordeal like the interview this afternoon. She has to get out and walk. She cannot bear to sit still. Mum noticed she was actually trembling earlier. She has no interest in food.

2. She is deathly pale and very exhausted from the slightest exertion. She has Crohn's disease so passes a lot of blood and mucus in the stool. This panics her as she fears she will die. At such times she insists her husband stays at home.

3. He had sudden nausea after coming off the roller coaster. He was so exhausted he broke into a cold sweat. He was so sensitive to movement we did not think we would get him home but he seemed alright lying in the back of the car almost stripped with his eyes closed in slumber!

4. He had much wind this morning with a greasy looking, pale stool that gurgled out noisily. It was Mum who said this because he does not say much although he looks at you intently, intelligently, and answers succinctly. He does

mention a heaviness in the stomach after eating. His thin, greasy face and lank hair and the warts on the hands give more of a clue to the remedy.

5. The child writhes with the colic. He is pouring with sweat. This is always worse at night. Sister says it's because he drinks milkshakes last thing at night. Next morning he may have a very slimy, smelly stool. He strains a great deal for this and is so exhausted afterwards he goes back to bed to sleep.

6. This irritable gentleman has severe gastric catarrh when he overeats but he cannot resist the pastries. If the room is warm he overheats so much he vomits them back up.

7. His wife came to complain about this patient because he has become impossible to live with. He is so irritable before meals if he is kept waiting. He is irritable afterwards because he is dopey and cannot remember things so he is worried he is not doing all the work he brought home with him. He spends ages in the toilet in the morning but may pass only volumes of wind. His abdomen is greatly distended.

8. He awoke this morning with an oppressive headache, a hangover. He had a celebration at that new restaurant last night. As soon as he moves he retches violently and gags but produces nothing. It is as if there were a stone in his abdomen, as if the meal were still lying there. He curses vociferously when the neighbour starts in his garden with a lawn mower.

9. The child has started to vomit almost every meal. There is profuse salivation and frequent hiccoughs. The problem seems mysterious until it goes as suddenly as it went but then it comes back again and Mum eventually twigs that Grandad has also come back with that smelly pipe of his and she is sure there is a connection.

10. The child has sore tummies frequently in the morning. There is no apparent cause. Mum is a bit concerned it is because he has started school as he is very shy with strangers and a bit reluctant to go. In fact he is so stubborn about this he has to be taken forcibly – almost. He is a podgy little boy with little appetite apart from chips. Mum also worries he is constipated. His stool consists of little round balls.

Test 7

1. When blowing the nose or sneezing, urine dribbles involuntarily. This may increase in cold winds. Once when she had a fright (burglars) she stopped urinating although sometimes she could go after drinking cold water. She is a dour person, always talking about what might happen to us if . . . . She was on about the atomic bomb again last week.

2. Although she has a constant desire to go she is passing very little urine and then there is an excruciating burning pain. She says she can almost feel the drops trickling along the urethra. She drinks a great deal of water to help but this seems to affect her throat which goes into spasm.

3. He wets the bed at night, usually in his first sleep. He does this if he has caught a chill but more often when he is worried about something, for example, last week before his history test. He gets really flustered before these tests because he may not remember. In fact his memory is very good but he cannot work under stress. He is a plodder best left to himself.

4. Frequent visits to the toilet to urinate end with a cutting pain. He seems to have caught a chill. He remembers it started in the thighs and he shivered violently whenever a part of the body was uncovered in warm air. He finds this most odd. Also, he noticed that he only sweats when he is sleeping. When he woke at 3 a.m. this morning he was covered in sweat but it stopped as soon as he woke.

5. She has had a chronic discharge of yellow-green mucus since puberty. She is a weedy sort with little energy who takes colds at the least exposure to cold, wet conditions. In earlier childhood she had a lot of earache on exposure to cold. She always went around with her hat on. She was a bedwetter until quite late on. Gran used to describe her as backward but really she was quite shy.

6. Urine seems to leak out at the least provocation, coughing, laughing, jumping up and down. After she has been at night she has to get back out of bed to go again. A lot of her symptoms are worse when she lies down. She is much worse in the cold and wet. The urinary symptoms can be awful after she gets her feet wet but she does not like to complain, she says. In fact although she may be meek with strangers she is very demanding of attention at home.

7. He is so easily excited and worked up about little things that do not affect others. So much energy wasted, his wife says. He dives in and out of the toilet with a severe burning pain during and after urination. He says he is better when he can get out and just walk off the energy.

8. He came in for help because he took fits during which he passes urine involuntarily. However, you notice that the urinary system alternates between passing great quantities and passing only small amounts. At times the patient's speech becomes incoherent as if drunk and he tends to bump into things. On questioning you discover this came about since his younger sister was born when he became consumed with jealousy.

9. After the child was exposed to extreme cold, he developed severe pain so he held in the urine. When it flowed it was very red and hot. The child is most anxious and holds himself before the urine flows. He is inconsolable. You notice he is in a cold sweat.

10. There is a constant urge and a continual flow probably from an enlarged prostate. He is a kind old gentleman though a little simple. His face is purplish, his abdomen is large. He almost dribbles as he speaks to you.

Test 8

1. It is a week before her period is due. The head feels full and oppressive. The pain on the forehead is much worse when she bends forwards to iron, or when she coughs (she has a little cold since she got soaked last week). She sits quietly in the chair not even moving her eyes.

2. This morning she has a throbbing headache on only half of her head, the left half. She blames it on the wine and coffee she had with her visitors last night. This morning when she woke the head was wet with sweat. She is still sweating a little now with the pain. She is very irritable at the least thing and was annoyed at the homoeopath's presence. Her husband says she does not know what she wants and drives him mad by asking for something and then not wanting it.

3. She had a heavy oppressive headache over her eyes which she described as hammering. She often has this in the morning before the periods. The vision is disturbed with zig-zags and she has nausea. Sleeping helps her but she has to keep her head up. Sometimes this headache comes when she tries to keep to her timetable. She is a conscientious worker, dislikes fuss and bother. Her workmates see her as rather prim and proper.

4. The woman has an oppressive headache as if a weight pressed on the top of the head. She has to be careful what she eats because any rich food will spark it off. She tends to be constipated and that makes the headache worse. She is more irritable then and can even become quite murderous when others contradict her. She knows she is right.

5. She has a pulsating, pounding headache before the period. The head is so heavy she says she cannot hold it up but she dare not lie down because it is so much worse. She goes out for a walk in the fresh air. This also helps the period pains, and it helps her emotions. She just is not herself before the period. Her moods swing and she cannot make her mind up about anything.

6. He has a heavy weight at the back of the head that appears to draw the head back. His face is a bit flushed, and he has nausea. Although he is hungry he is not interested in food. He sits miserable and groaning, and very chilly.

7. There is a heavy dullness about the forehead since he got up this morning. He stood at the bus stop yesterday in the rain without a hat on. Possibly a cold is developing. Although he wants to rest quietly he cannot sit down beside the fire without increasing the headache. He is completely off his food and is not at all thirsty.

8. His headache feels as if there were a nail pushed into the forehead. He rolls it backwards for relief. This makes the dizziness slightly worse because he is looking upwards. This may have been caused by the fried onions he had for breakfast.

9. He was so chilled yesterday after he went swimming because he was so hot! Fool he says. His head pain feels as if something were pressing heavily on his forehead. Funnily, he is better when he is talking.

10. With this headache he has pain behind the eyes, so he just does not want to move. He likes his wife to rub his temples but very gently as quick movements irritate him. Sometimes the headache is so severe he has to lie down as if to step out of it. Then he can become very chilly and needs to be kept warm.

Test 9

1. She has the most awful bearing down pain in the uterus and the period has not even started. When it does start she knows it will be very heavy. She is so irritable because she cannot fit all her jobs in. She wishes her husband would help or at least the kids would stay out of the way. She knows she does not really hate them but it requires so much energy and she just cannot be bothered. Yet, if she could get going she always feels better.

2. Her breasts feel so full and heavy before the period. Sometimes they are better once the flow starts but she can get nose bleeds sometimes, and the period is then delayed or may not come. Usually the period is dark and heavy. Her abdomen feels full and heavy. She has little energy and is irritable if hassled.

3. She has copious discharge that looks like white of egg. Sometimes it just gets worse and there is no period. Her husband complains she is a bit cut off from him but she says she simply does not want intercourse because it is painful. Her vagina is dry, despite the leucorrhoea.

4. The period comes early and is composed of bright red stringy bleeding. This is similar to the nosebleeds which she sometimes gets instead of menses. She is a very excitable character who is always talking about her boyfriends – yes, she has more than one. She is a day dreamer who is always romanticizing her encounters.

5. She has a numb pain in the right ovary. The period has not yet arrived. When it does, that ovary pain may become burning and stinging. She has suspicions that the doctor is not telling her everything. She does not understand why she keeps on dropping things around period time.

6. Her flow is intermittent with strong cramps that extend over the whole body. She is even more irritable at period time so the family avoid her a little. This does not please her as she cannot then keep them up to the mark, they start to backslide without her to organize them.

7. The period blood is almost black and there is little of it. She has very severe labour-like pains until the flow is properly established. The flow also relieves the constipation. During the menses there is a throbbing pain in the anus. The abdomen is enormous and she needs to support it firmly but is irritated by anything around the middle that does not offer firm support.

8. Her periods flow only during the day. The pains in the back and thighs are described as tearing. During the period her pessimism is increased greatly. She is always on about the state of the world and what is going to happen to all of us.

9. Her periods are always late. Sometimes they do not come at all. When this happens she might have a discharge instead. This comes in gushes and causes rawness. There may be a severe back pain as if the back were broken. The period can be delayed, or suppressed, when she gets her feet wet.

10. Her periods often only last for one day. The pain is better when she gets out and walks in the open air, and oddly is worse for warmth. Often she has a cold with the period. This comes with a runny nose and watery eyes, and a catarrhal headache.

Test 10

1. In the fever the skin is very dry, bright red and hot. You can feel the heat without even touching the skin. It is possible he got a little sunstroke this afternoon. The head feels as if it would burst and the patient is sensitive to noise and light. He wants to be left alone.

2. The baby's head is covered with thick crusty eruptions. He does not complain. He is such a placid child. He sits there smiling and watching all that goes on. Big sister says he is like a painted balloon with a big red head and little body – oh, except for his rather large abdomen. He loves his food and sucks greedily. He is so overweight.

3. Despite his age he still has acne. The round lumps are as benign as he is. He is so bashful he is like a gnome that hides from strangers. His tonsils and cervical glands are enormous, and have been for a very long time. Although he has frequent colds the glands never become nasty. It is his feet that are nasty – they are very sweaty.

4. His face is covered with large pustules which exude yellowish-white pus. His brother says he should stop eating so much. He simply gorges, anything but pork. His tongue has a thick white coating and he is often constipated. The stool is large lumps strung together with thick wads of mucus.

5. The skin is covered with a raw red rash of little red pimples. They are less itchy when the skin is cooled. His wife says there is little that can be done until he stops drinking a bottle of whisky every day. He grunts angrily at her and goes through to his study where he promptly nods off.

6. Her face is covered in acne with such large pustules they must be described as like boils. They itch in turn. She also suffers badly from wind which smells of rotten eggs. Her breath is little better when she burps continuously. She can be quite dopey especially after alcohol which she consumes immoderately.

7. He has a very itchy rash around the scrotum. The area is red and swollen. When worse it produces little vesicles which exude moisture which dries to form crusts. Sometimes the hair follicles are attacked – a little pus is produced at the root of the hair which then drops off. He does not like to wet this part as the itch is then worse.

8. The skin is red and shining as if burnt. It feels as if a million insects were crawling all over it. This has been there since Mum died. She still has nightmares about her and wakes screaming but does not recognize anyone and is unable to take any comfort. She does not understand what happened, so is frightened.

9. He has eczema on the fold of the skin. It started on the wrists and now covers the elbows and back of the knees, slightly worse on the left side. It itches very violently especially when he is in bed at night or after a shower. There is almost nothing he can do to relieve it. If he scratches it swells and bleeds, burning intensely. It makes him very irritable, finding fault with everyone and everything. He has little respect for others. Sister he says he is arrogant and self-centred.

10. Her eczema is very dry and scaly. Great areas are laid raw. There is a burning sensation much worse after she has consumed alcohol the night before or after a few cigarettes. She is very conscious of her appearance and is thickly covered in make-up to disguise the skin. It really seeps away at her confidence. This is a pity as she looks so elegantly dressed and sophisticated in manner. She is very fussy about where all the scales drop too, and apologetically brushes them up before she leaves.

Answers to Test-cases

Test 1
1. Mercurius.
2. Sulphur.
3. Gelsemium.
4. Bryonia.
5. Lachesis.
6. Silicea.
7. Causticum.
8. Phosphorus.
9. Belladonna.
10. Rhus toxicodendron.

Test 2
1. Silicea.
2. Hepar sulphuris.
3. Chamomilla.
4. Aconite.
5. Mercurius.
6. Pulsatilla.
7. Sulphur.
8. Belladonna.
9. Lachesis.
10. Lycopodium.

Test 3
1. Lycopodium.
2. Belladonna.
3. Chamomilla.
4. Ignatia.
5. Baryta carbonica.
6. Phosphorus.
7. Nux vomica.
8. Pulsatilla.
9. Arsenicum.
10. Calcarea carbonica.

Test 4
1. Argentum nitricum.
2. Silicea.
3. Ruta graveolus.
4. Rhus toxicodendron.
5. Sulphur.
6. Sepia.
7. Natrum muriaticum.
8. Ledum.
9. Symphytum.
10. Cantharis.

Test 5
1. Rhus toxicodendron.
2. Phosphorus.
3. Gelsemium.
4. Ignatia.
5. Lachesis.
6. Bryonia.
7. Causticum.
8. Mercurius.
9. Dulcamara.
10. Belladonna.

Test 6
1. Argentum nitricum.
2. Arsenicum.
3. Tabacum.
4. Thuja.
5. Mercurius.
6. Antimonium crudum.
7. Lycopodium.
8. Nux vomica.
9. Ignatia.
10. Calcarea carbonica.

Test 7
1. Causticum.
2. Cantharis.
3. Calcarea carbonica.
4. Thuja.
5. Silicea.
6. Pulsatilla.
7. Argentum nitricum.
8. Hyoscyamus.
9. Aconite.
10. Baryta carbonicum.

Test 8
1. Bryonia.
2. Chamomilla.
3. Natrum muriaticum.
4. Nux vomica.
5. Pulsatilla.
6. Graphites.
7. Antimonium crudum.
8. Thuja.
9. Dulcamara.
10. Rhus toxicodendron.

Test 9
1. Sepia.
2. Bryonia.
3. Natrum muriaticum.
4. Phosphorus.
5. Apis mellifica.
6. Nux vomica.
7. Lachesis.
8. Causticum.
9. Graphites.
10. Euphrasia.

Test 10
1. Belladonna.
2. Calcarea carbonica.
3. Baryta carbonica.
4. Antimonium crudum.
5. Ledum.
6. Arnica.
7. Rhus toxicodendron.
8. Stramonium.
9. Sulphur.
10. Arsenicum.

Modality Tests

These are useful facts to have at your fingertips. Use the Repertory to check your answers. There is more than one remedy possible for each question. Award yourself a point for each remedy that appears in black-letter type or italics in the Repertory. Take away a point for each incorrect answer. No points are given for remedies that appear in ordinary type in the repertory.

You can use these tests repeatedly to build up your memory.

Test 1
1. < cold, wet weather.
2. < windy weather.
3. < change of temperature.
4. < change of temperature from cold to warm.
5. < change of weather.
6. > continued motion.
7. < standing.
8. < fasting.
9. < after sleep.
10. < every 2nd day.
11. < lying down.
12. > lying down.
13. < dry weather.
14. > open air.
15. < noise.
16. < jar.
17. < after head injury.
18. < masturbation.
19. > exertion.
20. < alcohol.

Test 2
1. < open air.
2. < tight clothing.
3. < on waking in the morning.
4. < on entering a cool place.
5. < autumn.
6. < motion.
7. Perspiration ameliorates.
8. < after coition
9. < after eating.
10. > after eating.
11. < consolation.
12. < before menses.
13. < after menses.
14. < bathing.
15. < sun.
16. < becoming heated.
17. < rising from seat.
18. < approach of a storm.
19. < rubbing the part.
20. < after breakfast.

Test 3
1. < vinegar.
2. < warm food.
3. > warm food.
4. < rich food.
5. < bread.
6. < salty food.
7. < fats.
8. < coffee.
9. < sweets.
10. < cold drinks.
11. > cold drinks.
12. < sour things.
13. < ice cream.
14. < sour, acid fruits.
15. < pork.
16. < salads.
17. < milk.
18. < onions.
19. < green vegetables.
20. < sight and smell of food.

Test 4
1. < stretching.
2. < touch.
3. < tobacco.
4. < ascending.
5. > gentle exercise.
6. < uncovering.
7. < vomiting.
8. < after getting soaked.
9. > pressure if firm.
10. < descending.
11. < bad news.
12. < grief.
13. < disappointed love.
14. < night watching.
15. < excitement.
16. > closing eyes.
17. < scratching.
18. < after stool.
19. < summer.
20. < slight touch.

Test 5
1. < 10 a.m.
2. < 11 a.m.
3. < noon.
4. < 3 p.m.
5. < 4 p.m.–8 p.m.
6. < 3 p.m.– 5 p.m.
7. < 3 p.m.–6 p.m.
8. < 5 p.m.–8 p.m.
9. < 9 p.m.
10. < twilight.
11. < midnight.
12. < before midnight.
13. < after midnight.
14. < 1–2 a.m.
15. < 2–4 a.m.
16. < 3 a.m.
17. < after sunrise.
18. < morning and evening.
19. < night.
20. < daytime.

Test 6
Sensations common to remedies
1. Benumbing pains.
2. A stick-like pain.
3. Pains move about all over.
4. As if a part would burst.
5. As of red-hot coals.
6. Shooting pains along the track of the nerves.
7. As if bruised.
8. Prickling pains from without inwards.
9. As if the bone were broken.
10. As if the bones were scraped.
11. Pain as from a nail driven inwards.
12. As of a constricting band.

(Test 6 continued)
13. Bearing down as if all would fall out.
14. Squeezing as if between two stones – usually abdomen.
15. Stunning, stupefying pain – usually head.
16. Stinging pains.
17. Radiating pains.
18. Pains that tingle.
19. No pain where if would be expected.
20. Boring pains in small parts.

Repertory exercise
1. Give other words for – aching, tightening, cutting, throbbing, tearing.
2. How else could you describe the sensation of a plug?
3. List all the sensations found in the General section of the Repertory.
   a) Give three ways in which the patient might speak of these.
   b) List the main remedies.

Bibliography

* Allen J H Keynotes and characteristics with comparisons Jain, New Delhi

Boger C M 1982 Boenninghausen's characteristics Jain, New Delhi

* Boger C M 1987 The synoptic key of the materia medica Jain, New Delhi

Castro M 1990 The complete homoeopathy handbook Macmillan, London

A Clarke J H 1977 Dictionary of materia medica (3 vols) Health Science Press, Devon

A Coulter C 1986 Portraits of homoeopathic medicines (2 vols) North Atlantic Books, California

Dewey W A 1980 Essentials of homoeopathic materia medica World Homoeopathic Links, New Delhi

Dewey W A 1985 Essentials of homoeopathic therapeutics Jain, New Delhi

A Farrington E A 1986 Comparative materia medica Jain, New Delhi

A Farrington E A 1988 Clinical materia medica Jain, New Delhi

* Gibson D 1987 Studies of homoeopathic remedies Beaconsfield, England

* Gutman W 1987 Homoeopathy Homoeopathic Medical, Bombay

Hamilton E 1862 The flora homoeopathica Bailliere, London

* Kent J T 1971 Lectures in homoeopathic materia medica Jain, New Delhi

Lockie A 1989 The family guide to homoeopathy Guild, England

* Nash E B 1985 Leaders in homoeopathic therapeutics Jain, New Delhi

A Neatby E A, Stonham T G 1948 A Manual of homoeopathic therapeutics Foxlee-Vaughan, London

Patersimilias 1974 The song of the symptoms Health Science Press, Devon

A Phatak S R 1977 Materia medica of homoeopathic remedies Sunarda Publications, Bombay

Roy M 1994 The principles of homoeopathic philosophy Churchill Livingstone, Edinburgh

* Tyler M Homoeopathic drug pictures Health Science Press, Devon

* Von Lippe A Keynotes and redline symptoms World Homoeopathic Links, New Delhi

A Whitmont E C 1980 Psyche and substance North Atlantic Books, California

* Recommended

A Advanced

Glossary of Terms

Acute disease
In homoeopathy the term refers to a self-limiting episode of illness from which the patient either recovers or dies.

Aggravation
The initial increase in the intensity of symptoms when the activity of the vital force is increased, e.g. by a remedy.

Allopathy
The practice of treating disease by reversing the symptoms, usually by giving a medicine that creates the opposite effect to that produced by the body in reacting to the disease.

Amelioration
A decrease in the intensity of symptoms which naturally follows the aggravation phase.

Causation
The exciting, or maintaining, causes that activate the inherent predispositions of an individual. The original morbific agent.

Characteristic
A typical symptom associated with a remedy or a person. Often it distinguishes the remedy or person.

Concomitant symptom
A symptom occurs at the same time as another symptom. There is seldom any relationship between the two except time.

Constitution
This term indicates that individuals can be classified according to the characteristic reaction pattern of their vital force, i.e. there are patterns of chronic illness.

Crude dose
A medicine which has not been potentized in any way.

Cure
The permanent removal of a patient's symptoms.

Diagnosis
A term used by the allopath in labelling patterns of symptoms into commonly occurring groups.

Exciting cause
A detrimental factor to which this individual is particularly sensitive so the predisposition, or weakness, of the vital force is exposed.

Herb
A plant with medicinal value. The term is not used to refer to the potentized preparation from this plant.

Herbalism
This is the use of medicinal plants to effect an improvement in health. These may be prepared in tincture, or dried, etc., but they are not potentized and the practice does not involve the use of the basic homoeopathic laws such as the Law of Similars, The Single Remedy, The Single Dose, the Minimum Dose or the Law of Cure.

Holistic
When the patient is treated in such a way that each symptom is related to the whole.

Homoeopathy
The practice of treating disease by administration of a medicine capable of producing the very same symptoms.

Keynote
A particularly characteristic symptom that identifies a remedy.

Maintaining cause
A detrimental factor inimicable to life which lowers the vitality of an individual, thus making him/her more susceptible to ill health.

Materia Medica
A collection of symptom pictures of homoeopathic remedies. A delineation of the possible action of a medicine, a list of symptoms it may produce or cure.

Miasms
A chronic affliction of the vital force from which it cannot recover.

Modality
That which effects change to a symptom.

Natural Medicine
A substance which is unprocessed, or changed, in any way. A process whereby the body's own reactions are enhanced as these are recognized as the quickest and safest way to cure.

Naturopathy
A process of cure using the natural reaction of the body to disease.

Nosode
A special remedy prepared from human disease tissue, e.g. Tuberculinum from a tuberculosis cyst.

Objective symptom
One that is observable through the senses.

Orthodox medicine
Also called Western Medicine. That commonly accepted in Europe, North America, Oceania, etc. as established practice. Based on allopathic procedures and an extensive search for objective data.

Point of change
The point at which a pattern of symptoms originates.

Polycrest
A remedy that is commonly found because it has such a wide range of symptoms.

Potency
The number of times a homoeopathic medicine has been diluted and succussed.

Potentization
The process of diluting and succussing a homoeopathic remedy.

Predispositions	Inherent weaknesses in the vital force which arise from miasms.
Prescribing symptom	An unusual or distinctive symptom that characterizes the patient, or his/her illness.
Prognosis	A forecast or prediction as to how the pattern of symptoms will change.
Prophylactic	Preventive treatment.
Prophylaxis	A remedy given with the intention of preventing a person catching that disease.
Prover	A person who takes a homoeopathic remedy with the intention of proving it.
Proving	When a homoeopathic medicine is taken by a healthy person to discover what symptoms it is capable of producing.
Pseudo-chronic disease	Originates from a maintaining cause and, as such, will disappear when the cause is removed.
Remedy	The name given to a homoeopathic medicine. It is seldom called a drug.
Repertory	A dictionary of the symptoms produced by homoeopathic remedies.
Rubric	An entry of a symptom in the Repertory, e.g. absent-minded in the *Mind* section of the Repertory.
Similimum	That remedy which can produce a symptom picture most similar to that of the patient.
Specific	A remedy common to a particular disease pattern that it may be thought of routinely and given if the symptoms match.
Subjective symptom	One that is experienced only by the patient.
Suppression	When the symptoms disappear but not according to the Law of Cure.
Susceptibility	The degree of sensitivity to the remedy or to the exciting cause.
Symptom	An awareness of discomfort or disease which is abnormal to the patient.
Symptom picture	May be applied to the patient, or to a remedy. It is the characteristic group of symptoms produced by either of these.
Tincture	Is a medicinal substance prepared in alcohol.
Total symptom picture	Contains the entire symptom picture of the patient.
Trituration	A chemical process that involves grinding down the material to a very fine powder.
Vital force	The process or intelligence which corrects and maintains the organism within a set pattern.
Vitalism	A system of medicine that recognizes that the organism is more than a collection of chemicals. It recognizes the principle of life.
Vitality	The amount of energy available to sustain life.
Zymotic	Of organic origin, i.e. through fermentation.

Index

MR. L. ROBINSON